BMA

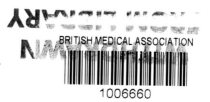

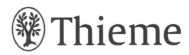

Meningiomas of the Skull Base

Treatment Nuances in Contemporary Neurosurgery

Paolo Cappabianca, MD
Professor and Chairman of Neurosurgery
Residency Program Director
Division of Neurosurgery
University of Naples Federico II
Naples, Italy

Domenico Solari, MD, PhD
Assistant Professor of Neurosurgery
Division of Neurosurgery
University of Naples Federico II
Naples, Italy

292 illustrations

Thieme
Stuttgart • New York • Delhi • Rio de Janeiro

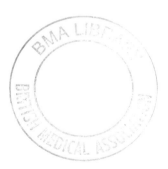

Library of Congress Cataloging-in-Publication Data

Names: Cappabianca, Paolo, editor. | Solari, Domenico, 1980- editor.

Title: Meningiomas of the skull base : treatment nuances in contemporary neurosurgery / [edited by] Paolo Cappabianca, Domenico Solari.

Description: Stuttgart ; New York : Thieme, [2018] | Includes bibliographical references and index. |

Identifiers: LCCN 2018024570 (print) | LCCN 2018024980 (ebook) | ISBN 9783132413023 | ISBN 9783132412866 | ISBN 9783132413023 (eBook)

Subjects: | MESH: Meningioma–surgery | Skull Base Neoplasms–surgery | Neurosurgical Procedures–methods

Classification: LCC RC280.B7 (ebook) | LCC RC280.B7 (print) | NLM WE 707 | DDC 616.99/481–dc23

LC record available at https://lccn.loc.gov/2018024570

© 2019 by Georg Thieme Verlag KG

Thieme Publishers Stuttgart
Rüdigerstrasse 14, 70469 Stuttgart, Germany
+49 [0]711 8931 421, customerservice@thieme.de

Thieme Publishers New York
333 Seventh Avenue, New York, NY 10001 USA
+1 800 782 3488, customerservice@thieme.com

Thieme Publishers Delhi
A-12, Second Floor, Sector-2, Noida-201301
Uttar Pradesh, India
+91 120 45 566 00, customerservice@thieme.in

Thieme Publishers Rio, Thieme Publicações Ltda.
Edifício Rodolpho de Paoli, 25º andar
Av. Nilo Peçanha, 50 - Sala 2508
Rio de Janeiro 20020-906 Brasil
+55 21 3172 2297 / +55 21 3172 1896

Cover design: Thieme Publishing Group
Typesetting by Thomson Digital, India

Printed in Germany by CPI Books GmbH   5 4 3 2 1

ISBN 978-3-13-241286-6

Also available as an e-book:
eISBN 978-3-13-241302-3

Important note: Medicine is an ever-changing science undergoing continual development. Research and clinical experience are continually expanding our knowledge, in particular our knowledge of proper treatment and drug therapy. Insofar as this book mentions any dosage or application, readers may rest assured that the authors, editors, and publishers have made every effort to ensure that such references are in accordance with **the state of knowledge at the time of production of the book.**

Nevertheless, this does not involve, imply, or express any guarantee or responsibility on the part of the publishers in respect to any dosage instructions and forms of applications stated in the book. **Every user is requested to examine carefully** the manufacturers' leaflets accompanying each drug and to check, if necessary in consultation with a physician or specialist, whether the dosage schedules mentioned therein or the contraindications stated by the manufacturers differ from the statements made in the present book. Such examination is particularly important with drugs that are either rarely used or have been newly released on the market. Every dosage schedule or every form of application used is entirely at the user's own risk and responsibility. The authors and publishers request every user to report to the publishers any discrepancies or inaccuracies noticed. If errors in this work are found after publication, errata will be posted at www.thieme.com on the product description page.

Some of the product names, patents, and registered designs referred to in this book are in fact registered trademarks or proprietary names even though specific reference to this fact is not always made in the text. Therefore, the appearance of a name without designation as proprietary is not to be construed as a representation by the publisher that it is in the public domain.

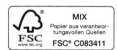

To our parents...

Paolo Cappabianca and Domenico Solari

Contents

11   Olfactory Groove Meningiomas 76

Daniel M. Prevedello, Alaa S. Montaser, Matias Gómez G., Bradley A. Otto, Ricardo L. Carrau

12   Middle Fossa Floor Meningiomas 87

Roberto Delfini, Benedetta Fazzolari, Davide Colistra

16 Cavernous Sinus Meningiomas 138
Antonio Bernardo, Philip E. Stieg

17 Reconstruction of the Skull Base 151
Sebastien Froelich, Domenico Solari, Moujahed Labidi, Shunya Hanakita, Anne Laure Bernat,
Philippe Herman, Paolo Cappabianca

18 Management of Recurrent Skull Base Meningiomas 161
Sheri K. Palejwala, Garni Barkhoudarian, Walavan Sivakumar, Daniel F. Kelly

19   Natural History and Adjunctive Modalities of Treatment 176

Peter F. Morgenstern, Jonathan Forbes, Theodore H. Schwartz

20   Complications in the Management of Skull Base Meningioma 185

Deopujari CE, Vikram S. Karmarkar

Foreword

The history of successful neurosurgical treatment of intracranial meningiomas began in 1884 with the removal of an olfactory groove meningioma by the Italian surgeon, Francesco Durante: details of such a remarkable surgery deserved publication in *The Lancet* in 1887. Since that time, the longstanding and alive debate concerning the best treatment strategy and understanding of the clinical and biological behavior of meningiomas has represented a challenging matter for the neurosurgical community. Indeed, because of their benign nature, total removal leads to effective cure and is still claimed as gold-standard treatment; however, the tumors' common involvement of surrounding skull base bone, dura, and neurovascular structures, and the tendency to recur in higher grades of histologic subtypes, makes complete removal challenging, sometimes risky or even impossible. To address skull base meningiomas with the goal of a radical resection, meningioma surgery has historically been performed through invasive surgical approaches with considerable associated morbidities; improvements in terms of both neurological outcome and extent of resection are the results of the continuous refinement of neurosurgical techniques.

The School of Naples has always dedicated extreme attention to meningiomas, and this book provides the latest testimony of it. On April 26 and 27, 1991, an International Meeting was held in Naples, entitled "Meningiomas: From Durante to Guidetti. Diagnostic and Therapeutic Aspects", to celebrate the first Italian who operated on a meningioma and Beniamino Guidetti, an unforgotten father of the Italian neurosurgery. The Neapolitan journey in the last three decades, from the transcranial pterional approach to the description of the endoscopic endonasal route as an innovative and feasible alternative, finally to the definition of the extended endoscopic endonasal transplanum approach, witnesses the inexhaustible seeking of the less invasive, safest, and more effective surgical strategies.

Nowadays, the surgical treatment philosophy for meningiomas is multifaceted, due, in part, to tremendous technological advancements that have been made in diagnostic and interventional radiology, as well as in surgical and radiation treatments, and above all in surgical techniques armamentarium, i.e., endoscopy, computer-assisted surgery, and radiosurgery. Additionally, recent development of molecular biology provides new information regarding outcome and perspective, thus leading to innovative, appropriate, and targeted adjuvant therapies to improve the quality of life.

In such a scenario, the editors are to be commended for their timely, due accomplishment: this book is intended to compile and disseminate the advances in regard to meningiomas of the skull base as per world renowned experts' opinion. Several chapters are aimed to collect the latest understanding about classification, intraoperative technology, and the role of radiotherapy. Other sections are dedicated to the conventional and advanced surgical management of meningiomas of the skull base according to the anatomical site. With this comprehensive content, the book is conceived not only to bring extensive updated understanding on the topic, but also to stimulate the thread of continuous learning, which represents a rewarding and challenging task for all modern neurosurgeons.

Finally, I wish to express my deep appreciation to all contributors for having made this book so fruitful and profitable.

Enrico de Divitiis
Professor Emeritus of Neurosurgery
University of Naples Federico II
Naples, Italy

Preface

Meningiomas are the second most frequent entity among intracranial tumors (incidence rate can go up to 36%), and are usually benign: every neurosurgeon has had the opportunity during his/her career to deal with many of these lesions.

Meningioma features have been deeply analyzed and reported in a myriad of scientific publications; however, the inner behavior has not yet been thoroughly understood. Exogenous factors influencing their growth, genes sequencing, and molecular patterns of development are supposed to disclose, in the forthcoming years, the actual biological aspects of meningiomas along with the mechanisms of their variability and attitudes.

This evolving body of information, indeed, has pushed a further refinement of the recent 2016 WHO classifications of meningiomas, the identification of new categories being necessary to fit lesions that were previously not properly categorized. Nevertheless, many more efforts have to be devoted before scientific speculations could enter clinical scenario and it will be possible to dig inside and treat the tumor cells directly.

So far, we have witnessed terrific advancements of surgical techniques and technological progress, together with a revolutionary process involving the therapeutic options for such disease, either surgical or medical; this inevitably yielded the possibility of defining safe treatment strategies for meningiomas, even those located at a hostile location such as the skull base.

In the last decades, a conspicuous number of surgical techniques to access meningiomas of the skull base have been described, defining more notable and effective procedures with lesser rate of morbidity, eventually improving patients' quality of life. Besides, radiotherapy and radiosurgery have entered the armamentarium of modern neurosurgery, providing control of the disease in cases of smaller lesions and/or where surgery cannot be radical.

However, the big leap affording the true advancement of the surgeon's dexterity is the pursuit of improving the vision quality. On the one hand, preoperative imaging studies have developed that provide clear definition of areas and fibers, while on the other, intraoperative visual detailing has been increased by means of technological advancements of microscopes, endoscopes, exoscopes, and the integrated, adaptive robot-controlled systems (ROVOT).

Most of us build our neurosurgical career receiving the privilege of studying the real pillars of knowledge in regard to meningiomas: *Meningiomas*, by Cushing and Eisenhardt; *Meningiomas of the Posterior Fossa*, by Castellano and Ruggiero; *Meningiomas*, by Al Mefty, etc.

This book is intended not only to set the bar of current skull base meningiomas management strategies, but also to provide new fuel to explore and define further options according to the actual anatomo-functional knowledge. We hope that this publication would boost enthusiasm for further researches the same way we had felt. Indeed, such undaunted study keeps fueling progresses among the scientific community, helps keep the mind healthy and, above all, helps one to look optimistically toward the future.

Last but not the least, we wish to express our gratitude to all the distinguished authors contributing to the book and to the staff of Thieme for the professional support.

Paolo Cappabianca, MD
Domenico Solari, MD, PhD

Contributors

Ossama Al-Mefty, MD, FACS, FAANS
Director of Skull Base Surgery
Brigham and Women's Hospital
Harvard Medical School
Department of Neurosurgery
Boston, Massachusetts, USA

Rami O. Almefty, MD
Resident
Department of Neurosurgery
Barrow Neurological Institute
Phoenix, Arizona, USA

Norberto Andaluz, MD
Professor of Neurosurgery
Department of Neurosurgery
University of Cincinnati (UC) College of Medicine
Comprehensive Stroke Center at UC Neuroscience
    Institute
Mayfield Clinic
Cincinnati, Ohio, USA

Jonathan Andrew Forbes, MD
Assistant Professor
Department of Neurosurgery
University of Cincinnati College of Medicine
Cincinnati, Ohio, USA

Filippo Flavio Angileri, MD, PhD
Associate Professor of Neurosurgery
Department of Biomedical and Dental Sciences and
    Morphofunctional Imaging
University of Messina
Messina, Italy

Michael L. J. Apuzzo, MD
Distinguished Adjunct Professor of Neurosurgery
Department of Neurosurgery
Yale School of Medicine
New Haven, Connecticut, USA
Adjunct Professor of Neurological Surgery
Senior Consultant
Department of Neurological Surgery
Weil Cornell Medical College
New York, New York, USA

Garni Barkhoudarian, MD, FAANS
Assistant Professor of Neurosurgery
Pacific Neuroscience Institute
John Wayne Cancer Institute
Santa Monica, California, USA

Antonino Bernardo, MD
Professor of Neurosurgery
Director—Microneurosurgery Skull Base and
    Surgical Innovation Training Center
Department of Neurological Surgery
Weill Medical College of Cornell University
New York, New York, USA

Anne Laure Bernat, MD
Assistant Professor
Department of Neurosurgery
Lariboisiere Hospital
Assistance Publique-Hôpitaux de Paris
Paris-Diderot University
Paris, France

Phillip A. Bonney, MD
Resident Physician
Department of Neurological Surgery
Keck School of Medicine
University of Southern California
Los Angeles, California, USA

Salvatore Massimiliano Cardali, MD, PhD
Associate Professor of Neurosurgery
Department of Biomedical and Dental Sciences and
    Morpho-Functional Imaging
Division of Neurosurgery
University of Messina
Messina, Italy

Marialaura Del Basso De Caro, MSc
Professor of Pathology
Department of Advanced Biomedical Sciences
Pathology Section
University of Naples Federico II
Naples, Italy

Ricardo L. Carrau, MD, FACS
Professor
Department of Otolaryngology—Head and Neck
    Surgery
Department of Neurological Surgery
The Ohio State University Wexner Medical Center
Columbus, Ohio, USA

Luigi Maria Cavallo, MD, PhD
Associate Professor
Division of Neurosurgery
Department of Neurosciences
Reproductive and Odontostomatological Sciences
University of Naples Federico II
Naples, Italy

Davide Colistra, MD
Resident of Neurosurgery
Neurosciences Department Neurosurgery Unit
Umberto I Hospital, "Sapienza" University of Rome
Rome, Italy

Alfredo Conti, MD, PhD, FEBNS
Associate Professor of Neurosurgery
University of Messina
Messina, Italy
Visiting Scientist
Charité—University Medicine Berlin
Berlin, Germany

Deopujari CE, MB, MS, MCh, MSc
Professor of Neurosurgery
Department Head
Department of Neurosurgery
Bombay Hospital Institute of Medical Sciences
Mumbai, India

Oreste de Divitiis, MD
Associate Professor
Department of Neurosciences and Reproductive and
    Odontostomatological Sciences
School of Medicine and Surgery
University of Naples Federico II
Napoli, Italy

Roberto Delfini, MD
Chairman
1st Chair of Neurosurgery
Sapienza University
Rome, Italy

Ian F. Dunn, MD
Associate Professor
Department of Neurological Surgery
Brigham and Women's Hospital
Harvard Medical School
Boston, Massachusetts, USA

Florian H. Ebner, MD
Associate Professor
Department of Neurosurgery
Eberhard-Karls-University
Tübingen, Germany

Benedetta Fazzolari, MD
Neurosurgeon
S.M. Goretti Hospital
Latina, Italy

Federico Frio, MD
Resident
Department of Neurosurgery
School of Medicine and Surgery
University of Naples Federico II
Napoli, Italy

Rosa Maria Gerardi, MD
Resident
Division of Neurosurgery
Department of Neurosciences and Reproductive and
    Odontostomatological Sciences
University of Naples Federico II
Naples, Italy

Antonino F. Germanò, MD
Professor and Chairman
Department of Neurosurgery
University of Messina School of Medicine
Messina, Italy

Felice Giangaspero, MD
Full Professor of Pathological Anatomy
Department of Radiological, Oncological and
    Anatomopathological Sciences
Sapienza University of Rome
Rome, Italy
IRCCS Neuromed
Pozzilli, Italy

Matias Gómez G., MD
Assistant Instructor
Department of Otolaryngology—Head and Neck
    Surgery
German Clinic of Santiago—Institute of
    Neurosurgery Dr Asenjo
Santiago, Chile

Danica Grujicic, MD
Head
Neurooncology Department
Clinic of Neurosurgery
Clinical Center of Serbia
Professor
Medical Faculty University of Belgrade
Belgrade, Serbia

Elia Guadagno, MD, PhD
Professor
Department of Advanced Biomedical Sciences
Pathology Section
University of Naples Federico II
Naples, Italy

Shunya Hanakita, MD, PhD
Skull Base Clinical Fellow
Department of Neurosurgery
Lariboisiere Hospital
Assistance Publique-Hôpitaux de Paris
Paris-Diderot University
Paris, France

Philippe Herman, MD, PhD
Chairman
ENT and Skull Base Department
Saint Louis-Lariboisière Hospital
Paris Diderot University
Paris, France

Rosanda Ilic, MD
Neurosurgeon
Clinic of Neurosurgery
Clinical Center of Serbia
Assistant
Medical Faculty University of Belgrade
Belgrade, Serbia

Vikram S. Karmarkar, MS, MRCSEd, DNB-Neurosurgery
Consultant Neurosurgeon and Assistant Professor
Department of Neurosurgery
Bombay Hospital Institute of Medical Sciences
Mumbai, India

Daniel F. Kelly, MD
Director
Pacific Neuroscience Institute Professor of Neurosurgery
John Wayne Cancer Institute Providence Saint John's Health Center
Santa Monica, California, USA

Jeyan Kumar, MD
Resident Physician
Department of Neurosurgery
University of Virginia Health System
Charlottesville, Virginia, USA

Moujahed Labidi, MD, FRCSC
Skull Base Clinical Fellow
Department of Neurosurgery
Lariboisiere Hospital
Assistance Publique-Hôpitaux de Paris
Paris-Diderot University
Paris, France

Edward R. Laws, Jr., MD, FACS
Professor of Neurosurgery
Harvard Medical School
Director
Pituitary/Neuroendocrine Center
Brigham and Women's Hospital
Boston, Massachusetts, USA

Gautam U. Mehta, MD
Skull Base Fellow
Department of Neurosurgery
University of Texas MD Anderson Cancer Center Houston
Houston, Texas, USA

Pietro Meneghelli, MD
Neurosurgery Fellow
Institute of Neurosurgery
University Hospital
Verona, Italy

Mihailo Milicevic, MD
Assistant Professor
Clinical Center of Serbia
Clinic of Neurosurgery
Medical Faculty University of Belgrade
Belgrade, Serbia

Alaa S. Montaser, MD
Research fellow
Department of Neurological Surgery
The Ohio State University Wexner Medical Centre
Columbus, Ohio, USA
Assistant lecturer
Department of Neurological Surgery
Ain Shams University
Cairo, Egypt

Peter F. Morgenstern, MD
Resident of Neurosurgery
Department of Neurological Surgery
New York Presbyterian Weill Cornell Medical Center
New York, New York, USA

Anil Nanda, MD, MPH, FACS
Professor and Chairman
Department of Neurosurgery
Louisiana State University Health Sciences Center
Shreveport, Louisiana, USA

Bradley A. Otto, MD
Assistant Professor
Department of Otolaryngology—Head and Neck
  Surgery
Department of Neurological Surgery
The Ohio State University Wexner Medical Center
Columbus, Ohio, USA

Sheri K. Palejwala, MD
Fellow
Minimally-Invasive Skull Base Neurosurgery
Neurological Surgery
John Wayne Cancer Institute Pacific Neuroscience
  Institute
Santa Monica, California, USA

Mohana Rao Patibandla, MBBS, MCh, iFAANS
Fellow
Endovascular Neurosurgery
Department of Neurological Surgery
University of Virginia Health System
Charlottesville, Virginia, USA

Devi Prasad Patra, MD, M.Ch, MRCSed
Clinical Fellow—Skull Base Neurosurgery
Department of Neurosurgery
LSU Health Science Center
Shreveport, Louisiana, USA

Daniel M. Prevedello, MD, FACS
Professor
Department of Neurological Surgery
The Ohio State University Wexner Medical Center
Columbus, Ohio, USA

Francesco Sala, MD
Professor of Neurosurgery
Department of Neurosciences
Biomedicine and Movement Sciences University
  Hospital
Verona, Italy

Dragan Savic, MD, PhD
Consultant Neurosurgeon
Clinical Center of Serbia
Clinic of Neurosurgery
Medical Faculty University of Belgrade
Belgrade, Serbia

Theodore H. Schwartz MD, FACS
David and Ursel Barnes Professor of Minimally
  Invasive Neurosurgery
Department of Neurosurgery, Otolaryngology
  and Neuroscience
Director, Anterior Skull Base and Pituitary Surgery
Director, Epilepsy Research Laboratory
Weill Cornell Medicine
New York Presbyterian Hospital
New York, New York, USA

Sebastien Froelich, MD
Professor and Chairman
Department of Neurosurgery
Lariboisiere Hospital
Assistance Publique-Hôpitaux de Paris
Paris-Diderot University
Paris, France

Jason P. Sheehan, MD
Professor
Neurosurgery and Radiation Oncology
Department of Neurological Surgery
University of Virginia Health System
Charlottesville, Virginia, USA

Walavan Sivakumar, MD
Associate Professor of Neurosurgery
John Wayne Cancer Institute
Department of Neurosurgery
Pacific Neuroscience Institute
Santa Monica, California, USA

Alberto Di Somma, MD
Resident Physician
Division of Neurosurgery
Department of Neurosciences
Reproductive and Odontostomatological Sciences
University of Naples Federico II
Naples, Italy

Teresa Somma, MD
Neurosurgeon
Department of Neurosciences and Reproductive
  and Odontostomatological Sciences
Division of Neurosurgery
University of Naples Federico II
Naples, Italy

Toma Yuriev Spiriev, MD, FEBNS
Neurosurgery Fellow
Department of Neurosurgery
Eberhard-Karls-University
Tübingen, Germany

Philip E. Stieg, MD, PhD
Chairman and Professor
Weill Cornell Medical College
Neurosurgeon-in-Chief
NewYork-Presbyterian Hospital
Professor of Neurosurgery
Consultant Neurosurgeon
Department of Orthopedic Surgery
Hospital for Special Surgery
Professor of Neurosurgery
Attending Neurosurgeon
Department of Neurological Surgery
Memorial Sloan Kettering Cancer Center
Attending Neurosurgeon
Department of Neurological Surgery
New York Presbyterian Queens
New York, New York, USA

Marcos Tatagiba, MD, PhD
Professor, Chairman, and Director
Department of Neurosurgery
University of Tübingen
Tübingen, Germany

Francesco Tomasello, MD
Professor of Neurosurgery
University of Messina
Messina, Italy
Honorary President of World
Federation of Neurosurgery (WFNS)
Milan, Italy
President of Network Innovation
Technology in neurosurgery (NITns)
Milan, Italy

Domenico La Torre, MD, PhD
Assistant Professor
Department of Neurosurgery
University of Messina
Messina, Italy

Gabriel Zada, MD, MS, FAANS
Associate Professor of Neurological Surgery and
  Otolaryngology
Department of Neurological Surgery
Keck School of Medicine
University of Southern California
Los Angeles, California, USA

Abbreviations

5-ALA	5-aminolevulinic acid
ACF	anterior cranial fossa
AEP	auditory evoked potentials
AICA	anterior inferior cerebellar artery
AKT1	v-akt murine thymoma viral oncogene homolog 1
AKT2	Protein kinase B
ASTRO	American Society for Radiation Oncology
BA	basilar artery
CBT	corticobulbar tract
CEA	carcinoembryonic antigen
CK18	Cytokeratin 18
CN	cranial nerve
CNS	central nervous system
COX-2	Cyclooxygenase 2
CPA	cerebellopontine angle
CSF	cerebrospinal fluid
CT	computed tomography
CTA	computed tomography angiography
CUSA	Cavitron Ultrasonic Surgical Aspirator
CV	craniovertebral
DNA	deoxyribonucleic acid
DSA	digital substraction angiography
DTI	diffusion tensor imaging
DVT	deep venous thrombosis
EBRT	external beam radiotherapy
ECA	external carotid artery
EEA	endonasal endoscopic approach
EGF	epidermal growth factor
EGFR	epidermal growth factor receptor
EMA	epithelial membrane antigen
EMG	electromyography
EOR	extent of resection
ERR	excess relative risk
$EtCO_2$	end tidal carbon dioxide
ETV	endoscopic thirdventriculostomy
FAS	fatty acid synthase
FLAIR	fluid-attenuated inversion recovery
FM	foramen magnum
FMEP	facial nerve motor evoked potentials
GFAP	glial fibrillary acidic protein
GSPN	greater superficial petrosal nerve
GTR	gross total resection
H&E	hematoxylin and eosin
HPC	haemangiopericytoma
IAC	internal auditory canal
IARC	International Agency for Research on Cancer
ICA	internal carotid artery
ICG	intravenous indocyanine green
ICP	intracranial pressure
IFN	interferon
IFN-α	interferon alpha
IGS	image-guided surgery
IONM	intraoperative neurophysiological monitoring

ITGB1	integrin beta-1
KLF4	Krupplelike factor 4
LMWH	low molecular weight heparin
MC	Meckel's cave
MCA	middle cerebral artery
MCF	middle cranial fossa
MEN1	multiple endocrine neoplasia type 1
MEP	motor evoked potentials
MMP2	Matrix Metalloprotease2
MRA	magnetic resonance angiography
MRI	magnetic resonance imaging
MRV	magnetic resonance venogram
N:C	nuclear to cytoplasmic ratio
NCCN	National Comprehensive Cancer Network
NF2	Neurofibromatosis type 2 gene
NMI	nuclear magnetic imaging
NSF	nasoseptal flap
OPN	osteopontine
OR	odds ratio
PAS-positive	periodic acidSchiff-positive
PCA	posterior cerebral artery
PCF	posterior cranial fossa
PCOS	polycystic ovary syndrome
PDGF	platelet-derived growth factor
PDGFR	platelet-derived growth factor receptor
PEEK	polyetheretherketone
PET	positron emission tomography
PFS	progression-free survival
PHH3	Phosphohistone-H3
PICA	posterior inferior cerebellar artery
PIK3CA	Phosphatidylinositol-4,5-biphosphate 3-kinase catalytic subunit alpha
PMMA	poly(methyl methacrylate)
PR	progesterone receptor
QUANTEC	Quantitative Analysis of Normal Tissue Effects in the Clinic
RISA	Retrosigmoid intradural suprameatal approach
RR	relative risk
RT	radiotherapy
SCA	superior cerebellar artery
SCC	semicircular canal
SEP	somatosensory evoked potentials
SFT	solitary fibrous tumor
SHH	sonic hedgehog
SOF	skull-base foramina
SPECT	single-photon emission computed tomography
SpO_2	oxygenation
SRS	stereotactic radiosurgery
SRT	stereotactic radiotherapy
SSTR2A	somatostatin receptor2A
STA	superficial temporal artery
Sv	sievert
SWMs	Sphenoid Wing Meningiomas
TERT	Telomerase reverse transcriptase
TRAF7	TNF receptor-associated factor 7
VA	vertebral artery
VEGF	vascular endothelial growth factor
VEGF-R	vascular endothelial growth factor receptor
VP	ventriculoperitoneal
WHO	World Health Organization

1 Introduction

Michael L. J. Apuzzo

1.1 Essential "Arrows" in the Technical Quiver: Fragments of Personal Memoirs

During the last generation, neurosurgery underwent a striking reinvention characterized by the phenomena specialization and subspecialization. This development was driven by need and the availability of technical adjuvants that allowed surgeries to meet the challenges afforded by neurological diseases.

One of the emerging areas of focused effort related to the discipline of cranial base surgery which engaged in problematical congenital, neoplastic, and vascular lesions in and around the skull base. Introduction of a few technical adjuvants and imaging modalities allowed the creation of capabilities for successfully approaching and dealing with these problems. This armamentarium emerged gradually over a four-decade period and laid the foundation for the new discipline. The author was fortunate to have frontline involvement in the introduction of a few of these tools.

The following paragraphs will offer fragments of the author's experiences in what were seminal moments.

1.2 Imaging (1973)

In 1973, following the completion of author's residency at Yale, *William F. Collins* (his chairman) encouraged him to travel from New Haven, Connecticut to Boston, Massachusetts to spend a week with *William Sweet*, a creative Harvard neurosurgeon who was engaged in transcutaneous electrocoagulation of fifth nerve structures through the foramen ovale for trigeminal neuralgia. These procedures were conducted in the *Radiology Department of the Massachusetts General Hospital* in a fluoroscopy room. Dr. Sweet was meticulous and rigorously controlled all the aspects of the procedure. However, the surrounding environment was unpredictable. Dr. Sweet was annoyed by the repetitive noise of activities in an adjacent area. Repeatedly, he uttered expletives regarding the "piece of junk" that was being installed next to his "sanctuary." A bit of investigation on his part disclosed that this was a British device—*(EMI) scanner*. This was a tool that would produce grainy images of the skull and intracranial content. It was in fact, the first imaging device (computed tomography [CT] scanner) of its kind to be installed in North America. A year later, he was in Los Angeles, California where industrious individuals had incorporated these devices into truck trailer boxes and offered imaging in hospital parking lots.

One of these individuals was Ernie Bates, a neurosurgeon from San Francisco, California. Ernie trained with Charlie Wilson at USC and finished a year before the author. He never practiced neurosurgery, but would go on to establish a business that would be listed on the New York Stock Exchange. Their paths would cross frequently as the years passed. A year later, a EMI scanner was installed on the fifth floor of the *Los Angeles County General Hospital*, only a few steps from the neurosurgical operating room, neurologic intensive care unit and his office. History was being made again as rudimentary stereotactic procedures included brachytherapy were undertaken under imaging control.

During the middle 1980s, with the introduction of *nuclear magnetic imaging (NMI)* later—*magnetic resonance imaging (MRI)*, it became apparent that imaging overlays in three-dimensional reconstructions of the brain and all intracranial contours would facilitate operative events. They worked with the *University of Southern California Film School*, filmmaker *George Lucas*, *Steve Jobs*, and *Industrial Light and Magic* to create early three-dimensional contours and reconstruction in what was termed the *"Operating Room of the Future"* in the *USC University Hospital* in 1991.

Setting the stage for what was to come, the concept was fueled by ideas and author's relationships with *Patrick Kelly (Rochester)*, *John Tew (Cincinnati)*, *Kintomo Takakura (Tokyo)*, *Kajime Honda (Kyoto)*, and *Kenichi Sugita (Nagoya/Matsumoto)*. It served as a global template.

1.2.1 The Operating Microscope (1955)

In 1921, Swedish otologists are credited with the introduction of the microscope into the surgical arena in otolaryngology. Although many ultimately defined the field, a small number of neurosurgeons were responsible for its introduction into intracranial surgery. *Theodore Kurze* in Los Angeles was an active member of this initial handful of pioneers. Ted was reluctantly introduced to the *Zeiss OPMI I Microscope* in the morgue at the Los Angeles County General Hospital by *Howard House* the notable otologist in the late 1950s. Ted along with *Leonard Malis* in New York and *"Peter Donaghy"* in Burlington, Vermont saw the potential value of the tool particularly in lesions of the cranial base. The author joined Ted as a junior staff person in 1973. By that time, he had long established a "sophisticated" microneurosurgery operating suite with one of the world's only overhead mountings. However, the rudiments of microsurgery were still evolving with basic issues such as scope sterility, tactics, intraoperative photography, and instrumentation being primitive. Retraction was clumsy and even head fixation was suboptimal. Author's early career as a "fellow" with Ted allowed them to evolve with refinement of the specialty ultimately developing the *"bag microscope cover,"* cortical protection material, irrigation solutions, dissection techniques, and more refined operative strategies and instrumentation with American, Swedish, German, Swiss, and Japanese colleagues.

Over the years, author worked with *V. Mueller, Aesculap, Zepplin*, and other microsurgical instrument development groups to create operative instruments that were both universal and procedure specific. They were based primarily on otology and ophthalmic concepts and were highlighted by close collaborations with *Al Rhoton (Gainesville), Bob Rand (Los Angeles), Taka Fukushima (Tokyo, Los Angeles)*, and *Kenny Sugita (Nagoya/Matsumoto)*. In parallel, Ted Kurze and author worked with *Jerry Urban* (Burbank) and Zeiss to develop operative photography and video capabilities that obviously were nonexistent in the early years.

For further documentation, detailed line drawings of key operative stages and maneuvers were developed with the remarkable max Brodel Institute trained illustrator *Diane Abeloff* for the classics *Surgery of the Third Ventricle and Brain Surgery: Complication Avoidance and Management*, text atlases. Most importantly, the operative strategies, techniques, and corridors that evolved were ultimately documented in *"Surgery of the Third Ventricle"* published in 1987, which was the result of more than 14 years of endeavors in microsurgical challenges.

1.2.2 Modern Endoscopy (1974)

Author's early years as a junior staff in Los Angeles, California had "many ups and downs." Like any young surgeon finding an identity in a new environment was difficult. The author often hoped for a personal discovery or an identity in what was a challenging and an unforgiving environment. His office was, in fact, the *Division's coffee room*! Their Division boosted many true "notables" in the young field—all accomplished—all contributors. One unique individual was the innovative Renaissance man esteemed bioengineer *Milton Heifetz*, the creator of the Heifetz aneurysm clip and other instrument nuances. He and author had a "connection." One day in his kindness, he presented the author with a metal box from *Storz*. It contained what were revolutionary endoscopes. He told the author that the company had asked him to work with these highly progressive prototype tools that were not currently in use in neurosurgery. They incorporated a new and unique lens system (*Hopkins*) that gathered light and presented remarkably clear images. Milt asked the author, *"Would you be willing to try them out?"* The author eagerly assumed the task and over an 18-month period applied the endoscopes to a myriad of procedures including cranial base surgery, aneurysm surgery, intraventricular surgery, pituitary surgery, and spinal procedures—all seminal work that was published in 1977 and led to modern endoscopy and its parameters that are exploited today—particularly in surgery of the cranial base.

1.2.3 Imaging Directed Stereotaxy and Navigation (1977)

Imaging-based navigation has its roots in imaging-based stereotaxic techniques defined in the late 1970s and 1980s. Once, the author saw the initial images in Boston and later worked in their CT scanner in Los Angeles, it became apparent that instrumentation that allowed translation of imaging data into a remote operative event was in the future. In 1977, while attending a ski meeting in Utah (*Richard Lende*), he saw a *plastic prototype* for a stereotactic system that could relate images to a remote operative event. Through persistence, he eventually learned that this model was the embryo of what would be the *Brown-Roberts-Wells Stereotactic System. Ted Roberts* the chairman at the *University of Utah* and the director of the project was enthusiastic to support author's involvement, but *Trent Wells*, the esteemed biomedical engineer, was not immediately receptive. *Edwin M. Todd (Todd/Wells Frame)*, a true Renaissance man and surgical innovator with a Yale background (*John Fulton's* Lab) and a member of USC neurosurgery faculty, interceded with Trent and the author's involvement was authorized—beginning a 30-year relationship with Trent that included the development in prototype testing, validation, and introduction of the *Brown-Roberts-Wells Stereotactic System* (#1), the *Cosman-Robert-Wells Stereotactic System* (#1), and the radiosurgical device *X-Knife* (#1). The author would eventually hold *the Edwin M. Todd, Trent H. Wells, Jr., Professorship at the Keck School of Medicine at the University of Southern California. The Brown-Roberts-Wells Stereotactic System and Cosman-Robert-Wells Stereotactic System* became the World's most universally employed devices and the *X-Knife remains in use today.*

Functionally, the *Brown-Roberts-Wells Stereotactic System* allowed for translation of individual patient imaging data into the operating room for point precision guidance in stereotactic and open surgical procedures. This opened the door for "frameless" systems that were developed with *Eric Cosman* of *Radionics* for navigation in intracerebral targets or at the cranial base. Later, *facial/cranial contouring* was developed similar to what was called *"Mode G"* bottom contouring navigation in nuclear submarine navigation, a method that the author had observed as submariner in the late 1960s.

The first radiosurgery procedures on a human (in North America) were performed with the *X-Knife* prototype at the *Kenneth R. Norris, Jr. Hospital and Research Institute* (USC)*, Los Angeles, California* and *Peter Bent Brigham Hospital (Harvard), Boston Massachusetts in 1984.*

1.2.4 Bipolar Forceps (1955)

Leonard Malis is credited with creating the first bipolar surgical forceps in 1955. In 1965, he performed what many consider to be the first microsurgical neurosurgical operation. He was both a friend and competitor of Ted Kurze. Both were New Yorkers with competitive spirits and uniquely similar operating styles. They were meticulous and laborious—acoustic neuroma surgery would be measured on a calendar! Having spent many hours with him in his operating room, Leonard was jovial and a lovely man with great patience with the author. He set a high standard of operative rigor and detail. The author feels privileged to count him as a mentor and an originator of many of his own personal operative approaches in strategy and technique. He was immensely proud of his contributions, but always strove to improve.

1.2.5 Ultrasonic Aspirator (1978)

In 1978, they received a prototype *ultrasonic aspirator (CUSA)* courtesy of neurosurgeon *Joseph Ransohoff*, chairman at New York University and a close friend of Ted Kurze. The unit was created by a Long Island firm and was shepherded into the clinical sector by *Eugene Flamm* in Joe's department. They were given the single prototype for a 3-month period after the New York University introduction. It was a miraculous tool and saved an enormous amount of time for them in a wide range of lesions. It remains an indispensable tool in neurosurgery and has been applied to a wider range of the surgical endeavor's catalog.

In retrospect, the author feels privileged to have been part of the instruments' initial introduction, evaluation, and promotional activities. As a former nuclear Submariner, the author was intrigued by the fact that the physics of cavitation had been established during the analysis of maritime propulsion systems in 1916. In nuclear submarines, the issue of cavitation was central. Other than potential damaging effects, the phenomenon created noise. The unique seven blade three story propellers for clandestine submarine operations was developed to reduce cavitation noise particularly at low resolutions.

1.2.6 Microanatomy (1973)

During the early days of microsurgery, there was limited comprehension of the anatomical substrate both normal and pathological with its distortions and nebulous nuances. These required definition as comfort grew with the microscopes application. The names of *Gazi Yasargil* and *Albert Rhoton* loomed large in providing comprehension and definition of what were quite murky areas. Their careers ran generally in parallel. Yasargil in Europe and Rhoton in North America, the author was privileged to be "close" to both particularly during his years as Editor of *Neurosurgery* where he encouraged Rhoton to publish and refine his collective work on microanatomy incorporated into operative events. *"Cranial Anatomy and Operative Approaches"* by Rhoton was published by *Neurosurgery* in 2007, under author's editorship—a landmark in the history of the specialty and a defining work with Yasargil's succession of *"Microsurgery"* monographs that he introduced in 1969. Yasargil was honored by the Journal in 1999, as one of two *"Neurosurgeons of the Century"* with Harvey Cushing. Working with Gazi, a longtime friend at that point in conjunction with that honor was a priceless experience for the author!

In combination, these "arrows in the surgeon's quiver" allowed the emergence of modern cranial base surgery. It is an endeavor that demands judgement and tactical nuance as much or more than simplistic neurosurgical "mechanics." The questions of when to *undertake*? How to *approach*? How to maintain technical *discipline* and appreciate a myriad of *end points*? and when is the exercise *over*? are central. These are key considerations for the surgeon as they face the individual patient and unique challenges.

The tangible "arrows" in the quiver allow and to a point define the opportunities for surgical exercise but strategy, discipline, and judgement are the *intangible* arrows that define the true essence of the accomplished surgeon.

Although the following chapters in this monograph will convey the "current" state of the art, it is essential to be aware of the "fact" that *molecular biology* and *genetics* as well as *immunology, nanotechnology,* and the application of *high-energy* forms appearing in their time and on the horizon will soon make these surgical exercises obsolete!

"Change" happens and all to be "modern" must first be victimized by time.

2 The Evolution of Surgery—the Soul of Neurosurgery

Edward R. Laws, Jr., Ian F. Dunn

Abstract

Meningiomas have been present in mankind since prehistoric times. This chapter records the history of this common tumor of the nervous system, its symptoms and signs, and its diagnosis and treatment. Many factors have evolved to make meningiomas a great intellectual and technical challenge, and a pivotal factor in the development of modern neurosurgery. They are a major focus of skull base surgery, and represent for many, as they did for Harvey Cushing, the soul of neurosurgery.

Keywords: meningioma, brain tumors, skull base surgery, microneurosurgery, endoscopic surgery, transsphenoidal surgery

2.1 Introduction: Early History

Evidence from prehistoric skulls indicates that meningiomas have been with us as long as humans have walked the earth. Descriptions in the literature of what probably were meningiomas date back as far as Plater's case of 1614 (▶ Table 2.1). It is likely that the first documented case of surgery for an intracranial meningioma was that of Berlinghieri in 1813, documenting treatment of a "sarcoma of the dura". Another Italian surgeon, Zenobi Pecchioli, described a similar procedure for successfully removing a "fungus of the dura mater" in 1835. Tito Vanzetti, surgeon for the Pope, exposed and removed a skull base tumor which probably was a meningioma in 1841.[1,2,3]

Traditionally, Sir William Macewen of Glasgow is credited with a successful craniotomy in 1879, for a skull base tumor arising from the roof of the left orbit, and presenting with seizures.[4] Other contributions included operations by Davide Giordano and Francesco Durante who used transfacial and trans-basal approaches, described in 1883 (▶ Fig. 2.1).[5] Durante also reported a craniotomy for the removal of a left olfactory groove meningioma in 1885.[5] In the United States, Frank Hartley of New York City described surgery for a meningioma in 1896. Robert

Weir and William W. Keene described successful surgical cases in 1887, in New York City and Philadelphia, respectively. In Berlin, Fedor Krause successfully diagnosed and excised a frontal skull base meningioma in 1905. Removal of meningiomas of the posterior fossa and the cerebellopontine angle were described by Sir Charles Ballance in 1894 (London) and by Fedor Krause in 1906 (▶ Table 2.2).

2.2 Nomenclature

Ultimately, the above accomplishments by some of the pioneer figures in neurosurgery were overshadowed by those of Dr Harvey Cushing (▶ Fig. 2.2) Many of these tumors had been given a series of descriptive names such as dural endothelioma, fibrous tumor of the dura, sarcomas, meningeal fibroblastomas, etc. It was Cushing who coined the name "meningioma" in 1922, and described this tumor as "the soul of neurosurgery". In his monograph of 1938, Harvey Cushing thoroughly recounted the origin of meningiomas as arising from the arachnoid cap cells of the Pacchionian granulations.[6] He described the distribution of these tumors along the venous sinuses and the dura of the skull base, and recognized that they usually were benign lesions that could be surgically excised. Dr Cushing stated, "There is nothing in the whole realm of surgery more gratifying than the successful removal of a meningioma with subsequent perfect functional recovery."[6]

In reviewing his early meningioma cases, Cushing said that the most common were meningiomas of the anterior skull base, divided among 29 olfactory groove meningiomas, 28 suprasellar meningiomas, and a few meningiomas of the orbital roof. Second most common were meningiomas of the sphenoid ridge, which occurred either as mass lesions or en plaque. He also described the less common meningiomas involving the cavernous sinus.[7]

Table 2.1 Early descriptions of meningioma

1614	Felix Plater, Switzerland: Autopsy
1730	Johann Salzmann, Germany: Autopsy
1743	Laurenz Heister, Germany: Unsuccessful Rx with caustic lime
1768	Olaf Acrel, Sweden: Unsuccessful attempt at surgery
1774	Antoine Louis, France: Unsuccessful attempt at surgery
1864	John Cleland, Scotland: Villous tumor of arachnoid

Table 2.2 Surgical pioneers: meningioma

1813	Andrea Berlingheri, Italy
1835	Zanobi Pecchioli, Italy
1879	William Macewen, Scotland
1885	Francesco Durante, Italy
1887	Robert F Weir, United States
1887	William W Keen, United States
1894	Charles Ballance, England
1905	Fedor Krause, Germany

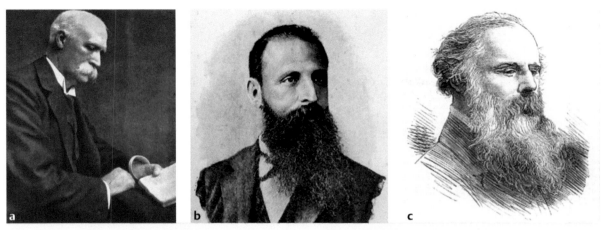

Fig. 2.1 (a) Sir William Macewen, (b) Francesco Durante, and (c) Tito Vanzetti—pioneers of meningioma surgery.

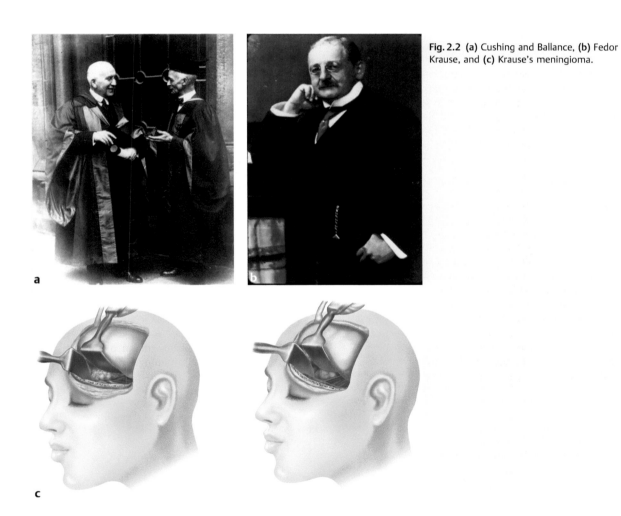

Fig. 2.2 (a) Cushing and Ballance, (b) Fedor Krause, and (c) Krause's meningioma.

2.3 Stages of Surgery for Meningiomas

The evolution of skull base surgery for meningiomas occurred in stages. These stages exemplified the various aspects of successful neurosurgery in general, and of successful skull base surgery in particular.

The initial challenges were those of making the diagnosis and localizing the lesion. Early cases were detected because of deformations of the skull and other external signs, including proptosis. Visual loss was an obvious sign, particularly when it was present as a bitemporal hemianopsia, or was associated with papilledema and optic atrophy, as in the Foster Kennedy syndrome, which also could include loss of olfaction. Cranial nerve deficits such as ptosis, anisocoria, diplopia, and loss of facial sensation, were identified as characteristic of meningiomas with cavernous sinus involvement. With the advent of roentgenography, tumors could be diagnosed by changes in the sellar bone and by blistering of bone and hyperostosis in the skull base, along with calcifications in some cases. Posterior fossa tumors were noted to cause tinnitus, hearing loss, and facial weakness or facial sensation disorders. Pituitary endocrinopathy was noted to occur with sellar and parasellar lesions. Seizures, and their location were also often important clues for the diagnosis of these tumors.

2.4 Initial Surgical Progress

Once diagnosed and localized, the next challenge was to expose the tumor accurately and safely. The initial exposures were transcranial, as described by the pioneers, and later by Sir Victor Horsley, Harvey Cushing, Walter Dandy with George Heuer, Charles Frazier, Herbert Olivecrona, Francesco Castellano, Beniamino Guidetti, Clovis Vincent, Pierre Wertheimer, Charles Elsberg, John Jane, and Collin McCarty (who described the essential "keyhole" placement for the frontotemporal craniotomy)[1,8,9,10,11,12,13,14,15,16] (Box 2.1), (► Fig. 2.3).

Box 2.1 Craniotomy for meningioma

Victor Horsley
- Charles Frazier
- George Heuer/Walter Dandy
- Harvey Cushing
- Charles Elsberg
- Herbert Olivecrona
- Collin MacCarty
- Ludwig Kempe
- John Jane Sr.
- Pierre Wertheimer
- Patrick Derome

2.5 Extracranial Approaches to Skull Base Lesions

A parallel series of skull base approaches using extracranial methods developed as well. Many of the pioneers, following Durante's lead, were the Viennese surgeons Hermann Schloffer (1907), and Anton von Eiselsberg, along with Theodor Kocher and Oscar Hirsch (► Fig. 2.4) Ultimately, the transnasal transsphenoidal approach became favored, and was advocated by Cushing, and by A. E. Halstead and Allen Kanavel of Chicago. They represented the first wave of transsphenoidal surgery that lapsed for some time after Dr Cushing abandoned it in 1926. The second wave began with Cushing's trainee, Norman Dott of Edinburgh, who persisted with the transsphenoidal technique.[17] He trained Gerard Guiot of Paris, who added much to the concepts and to details of the techniques (► Fig. 2.5) Guiot, in turn, trained Jules Hardy of Montréal. Dr. Guiot is credited with the introduction of video fluoroscopy in this operation, and he also

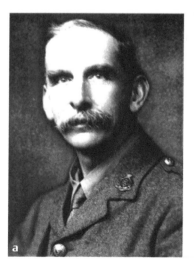
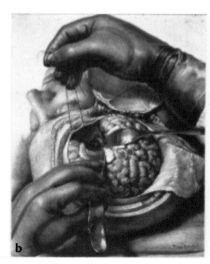

Fig. 2.3 (a) Victor Horsley and **(b)** Heuer/Dandy approach.

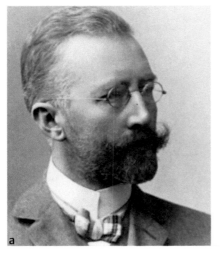

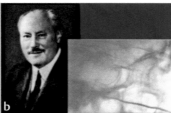

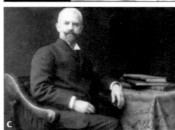

Fig. 2.4 (a) Schloffer, **(b)** Oskar Hirsch, and **(c)** Von Eiselsberg.

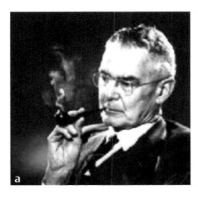

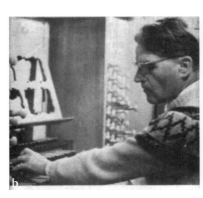

Fig. 2.5 (a) Norman Dott and **(b)** Gerard Guiot.

performed the first endoscopic approach to the pituitary in 1963. Dr Hardy introduced the use of the operating microscope for pituitary surgery, and demonstrated its effectiveness in performing hypophysectomy and also for the selective removal of pituitary microadenomas[18] (Box 2.2).

Box 2.2 The microsurgical era in meningioma surgery

Dwight Parkinson
- Vinko Dolenc
- Laligam Sekhar
- M. Gazi Yasargil
- Leonard Malis
- John Fox
- Ossama Al-Mefty
- Albert Rhoton
- Robert Spetzler
- Kenchiro Sugita
- Hakuba, A.
- Kawase, T.
- Bernard George
- Perneczky, A.

2.6 Microneurosurgery

The entire field of skull base surgery was revolutionized in the 1960s by the advent of the use of the operating microscope, and the consequent development of microsurgical dissection[19,20,21,22,23,24,25] (▶ Fig. 2.6). These advances in technique dramatically altered the outcomes for patients with a variety of brain lesions. In addition, both these methods and these concepts were applicable to skull base approaches either by craniotomy[26,27,28,29,30,31] or by extracranial methods including transnasal transsphenoidal approaches[32,33,34,35,36,37] (▶ Table 2.3) The technical advances associated with micro-neurosurgery enabled novel concepts of microsurgical anatomy. As structures and relationships that have never been noted previously came into plain view, it enabled a new level of precision in the surgical removal of skull base tumors, particularly meningiomas. Great enthusiasm followed the demonstration of improved surgical results, fewer complications, and better outcomes for the patients.

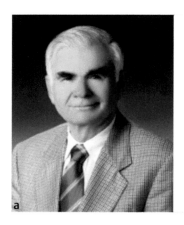
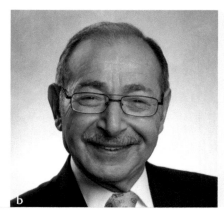

Fig. 2.6 (a) Yasargil and (b) Al-Mefty.

Table 2.3 Extracranial approaches to skull base meningiomas

1880	William Macewen: Orbital roof tumor with proptosis
1883	Francesco Durante: Transpalatal for sinus extension
1807–1927	Transsphenoidal pioneers: Schloffer, von Eiselsberg, Hirsch, Kocher, Cushing, AE Halstead, Kanavel
1927–1969	Persisting extracranial approaches: Dott, Guiot, Hardy
1969–1998	The microsurgical era: Hardy, Tindall, VanGilder, Wilson, Laws, Giovanelli, Derome, Apuzzo, Weiss, Fahlbusch, Teasdale, Stevenaert, Rhoton, etc
1995–2017	The endoscopic era: Sethi/Pillay, Jho/Carrau, DeDivitiis/Cappabianca, Kassam, Schwartz, Frank, Kelly, Jane Jr., etc
2001–2017	Extended approaches for skull base lesions: Kaptain (Laws), Cappabianca, Frank, Jane Jr. Kassam

2.7 Refined Skull Base Approaches and Anatomical Studies

Meningiomas clearly were a focus of new developments that helped to enhance the field of skull base surgery. A primary factor in the development of the subspecialty of skull base surgery, was an emphasis on the anatomy of the central nervous system and its afflictions, primarily in the form of tumors, and most notably in dealing with meningiomas. New understanding of pathophysiological anatomy, and advances in neuroanesthesia allowed for novel approaches without the previous trauma related to brain retraction. The concept of minimal approaches to skull base tumors flourished. Studies of the anatomy of the cavernous sinus by Parkinson,[38] Dolenc,[39] and others led to new pathways for reaching difficult tumors in an atraumatic fashion. Further knowledge regarding the cerebrovascular system, coupled with the new microsurgical

techniques allowed for more accurate tumor resection, and the preservation or restoration of blood flow to the brain. New microsurgical approaches included the splitting of the Sylvian fissure in the pterional frontotemporal approach, extradural and intradural approaches to the middle fossa and the tentorial margin,[40,41,42,43,44] and temporal bone pathology. Transpetrosal approaches became practical and efficient for petroclival tumors.[45] For skull base tumors in the posterior fossa, middle fossa and translabyrinthine approaches developed, as did skeletonization of the sigmoid sinus and the jugular foramen.[46,47] Transcondylar approaches assisted in the management of tumors of the foramen magnum.[48]

2.8 Allied Advances in Meningioma Management

It should be recognized that none of the aforementioned advances in technique and concepts could have been possible without continuing improvement in associated fields. Perhaps the most essential of these was in neuroimaging. Beginning with plain X-rays, ventriculograms, pneumoencephalograms, angiography, nuclear scans, computed tomography scans and magnetic resonance imaging, the information available for the surgeon keeps increasing in precision and value. Techniques of anesthesia and protection of the brain, along with intraoperative monitoring, have added additional capability to the successful removal of skull base tumors. Techniques and methods of pathologic investigation of the tumors removed continue to add new and valuable information about the pathogenesis and ultimate treatment of these lesions.

2.9 Modern Surgical Management

The challenge of meningiomas involving the anterior skull base continues to provoke new concepts and new

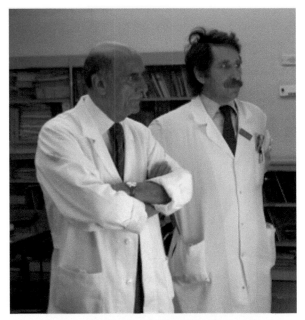

Fig. 2.7 Endoscopic pioneers: DeDivitiis and Cappabianca.

methods of treatment. The introduction of the operating microscope and the transsphenoidal and other extended transnasal approaches has revolutionized the management of lesions in the region of the pituitary fossa. Subsequently, another wave of enthusiasm developed with the advent of the operating endoscope in the 1990s.[49,50,51] The success of the endoscopic methods for pituitary based tumors widened significantly, to encompass meningiomas involving areas beyond the sellar region and cavernous sinuses (▶ Fig. 2.7) Increasingly, other selected meningiomas of the skull base, originating from the tuberculum sellae, planum sphenoidale, and olfactory groove, have become amenable to transnasal and transcranial endoscopic resection.[52] In using these approaches, surgeons incorporate the basic principles that have evolved as essential elements of successful skull base surgery (Box 2.3). The initial enthusiasm for these novel techniques continues, and has led to even more in the way of novel approaches to difficult skull base lesions. Surgeons continue to explore "the edge of the envelope,"[53] and in doing so continue to enhance the surgical capabilities of dealing with meningiomas of the skull base.

References

[1] Guidetti B, Giuffrè R, Valente V. Italian contribution to the origin of neurosurgery. Surg Neurol. 1983; 20(4):335–346

[2] Artico M, Pastore FS, Fraioli B, Giuffrè R. The contribution of Davide Giordano (1864–1954) to pituitary surgery: the transglabellar-nasal approach. Neurosurgery. 1998; 42(4):909–911, discussion 911–912

[3] Priola SM, Raffa G, Abbritti RV, et al. The pioneering contribution of italian surgeons to skull base surgery. World Neurosurg. 2014; 82 (3–4):523–528

[4] al-Rodhan NR, Laws ER, Jr. Meningioma: a historical study of the tumor and its surgical management. Neurosurgery. 1990; 26(5):832–846, discussion 846–847

[5] Durante F. Contribution to endocranial surgery. Lancet. 1887 2: 654–655

[6] Cushing H. Meningiomas, their classification, regional behaviour, life history, and surgical end results. New York, NY: Hafner; 1938

[7] Cushing H. Intracranial tumors. Notes upon a series of two thousand verified cases with surgical-mortality percentages pertaining thereto. Springfield, IL: Charles C Thomas Publisher Limited; 1932. pp. 154

[8] Horsley V. On the technique of operations on the central nervous system. BMJ. 1906; 2:411–423

[9] Cushing H. The pituitary body and its disorders: clinical states produced by disorders of the hypophysis cerebri. Philadelphia and London: JB Lippincott company; 1912

[10] Dandy WE. A new hypophysis operation. Johns Hopkins Hospital Bulletin.. 1918; 29:154–155

[11] Heuer GJ. Surgical experiences with an intracranial approach to chiasmal lesions. Arch Surg. 1920; 1:368–381

[12] Frazier CH. Choice of method in operations upon the pituitary body. Surg Gynecol Obstet. 1919; 29:9–16

[13] Luft R, Olivecrona H. Experiences with hypophysectomy in man. J Neurosurg. 1953; 10(3):301–316

[14] Castellano F, Ruggiero G. [Surgery of meningioma of the posterior cranial fossa]. Minerva Chir. 1951; 6(19):537–542

[15] MacCarty CS. The surgical treatment of meningiomas. Springfield, IL: Charles C Thomas Publishers Limited; 1961. pp. 57–60

[16] Jane JA, Park TS, Pobereskin LH, Winn HR, Butler AB. The supraorbital approach: technical note. Neurosurgery. 1982; 11(4):537–542

[17] Lanzino G, Laws ER, Jr. Pioneers in the development of transsphenoidal surgery: Theodor Kocher, Oskar Hirsch, and Norman Dott. J Neurosurg. 2001; 95(6):1097–1103

[18] Kanter AS, Dumont AS, Asthagiri AR, Oskouian RJ, Jane JA, Jr, Laws ER, Jr. The transsphenoidal approach. A historical perspective. Neurosurg Focus. 2005; 18(4):e6

[19] Rand RW, Jannetta PJ. Microneurosurgery: application of the binocular surgical microscope in brain tumors, intracranial aneurysms, spinal cord disease, and nerve reconstruction. Clin Neurosurg. 1968; 15:319–342

[20] Rand RW, Kurze T. Micro-neurosurgical resection of acoustic tumors by a transmeatal posterior fossa approach. Bull Los Angel Neuro Soc. 1965; 30:17–20

[21] Donaghy RM, Yasargil G. Microangeional surgery and its techniques. Prog Brain Res. 1968; 30:263–267

[22] Malis LI. Instrumentation and techniques in microsurgery. Clin Neurosurg. 1979; 26:626–636

[23] Hardy J. La chirurgie de l'hypophyse par voie trans-sphénoidale ouverte. Etude comparative de deux modalités techniques [French]. Ann Chir. 1967; 21(15):1011–1022

[24] Handa H. Microneurosurgery. Tokyo: Igaku Shoin; 1975

[25] Rhoton AL. Cranial anatomy and surgical approaches. Philadelphia, PA: Lippincott Williams and Wilkins; 2007

[26] Konovalov AN, Fedorov SN, Faller TO, Sokolov AF, Tcherepanov AN. Experience in the treatment of the parasellar meningiomas. Acta Neurochir Suppl (Wien). 1979; 28(2):371–372

[27] Al-Mefty O, Holoubi A, Rifai A, Fox JL. Microsurgical removal of suprasellar meningiomas. Neurosurgery. 1985; 16(3):364–372

[28] Symon L. Aspects of the management of skull base tumors. Clin Neurosurg. 1990; 36:48–70

[29] Sundt TM, Jr. Neurovascular microsurgery. World J Surg. 1979; 3(1):53–65, 127

[30] Sugita K, Kobayashi S, Mutsuga N, et al. Microsurgery for acoustic neurinoma—lateral position and preservation of facial and cochlear nerves. Neurol Med Chir (Tokyo). 1979; 19(7):637–641

[31] Suzuki K. Microneurosurgical Atlas. Springer-Verlag; 1985

[32] Guiot GTB. L'exerese des adenomes de l'hypophyse par voie transsphenoidale. Masson Paris. 1958. pp. 165–180

[33] Mason RB, Nieman LK, Doppman JL, Oldfield EH. Selective excision of adenomas originating in or extending into the pituitary stalk with preservation of pituitary function. J Neurosurg. 1997; 87(3):343–351

[34] Wilson CB. Surgical management of pituitary tumors. J Clin Endocrinol Metab. 1997; 82(8):2381–2385

[35] Tindall GT, Tindall SC. Surgery of the pituitary gland. Curr Probl Surg. 1981; 18(10):609–679

[36] Fahlbusch R, Buchfelder M. Transsphenoidal surgery of parasellar pituitary adenomas. Acta Neurochir (Wien). 1988; 92(1–4):93–99

[37] Powell M. Microscope and endoscopic pituitary surgery. Acta Neurochir (Wien). 2009; 151(7):723–728

[38] Parkinson D. A surgical approach to the cavernous portion of the carotid artery. Anatomical studies and case report. J Neurosurg. 1965; 23(5):474–483

[39] Dolenc VV. Surgery of vascular lesions of the cavernous sinus. Clin Neurosurg. 1990; 36:240–255

[40] Hakuba A, Tanaka K, Suzuki T, Nishimura S. A combined orbitozygomatic infratemporal epidural and subdural approach for lesions involving the entire cavernous sinus. J Neurosurg. 1989; 71(5 Pt 1): 699–704

[41] Kawase T, Shiobara R, Toya S. Anterior transpetrosal-transtentorial approach for sphenopetroclival meningiomas: surgical method and results in 10 patients. Neurosurgery. 1991; 28(6):869–875, discussion 875–876

[42] Dolenc VV. Frontotemporal epidural approach to trigeminal neurinomas. Acta Neurochir (Wien). 1994; 130(1–4):55–65

[43] Al-Mefty O, Smith RR. Tailoring the cranio-orbital approach. Keio J Med. 1990; 39(4):217–224

[44] Al-Mefty O, Anand VK. Zygomatic approach to skull-base lesions. J Neurosurg. 1990; 73(5):668–673

[45] Gross BA, Tavanaiepour D, Du R, Al-Mefty O, Dunn IF. Evolution of the posterior petrosal approach. Neurosurg Focus. 2012; 33(2):E7

[46] House WF. Surgical exposure of the internal auditory canal and its contents through the middle, cranial fossa. Laryngoscope. 1961; 71: 1363–1385

[47] Samii M, Gerganov VM. Surgery of extra-axial tumors of the cerebral base. Neurosurgery. 2008; 62(6) Suppl 3:1153–1166, discussion 1166–1168

[48] George B, Lot G. Anterolateral and posterolateral approaches to the foramen magnum: technical description and experience from 97 cases. Skull Base Surg. 1995; 5(1):9–19

[49] Jho HD, Carrau RL. Endoscopic endonasal transsphenoidal surgery: experience with 50 patients. J Neurosurg. 1997; 87(1):44–51

[50] Cappabianca P, Alfieri A, de Divitiis E. Endoscopic endonasal transsphenoidal approach to the sella: towards functional endoscopic pituitary surgery (FEPS). Minim Invasive Neurosurg. 1998; 41(2):66–73

[51] Kassam A, Snyderman CH, Mintz A, Gardner P, Carrau RL. Expanded endonasal approach: the rostrocaudal axis. Part I. Crista galli to the sella turcica. Neurosurg Focus. 2005; 19(1):E3

[52] Fries G, Perneczky A. Endoscope-assisted brain surgery: part 2-analysis of 380 procedures. Neurosurgery. 1998; 42(2):226–231, discussion 231–232

[53] Zada G, Du R, Laws ER, Jr. Defining the "edge of the envelope": patient selection in treating complex sellar-based neoplasms via transsphenoidal versus open craniotomy. J Neurosurg. 2011; 114(2):286–300

3 Inside the Pathology

Marialaura Del Basso De Caro, Elia Guadagno, Felice Giangaspero

Abstract

Meningiomas represent a group of neoplasms deriving from the arachnoidal cap cells and showing a wide range of morphologic aspects. According to the 2016 WHO classification, three grades of malignancies are recognized: grade I, with a low recurrence rate (7–25%), grade II with a significant increased risk of recurrence (29–52%) and decrease in survival, and grade III, truly malignant lesions, with an increased risk not only of recurrence (50–94%), but also of distant metastasis and death from disease.

The present chapter deals with meningiomas of the skull base that is a complex anatomical region that forms the floor of the cranial cavity and whose proximity to cranial nerves and important vasculature make surgical treatment more challenging. As gross total resection is not always achieved, it is wise to identify the factors that are able to precisely predict the recurrence in meningiomas of this site. Moreover, grades II and III meningiomas are very infrequent in the skull base region. Therefore, grading and extent of resection may not be considered enough strong predictors of recurrence in this site.

In one of the largest modern series of patients surgically treated for meningiomas, with a long follow-up time, a diverging pattern of recurrence was observed in skull base compared with non–skull base tumors, suggesting that they may be genetically different.

Herein molecular features and biological factors that have been explored in both types of meningiomas are thoroughly described.

Keywords: skull base, meningiomas, recurrence

3.1 Skull Base: Elements of Anatomy and Embryology

The skull base is a complex anatomical region that forms the floor of the cranial cavity. The knowledge of this structure is essential to understand the difficulties of surgical procedures in this site.[1] Because of its embryology, it represents a key player in the development of adjacent structures as the brain, the neck, and craniofacial skeleton.[2,3]

It develops mainly in the midline, where it is composed of basioccipital, sphenoid, ethmoid, and frontal bones, and it extends laterally, with paired temporal bones. The intracranial portion of the skull base is generally divided into three regions: the anterior, the middle, and the posterior cranial fossa (ACF, MCF, and PCF, respectively).

Anteriorly, the ACF is limited by the posterior wall of the frontal sinus; the posterior limit is marked by the anterior clinoid processes and the planum sphenoidale, while the frontal bones form the lateral walls. The floor of the ACF is made of the orbital portion of the frontal bone and, in the center, by the ethmoid bone, with its cribriform plate that is passed by the olfactory tracts. Therefore, the ACF region takes contact with delicate structures as the olfactory bulb, the optic nerves, the supracavernous internal carotid artery, the superior and inferior orbital fissures that convey cranial nerves and veins.

The anterior limit of the MCF is formed by the greater wings of the sphenoid which extend laterally and upward to meet the temporal bones and part of the parietal bones. The body of the sphenoid bone forms the center of the MCF and is composed of the sella turcica, a prominent concave structure that guests the hypophysis and that is delimited at both sides by the cavernous sinuses. The latter are crossed by the internal carotids and the abducens nerves bilaterally; maxillary, ophthalmic, trochlear, and oculomotor nerves run within their lateral walls. The petrous portion of the temporal bone limits the MCF posteriorly; it houses the trigeminal ganglion in the Meckel cave, a duplication of the dura that lies in its anteromedial tip.

The anterior portion of the PCF is formed by the basal portion of the occipital bone and the basisphenoid, while the posterior surfaces of the petrous temporal bones and the lateral aspect of the occipital bones form the lateral wall.

The skull base is an intriguing structure also because of its distinct embryologic origins. While the anterior region origins from the neural crest, just like other facial bones, the posterior region derives from the paraxial mesoderm and the division of these two areas is marked by the middle of the basisphenoid. Endochondral ossification is the mechanism by which the skull base takes origin from a cartilage plate (chondrocranium) that later is replaced by bones, unlike other craniofacial bones that derive from intramembranous ossification. SOX9 transcription factor is essential in the neural crest chondrogenesis of the skull base,[4] in SOX9-knockout mice, the sphenoid bone is missing.

3.2 Surgical Resectability

Several different neoplastic processes can manifest in the skull base, with different distribution in the anterior, middle, and posterior regions, respectively (▶ Table 3.1). Meningiomas can occur in the whole skull base and all their aspects will be thoroughly treated in this chapter. Even though they mostly are benign lesions, in this site, complex anatomy and proximity to cranial nerves and important vasculature make surgical treatment of skull base meningiomas more challenging. However, modern

Table 3.1 Neoplastic lesions involving each topographic region of the skull base

Anterior	Central	Posterior
Sinonasal carcinoma	Chordoma	Schwannoma
Metastatic lesions	Chondrosarcoma	Endolymphatic sac tumor
Sinonasal undifferentiated carcinoma	Ecchordosis physaliphora	**Meningioma** of the jugular foramen
Juvenile nasal angiofibroma	Pituitary macroadenoma	Skull base metastases
Sinonasal melanoma	Craniopharyngioma	Arachnoid granulation (dural sinus)
Hemangiopericytoma/fibrous solitary tumor	Schwannoma	Glomus jugulare paraganglioma
Non-Hodgkin's lymphoma	**Meningioma**	Chordoma/chondrosarcoma
Nerve sheath tumor	Skull base metastases	Plasmacytoma
Esthesioneuroblastoma	Hemangiopericytoma/fibrous solitary tumor	Giant cell tumor
Meningioma	Multiple myeloma	
	Non-Hodgkin's lymphoma	

imaging techniques CT, MRI, positron emission tomography [PET]) provide precise anatomical detail[5] that may be of help in planning surgery. Furthermore, neuromonitoring and microsurgical instruments have greatly improved surgical resectability of skull base meningiomas.[6] In the surgery of ACF and MCF lesions, the preservation of visual functions is crucial, much to affect the selection of the best therapeutic approach. In case of lesions of the cavernous sinus, stereotactic radiotherapy in addition to subtotal resection has been regarded an acceptable treatment that preserves cranial nerves functions.[7] PCF meningiomas represent the most challenging tumor, especially the petroclival, due to the proximity to neurovascular structures. In the past, most of them were considered unresectable.

3.3 Meningiomas

3.3.1 Definition and Epidemiology

Meningiomas represent a group of neoplasms deriving from the arachnoidal cap cells and showing a wide range of morphologic aspects. They account for 36% of all brain tumors and only for 2.8% in pediatric population.[8] Most of them are sporadic, but a history of prior radiation is the only predisposing environmental risk factor that has been recognized. Chemical, dietary factors, occupation, head trauma, and the use of mobile phone have all been investigated as possible risk factors, but no conclusive evidences have been provided in this regard.[9]

3.3.2 Histopathology

Intracranial meningiomas occur preferentially on the parasagittal structures of the cerebral convexities such as the falx and the venous sinus, but they frequently involve also skull base structures such as olfactory grooves, sphenoid ridges, para-/suprasellar regions, optic nerve sheaths, petrous ridges, tentorium, and posterior fossa.

The 2016 WHO classification[10] recognized three grades of malignancy based on morphologic parameters. Grade I

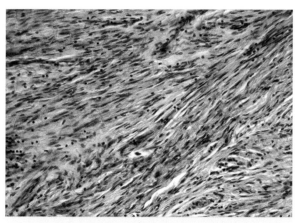

Fig. 3.1 Fibrous meningioma. The neoplasm is composed of spindled cells forming parallel, storing, and interlacing bundles in a collagen-rich matrix. (Hematoxylin and Eosin stain, 20x magnification.)

meningiomas, which represent the majority, are benign tumors with a low recurrence rate (7–25%); grade II represents an intermediate category with a significant increased risk of recurrence (29–52%) and decrease in survival; grade III, truly malignant lesions, has an increased risk not only of recurrence (50–94%), but also of distant metastasis and death from disease.

Among **grade I** meningiomas, nine histological variants are included:

- **Meningothelial**: A frequent variant, characterized by lobules of medium-sized epithelioid tumor cells, delimited by collagenous septa. Indistinct cell borders explain the term "syncytial meningioma" that was used in the past. Occasional atypical cells may be observed, but they have no prognostic relevance.
- **Fibrous**: Intersecting fascicles, also showing a storiform pattern, of fibroblast-like spindle cells are characteristic of this variant. There is often a prominent collagen deposition (▶ Fig. 3.1).

- **Transitional**: The most common variant, composed of a mixture of meningothelial and fibrous types. Whorls are well represented, often in association with psammoma bodies (► Fig. 3.2).
- **Psammomatous**: Common variant in the spinal cord of older women; psammoma bodies represent over half of the tumor and over time their confluence evolves into calcifications that may obscure meningothelial cells (► Fig. 3.3).
- **Angiomatous**: Meningiomatous cells are intermingled with numerous (exceeding 50% of the total tumor volume) small- to middle-sized blood vessels, that are thin- or thick walled, and variably hyalinized; tumor cells with degenerative nuclear atypia may be observed but almost all cases are benign. Angioblastic

meningioma is another entity and is the term that was referred in the past to solitary fibrous tumor/hemangiopericytoma (SFT/HPC), a tumor that may exhibit aggressive behavior (see below) (► Fig. 3.4).
- **Microcystic**: Neoplastic cells have thin elongated processes that are arranged in a cobweb-like background due to the collection of intercellular clear fluid and often display nuclear degenerative atypia. Hypervascularity may be observed (► Fig. 3.5).
- **Secretory**: Pseudopsammoma bodies are pathognomonic morphologic features, consisting of intracellular lumina containing periodic acid–Schiff-positive (PAS-positive) eosinophilic secretions (► Fig. 3.6), which are also positive to carcinoembryonic antigen (CEA). It may be explained as an advanced form

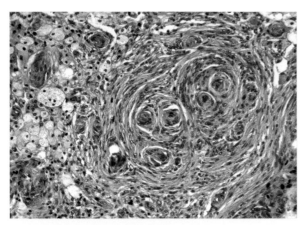

Fig. 3.2 Transitional meningioma. Histological variant containing meningothelial and fibrous patterns, as well as transitional features. Focal xanthomatous degeneration may be observed on the left side. (Hematoxylin and Eosin stain, 20x magnification.)

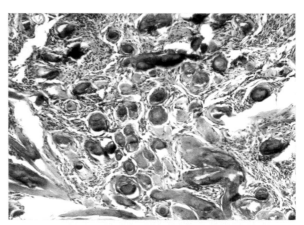

Fig. 3.3 Psammomatous meningioma. In this variant, psammoma bodies are predominant over tumor cells. (Hematoxylin and Eosin stain, 10x magnification.)

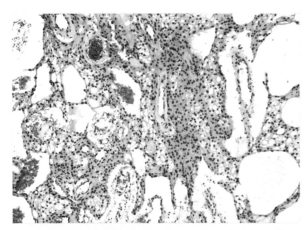

Fig. 3.4 Angiomatous meningioma. Numerous blood vessels characterize this histological variant and are intermixed with meningothelial meningioma cells. (Hematoxylin and Eosin stain, 10x magnification.)

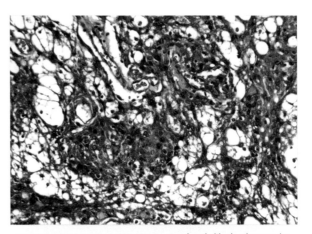

Fig. 3.5 Microcystic meningioma. A cobweb-like background is provided by cells with thin, elongated processes. (Hematoxylin and eosin stain, 20x magnification.)

of epithelial differentiation; cells surrounding them usually react to cytokeratin. Very rare is the pure form; this morphologic aspect usually develops inside a meningothelial or transitional meningioma. Secretory meningiomas may have a particular clinical relevance because they can cause severe cerebral edema more frequently than other variants.

- **Lymphoplasmacyte-rich**: In this variant, a dense infiltrate of lymphocytes and plasma cells exceeds the neoplastic proliferation so that to obscure it. It may also be referred with the definition of "inflammation-rich meningioma."
- **Metaplastic**: This variant, while retaining immunohistochemical and ultrastructural features of meningothelial cells, may include areas of cartilaginous, osseous (▶ Fig. 3.7), lipomatous, myxoid, and xanthomatous tissue, either singly or in combination.

Three subtypes of meningiomas are of **grade II**:
- **Atypical**: Despite the name, cellular atypia is not a diagnostic feature. The diagnosis is made when one of the three major criteria is satisfied:
- High mitotic index (≥ 4 mitoses/10 HPF) (▶ Fig. 3.8).
- Brain invasion (presence of irregular, tongue-like protrusions of tumor cells that infiltrate the parenchyma, without the interposition of leptomeninges) (▶ Fig. 3.9) in meningiomas that otherwise appear benign.
- At last three of five morphologic parameters (sheeting architecture, presence of small cells with high nuclear/

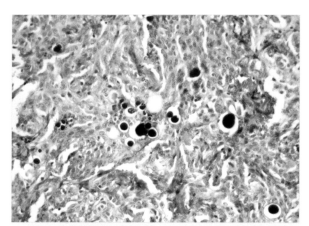

Fig. 3.6 Secretory meningioma. Focal epithelial differentiation consists of intracellular lumina containing periodic acid–Schiff-positive pseudopsammoma bodies. (Periodic acid–Schiff histochemical stain, 20x magnification.)

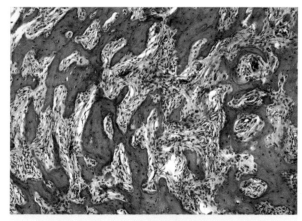

Fig. 3.7 Metaplastic meningioma. Osseous metaplastic tissue makes part of the neoplasm. (Hematoxylin and Eosin stain, 10x magnification.)

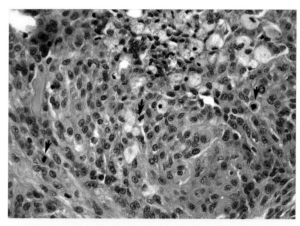

Fig. 3.8 Atypical meningioma. High mitotic rate (*arrows*) was detected throughout this atypical meningothelial meningioma. (Hematoxylin and Eosin stain, 40x magnification.)

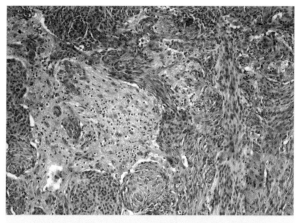

Fig. 3.9 Brain infiltration. Irregular tongue-like protrusions of tumor cells infiltrate the underlying brain parenchyma, without intervening meninges (Hematoxylin and Eosin stain, 10x magnification.)

cytoplasmic ratio, hypercellularity, prominent nucleoli, and spontaneous necrosis) (▶ Fig. 3.10).
- **Chordoid**: Its name derives from the striking resemblance to chordoma, a bone tumor composed by ribbons or cords of epithelioid to spindle cells arranged in a basophilic mucoid matrix; foamy or vacuolated "physaliphorous-like" cells are also present (▶ Fig. 3.11). Pure forms are rare; they are usually intermingled with more typical meningioma tissue. The presence of a well-developed chordoid pattern has been associated with an aggressive behavior.
- **Clear cell**: Usually of the spinal cord or of the PCF, they are composed by sheets of polygonal clear cells, whose aspect is due to cytoplasmic glycogen accumulation, that is positive to PAS diastase (▶ Fig. 3.12). Psammoma bodies and whorls formation are rare. Interstitial and perivascular collagen deposition is a distinctive feature;

in cases of coalescence, large acellular zones of hyalinization or amianthoid-like collagen may be observed.

Grade III lesions are comprehensive of three variants:
- **Anaplastic (malignant)**: Lesion displaying malignant cytology (carcinoma-, melanoma- or high-grade sarcoma-like) and/or elevated mitotic activity (≥ 20 mitoses/10 HPF). The meningothelial nature of neoplastic cells needs to be confirmed by a history of meningioma and/or immunohistochemical, ultrastructural, and/or genetic support when these diagnostic aspects have diffuse distribution. Useful diagnostic features are geographic necrosis and Ki67 proliferation index greater than 20% (▶ Fig. 3.13).
- **Papillary**: Tumor with a predominant pseudopapillary pattern, composed by discohesive epithelioid tumor

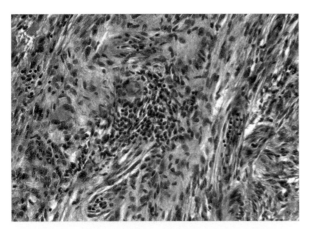

Fig. 3.10 Atypical meningioma. In this field, small cells, with a high nuclear-to-cytoplasmic ratio, were observed. (Hematoxylin and Eosin stain, 20x magnification.)

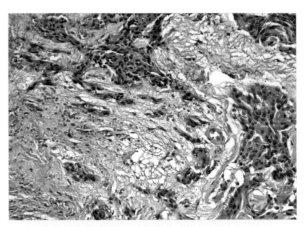

Fig. 3.11 Chordoid meningioma. Ribbons and cords of eosinophilic cells are arranged in a basophilic mucous-rich stroma. (Hematoxylin and Eosin stain, 20x magnification.)

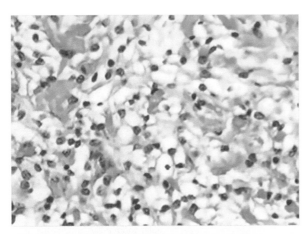

Fig. 3.12 Clear cell meningioma. Rounded clear cells are intermixed with collagenized stroma. (Hematoxylin and Eosin stain, 20x magnification.)

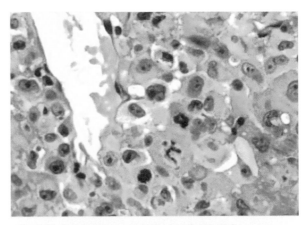

Fig. 3.13 Anaplastic meningioma (grade III). Malignant cytology, associated with high mitotic activity, also atypical, are diagnostic elements for this tumor category. (Hematoxylin and Eosin stain, 40x magnification.)

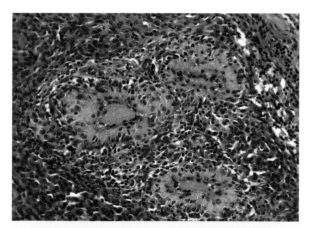

Fig. 3.14 **Papillary meningioma.** An evident perivascular pseudopapillary pattern characterizes most of the tumor. (Hematoxylin and Eosin stain, 20x magnification.)

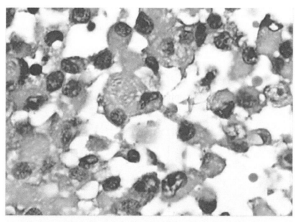

Fig. 3.15 **Rhabdoid meningioma.** Eccentric nucleus, with vesicular chromatin and a central nucleolus, and an evident eosinophilic paranuclear inclusion are pathognomonic aspects of this variant. (Hematoxylin and Eosin stain, 40x magnification.)

cells with perivascular arrangement. These aspects are frequently associated with other histological features of anaplasia. The diagnosis of papillary meningioma may be done when the architectural pattern is dominant (> 50%) (▶ Fig. 3.14).

- **Rhabdoid**: Neoplastic cells are characterized by eccentric nuclei, open chromatin, a prominent nucleolus, and an eosinophilic paranuclear inclusion (▶ Fig. 3.15). This morphology must represent more than a half of the whole tumor. When it is focally present, the neoplasm has to be graded as normally. Most of rhabdoid meningiomas have also other additional malignant features, as high mitotic index, necrosis, and anaplasia. Occasionally, the combination with papillary architecture may be observed.

Other unrecognized morphologic variants: Meningiomas with oncocytic, mucinous, sclerosing, whorling-sclerosing, glial fibrillary acidic protein (GFAP)-expressing, and granulofilamentous inclusion-bearing features. These variants are not well recognized because of their rarity.

3.3.3 Immunohistochemistry

Meningiomas are constantly positive for vimentin; other markers such as epithelial membrane antigen (EMA), S100, and somatostatin receptor, are also expressed in a high percent of cases. Although none of these markers is specific, immunohistochemistry is a valid tool for differential diagnosis with many other neoplasms and for the evaluation of prognostic factors (▶ Table 3.2).

3.3.4 Molecular Features

Molecular diagnosis is topical in brain tumors (e.g., gliomas, embryonal tumors), but in meningiomas no conclusive data have been obtained about the prognostic significance of the genotype.[27] However, genetic status has been extensively investigated in these tumors.

The most common genetic aberration in meningiomas is the monosomic loss of chromosome 22[28] (in 49% of grade I and in 85% of grade II meningiomas). Many other chromosome losses have been reported and their increased frequency has been associated with increasing histological grade; indeed, also losses of chromosomes 14q (60%) and 1p (55%) are detected in grade II meningiomas,[29] while in grade III, additional losses are reported (18q in 75%, 6q in 63%, 10q in 63%, 11p in 50%, 7p in 38%, and 4p in 38%) besides 22 (75%), 1p (75%), and 14q (38%).

There is a kind of molecular hierarchy in which the loss of chromosome 22 represents a starting event to which are added all other events. 1p loss would be a decisive step toward tumor progression.

Neurofibromatosis type 2 gene (NF2) is on chromosome 22 and is a tumor suppressor gene that can be mutated in sporadic (60%) and NF2-related meningiomas.

In order to gain further insight into molecular mechanisms of tumorigenesis in meningiomas, next-generation techniques have been applied.[27,30,31] Two main groups were identified:

- **NF2 meningiomas**: This is the most frequent one. Fibrous meningiomas are the majority of NF2 type and more than 60% of this group are located in the convexity of the skull, parasagittal region, and falx cerebri. About 34% are grades II and III.
- **Non-NF2 meningiomas**: Include six main subgroups:[27]
  - **TRAF7/KLF4**: Meningiomas with mutations of both TNF receptor–associated factor 7 (TRAF7) and Kruppel-like factor 4 (KLF4). Secretory is the most characteristic histological subtype. They are always WHO grade I tumors.

Table 3.2 Immunohistochemical markers in meningiomas

Markers	Utility	References
	Diagnostics	
EMA (epithelial membrane antigen)	Positive in 50–100% of meningiomas	[10]
CK18 (cytokeratin 18)	Commonly positive in meningiomas	[11]
CEA (carcinoembryonic antigen)	Pseudopsammoma bodies and their surrounding cells (CK + and vimentin−) are positive in secretory variant	[12]
Claudin-1	Positive in 50% of meningiomas but negative in solitary fibrous tumor/hemangiopericytoma and vestibular schwannoma	[13]
S100	Useful for differential diagnosis with schwannoma, although 90% of fibrous meningiomas are positive	[13]
CD34	Positive in all solitary fibrous tumor/hemangiopericytoma, in 40% of fibrous meningiomas and 60% of atypical meningiomas	[14]
STAT6	Positive in all solitary fibrous tumors/hemangiopericytomas and negative in all meningiomas	[15]
Brachyury	Useful in the differential diagnosis between chordoma (positive) and chordoid meningioma	[16]
	Prognostic	
PHH3 (phosphohistone-H3)	A mitosis-specific marker that may facilitate rapid reliable grading of meningiomas	[17]
Ki67-MIB1	Proliferation marker, useful in predicting the recurrence risk; in case of labeling index < 4%, 4–20%, or > 20% the risk of recurrence is like grades I, II, and III meningiomas, respectively. A definitive cutoff was not identified	[18]
PR (progesterone receptor)	Positive in most of grade I meningiomas, negative or less expressed in grade II or III. Inversely correlated with Ki67	[19]
FAS (fatty acid synthase), osteopontin protein, AKT2 (protein kinase B)	More expressed in brain invasive and recurrent meningiomas. Prominent in grade II or III, compared with grade I and, among grade I, in those with a higher Ki67	[20,21,22]
COX-2 (Cyclooxygenase 2)	Strong or moderate expression strongly correlated with worse prognosis	[23]
NY-ESO-1 (a cancer/testis gene product)	High expression is correlated with higher tumor grade, worse disease-free survival, and overall survival	[24]
CD163	Its expression is correlated with histological atypical parameters	[25]
SSTR2A (somatostatin receptor 2A)	High expression is correlated with high grade and high Ki67 positivity	[26]

- **TRAF7/AKT1**: They harbor mutations in both TRAF7 and v-akt murine thymoma viral oncogene homolog 1 (AKT1), not in other genes. Meningothelial and transitional histotypes are commonly seen. Most of them are located in ACF and MCF (75%). Mostly benign.
- **SMO**: With the most frequent mutations (L412F and W535L) of smoothened frizzled family receptor, even in case of concomitant NF2 loss. Located in the ACF in 50% of cases. Always benign.
- **Others**: Mutations in TRAF7, AKT1, KLF4, and/or PIK3CA (phosphatidylinositol-4,5-biphosphate 3-kinase catalytic subunit alpha). Most cases are grade I.
- **Complex**: When two points are satisfied, as mutations in TRAF7, AKT1, KLF4, and/or PIK3CA and NF2 aberration (loss and/or mutation). Histologically, intermediate between NF2 type and benign meningiomas.
- **None**: Without any mutations of the six genes or NF2 loss.

Loss of **CDKN2A** and **CDKN2B** has been associated with progression to grade III meningiomas. Moreover, specific aberrations are common to specific histotypes:
- Germline **SMARCE1** loss causes pediatric and familial clear cell meningiomas.[32]
- **BRAF V660E** mutation has been detected in cases of rhabdoid meningiomas.[33]
- Polysomy of **chromosomes 5, 13, and 20** has been described in angiomatous meningiomas.[34]

Point mutations (C228 T and C250T) in telomerase reverse transcriptase (**TERT**) promoter lead to TERT transcriptional activation by two- to fourfolds, that is, statistically associated with shorter time to progression in meningiomas.[35]

3.3.5 Prognostic Factors

The identification of prognostic factors in meningiomas is of help in determining the need for close radiological observation at shorter intervals, or the need for radiotherapy as an adjuvant treatment in the early postoperative period. To date, the grading and the extent of tumor resection[36] are considered the most reliable predictors of tumor recurrence. Other factors have been reported[37]: skull base location, tumor size, calcifications, cavernous sinus invasion, MIB-1 index, loss of chromosome 1p, and other biological factors (see ▶ Table 3.2).

3.4 Solitary Fibrous Tumor/Hemangiopericytoma

SFT/HPC is the more frequent mesenchymal, nonmeningothelial tumor arising in the meninges. For a long period, it has been diagnosed as an angiomatous variant of meningiomas. SFT/HPC is today a distinct pathologic and molecular entity.[12] Histologically, it is a fibroblastic type of mesenchymal tumor characterized by a rich vascular branching network. Two major histological patterns can be recognized: (a) SFT type, characterized by low cellularity, discrete borders, hyalinized vessels, abundant collagenous fibers, and very low mitotic figures; (b) HPC type, a highly cellular tumor with prominent branching vessels. The SFT/HPC has NAB2/STAT6 fusion as molecular signature. Immunohistochemical detection of nuclear positivity for STAT6 is very useful to differentiate SFT/HPC from meningiomas. The WHO classification proposes a three-tiered grade system: grade I, applied to classic SFT type of tumor, grade III to the HPC type with high mitotic index (>5/10 HPF) and necrosis, and grade II, to a mixture of the two types with mitoses greater than 5/10 HPF. The clinical behavior of SFT type is generally benign after gross total resection, whereas HPC type has a high rate of recurrence (>75% at 10 years) and may also metastasize extracranially to bone, lungs, and liver.

3.5 Meningiomas of the Skull Base

Skull base meningiomas represent a challenge for the surgeon by virtue of their contact with vital structures like cranial nerves, brainstem, and major blood vessels. In the management of these tumors, an equilibrium between maximal resection and minimal dysfunction must be pursued, therefore, gross total resection is not always achieved. Additional radiation therapy for residual tumor could be considered in some cases, not without bearing in mind the proximity of these tumors to eloquent and radiosensitive tissue. It is therefore wise to identify the factors that are able to precisely predict the recurrence in meningiomas of this site.

A few studies[37,38] have reported that grades II and III meningiomas are very infrequent in the skull base region. It may be because of a different embryologic origin of meninges covering the convexities from those covering

the brainstem, or because the close proximity to critical structures makes these lesions rapidly symptomatic, depriving them of the time needed to acquire new mutations. Therefore, grading and extent of resection may not be considered enough strong predictors of recurrence in this site.

No statistical differences in progression-free survival (PFS) have been found[37] between cases treated with gross total resection and those treated with subtotal resection followed by radiation therapy, which may be considered a valid treatment alternative. It was much lower in cases treated with subtotal resection without radiation therapy. However, peritumoral edema, radiation necrosis, and secondary tumors represent important side effects of radiation therapy.[39]

Therefore, the identification of factors affecting biological aggressivity of skull base meningiomas is of paramount importance. In this context, a significant association[37] has been observed between a high MIB-1 (>3%) or p53 reactivity and PFS, also in case receiving gross total resection.

By dividing skull base regions into central (including tuberculum sellae, anterior clinoid process, cavernous sinus, cerebellopontine angle, petroclival region or clivus, jugular foramen, and foramen magnum) and peripheral (olfactory groove, planum sphenoidale, middle and lateral sphenoid wings, spheno-orbital region, MCF, posterior pyramis), the recurrence rate is higher in the former; a possible explanation may be that complete excision is more feasible in the latter, compared to the former.[40] No differences in biology of central and peripheral skull base meningiomas may be safely mentioned.

A subset of meningiomas has preferential bony tropism, with a particular tendency to infiltrate the bone, neural and soft tissue, and to create hyperostosis. In the skull base, this aspect represents a further recurrence risk factor, in addition to the location. The expression profile of three bone-modulating factors, matrix metalloprotease 2 (MMP2), osteopontine (OPN), and integrin beta-1 (ITGB1), has been investigated[41] in two subgroups of skull base bone-invasive meningiomas (spheno-orbital and transbasal anterior skull base meningiomas). No association between meningioma subtype and MMP2, OPN, or ITGB1 have been found. Only the ITGB1 showed a significant higher expression in transbasal bone-invasive versus anterior skull base noninvasive meningiomas, mainly located in the tumor vasculature. These results are suggestive of a possible role of anatomical location in regulating bone tropism, osteolytic activity, and vascular remodeling in meningiomas, and also of the potentiality to use ITGB1 expression as therapeutic target.

In one of the largest modern series[42] of patients surgically treated for meningiomas, with a long follow-up time (100 months), a diverging pattern of recurrence was observed in skull base compared with non–skull base tumors, suggesting that they may be genetically different.

3.5.1 Skull Base Meningiomas in Pediatric Age

Meningiomas in pediatric age differ significantly from the adult counterpart because of male predilection, cystic change, higher frequency of neurofibromatosis and high-grade meningiomas, lack of dural attachment, and genotypical and phenotypical aggression.[43] In children, intracranial meningiomas account for 0.4 to 4.6% of brain tumors and skull base lesions represent 27% of all meningiomas. Similar WHO grade distribution is observed at both skull base and non–skull base meningiomas in pediatric age; this means that skull base meningiomas have a lower benign histology rate[44] and a higher incidence of recurrence, compared to adult population.

3.6 Future Perspectives

Surgical resection is expected to remain the main therapeutic option for skull base meningiomas and during the last 15 years several innovations in surgical techniques have been developed.[45] However, a multimodal approach would be desirable in most aggressive and unresectable cases. In this context, molecular and biological features are to be further investigated in order to implement a tailored targeted therapy.

References

[1] Di Ieva A, Bruner E, Haider T, et al. Skull base embryology: a multidisciplinary review. Childs Nerv Syst. 2014; 30(6):991–1000

[2] McBratney-Owen B, Iseki S, Bamforth SD, Olsen BR, Morriss-Kay GM. Development and tissue origins of the mammalian cranial base. Dev Biol. 2008; 322(1):121–132

[3] Nie X. Cranial base in craniofacial development: developmental features, influence on facial growth, anomaly, and molecular basis. Acta Odontol Scand. 2005; 63(3):127–135

[4] Mori-Akiyama Y, Akiyama H, Rowitch DH, de Crombrugghe B. Sox9 is required for determination of the chondrogenic cell lineage in the cranial neural crest. Proc Natl Acad Sci U S A. 2003; 100(16):9360–9365

[5] Choudhri AF, Parmar HA, Morales RE, Gandhi D. Lesions of the skull base: imaging for diagnosis and treatment. Otolaryngol Clin North Am. 2012; 45(6):1385–1404

[6] Goto T, Ohata K. Surgical resectability of skull base meningiomas. Neurol Med Chir (Tokyo). 2016; 56(7):372–378

[7] Pichierri A, Santoro A, Raco A, Paolini S, Cantore G, Delfini R. Cavernous sinus meningiomas: retrospective analysis and proposal of a treatment algorithm. Neurosurgery. 2009; 64(6):1090–1099, discussion 1099–1101

[8] Dolecek TA, Propp JM, Stroup NE, Kruchko C. CBTRUS statistical report: primary brain and central nervous system tumors diagnosed in the United States in 2005–2009. Neuro-oncol. 2012; 14 suppl 5:v1–v49

[9] Flint-Richter P, Mandelzweig L, Oberman B, Sadetzki S. Possible interaction between ionizing radiation, smoking, and gender in the causation of meningioma. Neuro-oncol. 2011; 13(3):345–352

[10] Perry A. Meningiomas. In: McLendon RE, Rosenblum MK, Bigner DD, eds. Russel and Rubinstein's Pathology of Tumours of the Nervous System. 7th ed. London, UK: Hodder Arnold; 2006:427–474

[11] Miettinen M, Paetau A. Mapping of the keratin polypeptides in meningiomas of different types: an immunohistochemical analysis of 463 cases. Hum Pathol. 2002; 33(6):590–598

[12] Perry A, Louis DN, Budka H, von Deimling A, Sahm F. Meningioma. In: Loius DN, Ohgaki H, Wiestle OD, et al, eds. WHO Classification of Tumours of the Central Nervous System. Revised 4th ed. Lyon: IARC; 2016

[13] Hahn HP, Bundock EA, Hornick JL. Immunohistochemical staining for claudin-1 can help distinguish meningiomas from histologic mimics. Am J Clin Pathol. 2006; 125(2):203–208

[14] Okada T, Fujitsu K, Ichikawa T, et al. A strongly CD34-positive meningioma that was difficult to distinguish from a solitary fibrous tumor. Ultrastruct Pathol. 2014; 38(4):290–294

[15] Schweizer L, Koelsche C, Sahm F, et al. Meningeal hemangiopericytoma and solitary fibrous tumors carry the NAB2-STAT6 fusion and can be diagnosed by nuclear expression of STAT6 protein. Acta Neuropathol. 2013; 125(5):651–658

[16] Barresi V, Caffo M, Branca G, Caltabiano R, Tuccari G. Meningeal tumors histologically mimicking meningioma. Pathol Res Pract. 2012; 208(10):567–577

[17] Ribalta T, McCutcheon IE, Aldape KD, Bruner JM, Fuller GN. The mitosis-specific antibody anti-phosphohistone-H3 (PHH3) facilitates rapid reliable grading of meningiomas according to WHO 2000 criteria. Am J Surg Pathol. 2004; 28(11):1532–1536

[18] Perry A, Stafford SL, Scheithauer BW, Suman VJ, Lohse CM. The prognostic significance of MIB-1, p53, and DNA flow cytometry in completely resected primary meningiomas. Cancer. 1998; 82(11): 2262–2269

[19] Guevara P, Escobar-Arriaga E, Saavedra-Perez D, et al. Angiogenesis and expression of estrogen and progesterone receptors as predictive factors for recurrence of meningioma. J Neurooncol. 2010; 98(3): 379–384

[20] Makino K, Nakamura H, Hide T, et al. Fatty acid synthase is a predictive marker for aggressiveness in meningiomas. J Neurooncol. 2012; 109(2):399–404

[21] Tseng KY, Chung MH, Sytwu HK, et al. Osteopontin expression is a valuable marker for prediction of short-term recurrence in WHO grade I benign meningiomas. J Neurooncol. 2010; 100(2):217–223

[22] Wang Q, Fan SY, Qian J, et al. AKT2 expression in histopathologic grading and recurrence of meningiomas. Eur J Surg Oncol. 2014; 40 (9):1056–1061

[23] Kang HC, Kim IH, Park CI, Park SH. Immunohistochemical analysis of cyclooxygenase-2 and brain fatty acid binding protein expression in grades I-II meningiomas: correlation with tumor grade and clinical outcome after radiotherapy. Neuropathology. 2014; 34(5):446–454

[24] Baia GS, Caballero OL, Ho JS, et al. NY-ESO-1 expression in meningioma suggests a rationale for new immunotherapeutic approaches. Cancer Immunol Res. 2013; 1(5):296–302

[25] Kanno H, Nishihara H, Wang L, et al. Expression of CD163 prevents apoptosis through the production of granulocyte colony-stimulating factor in meningioma. Neuro-oncol. 2013; 15(7):853–864

[26] Barresi V, Alafaci C, Salpietro F, Tuccari G. Sstr2A immuno-histochemical expression in human meningiomas: is there a correlation with the histological grade, proliferation or microvessel density? Oncol Rep. 2008; 20(3):485–492

[27] Yuzawa S, Nishihara H, Tanaka S. Genetic landscape of meningioma. Brain Tumor Pathol. 2016; 33(4):237–247

[28] Ragel BT, Jensen RL. Molecular genetics of meningiomas. Neurosurg Focus. 2005; 19(5):E9

[29] Lee Y, Liu J, Patel S, et al. Genomic landscape of meningiomas. Brain Pathol. 2010; 20(4):751–762

[30] Clark VE, Erson-Omay EZ, Serin A, et al. Genomic analysis of non-NF2 meningiomas reveals mutations in TRAF7, KLF4, AKT1, and SMO. Science. 2013; 339(6123):1077–1080

[31] Brastianos PK, Horowitz PM, Santagata S, et al. Genomic sequencing of meningiomas identifies oncogenic SMO and AKT1 mutations. Nat Genet. 2013; 45(3):285–289

[32] Smith MJ, Wallace AJ, Bennett C, et al. Germline SMARCE1 mutations predispose to both spinal and cranial clear cell meningiomas. J Pathol. 2014; 234(4):436–440

[33] Mordechai O, Postovsky S, Vlodavsky E, et al. Metastatic rhabdoid meningioma with BRAF V600E mutation and good response to

personalized therapy: case report and review of the literature. Pediatr Hematol Oncol. 2015; 32(3):207–211

[34] Abedalthagafi MS, Merrill PH, Bi WL, et al. Angiomatous meningiomas have a distinct genetic profile with multiple chromosomal polysomies including polysomy of chromosome 5. Oncotarget. 2014; 5(21):10596–10606

[35] Sahm F, Schrimpf D, Olar A, et al. TERT promoter mutations and risk of recurrence in meningioma. J Natl Cancer Inst. 2015; 108(5)

[36] Simpson D. The recurrence of intracranial meningiomas after surgical treatment. J Neurol Neurosurg Psychiatry. 1957; 20(1):22–39

[37] Ohba S, Kobayashi M, Horiguchi T, et al. Long-term surgical outcome and biological prognostic factors in patients with skull base meningiomas. J Neurosurg. 2011; 114(5):1278–1287

[38] Sade B, Chahlavi A, Krishnaney A, Nagel S, Choi E, Lee JH. World Health Organization Grades II and III meningiomas are rare in the cranial base and spine. Neurosurgery. 2007; 61(6):1194–1198, discussion 1198

[39] Lee JY, Niranjan A, McInerney J, Kondziolka D, Flickinger JC, Lunsford LD. Stereotactic radiosurgery providing long-term tumor control of cavernous sinus meningiomas. J Neurosurg. 2002; 97(1):65–72

[40] Nakao N, Ohkawa T, Miki J, et al. Analysis of factors affecting the long-term functional outcome of patients with skull base meningioma. J Clin Neurosci. 2011; 18(7):895–898

[41] Salehi F, Jalali S, Alkins R, et al. Proteins involved in regulating bone invasion in skull base meningiomas. Acta Neurochir (Wien). 2013; 155(3):421–427

[42] Mansouri A, Klironomos G, Taslimi S, et al. Surgically resected skull base meningiomas demonstrate a divergent postoperative recurrence pattern compared with non-skull base meningiomas. J Neurosurg. 2016; 125(2):431–440

[43] Gump WC. Meningiomas of the pediatric skull base: a review. J Neurol Surg B Skull Base. 2015; 76(1):66–73

[44] Li Z, Li H, Jiao Y, et al. A comparison of clinicopathological features and surgical outcomes between pediatric skull base and non-skull base meningiomas. Childs Nerv Syst. 2017; 33(4): 595–600

[45] Sekhar LN, Juric-Sekhar G, Brito da Silva H, Pridgeon JS. Skull base meningiomas: aggressive resection. Neurosurgery. 2015; 62 suppl 1: 30–49

4 Exogenous Factors Affecting Meningiomas

Moujahed Labidi, Anne Laure Bernat, Sebastien Froelich

Abstract

On rare occasions, intracranial meningiomas are associated with genetic syndromes or occur in familial clusters. However, the vast majority of meningiomas are sporadic. A few environmental (or exogenous) factors have been associated with the occurrence of these tumors. In this review, we will see that the most clearly established risk factor for the development of intracranial meningiomas is ionizing radiation. In fact, there is strong evidence in support of this causal relationship from studies involving survivors of exposure to irradiation from atomic bombs, childhood cancer survivors, and patients previously irradiated for tinea capitis. Similarly, there are now data in support of a direct effect of female sex hormones on meningioma growth. As a matter of fact, exogenous hormone intake, especially progestational agents, has to be specifically inquired about when assessing a patient with a newly diagnosed meningioma. In such cases, hormonal therapy cessation may be the only required intervention in the management of these tumors.

Other probable or suspected risk factors for the development of meningioma discussed in this chapter are radiofrequency electromagnetic fields, such as those emitted by mobile phones, obesity, and exposure to iron. We will also review evidence indicating that there may be a protective association between smoking and diabetes, and meningioma.

Keywords: exogenous factors, ionizing radiation, female sexual hormones, radiofrequency electromagnetic fields

4.1 Introduction

Meningiomas account for approximately 35% of all primary intracranial tumors.[1] In some rare situations, meningiomas occur in association with genetic syndromes. Among these, the most frequently encountered is neurofibromatosis type II, but there are few others, namely ataxia telangiectasia syndrome, Gorlin syndrome, Rubinstein-Taybi syndrome, etc. There have also been reports of familial clustering of intracranial meningiomas, in the absence of a genetic syndrome.[2,3]

However, most meningiomas are sporadic and their etiology remains largely unknown. In this chapter, we will review the most recent evidence on exogenous factors that may act as risk factors for the development of intracranial meningiomas. Understanding this data is key in the hypothesis-generation of pathophysiological mechanisms of meningioma induction and growth. Among the suspected risk factors, we will focus this review on (1) ionizing radiation, (2) exogenous hormones, (3) radiofrequency magnetic fields (emitted by cellular phones), (4) metabolic syndrome, (5) occupational exposures, (6) smoking, (7) immunity, and (8) trauma.

4.2 Ionizing Radiation

Moderate to high dose ionizing radiation is the most clearly established risk factor for the development of intracranial meningiomas. In fact, there is strong evidence in support of this causal relationship from studies involving survivors of exposure to irradiation from atomic bombs, childhood cancer survivors, and patients previously irradiated for tinea capitis.

The two largest studies on the subject of childhood cancer survivors, the *USA Childhood Cancer Survivor Study* (CCSS) and the *British Childhood Cancer Survivor Study* (BCCSS) both reported a significant increase in the rate of secondary malignancies, including intracranial meningiomas. In the American study, the cumulative incidence of secondary malignancy at 30 years after primary diagnosis was 20.5%, including a 3.1% increase in meningioma incidence alone.[4] Moreover, in the British study, the risk of having a meningioma after radiation was linearly related to the radiation dose received. The adjusted relative risk (RR) of meningioma among those irradiated with doses of at least 40 Grays (Gy) was 479 times that of unexposed control cases.[5]

In the Japanese *Life Span Study of Atomic Bomb Survivors*, the mean dose to the brain during this one-time exposure to radiation was 0.078 to 10 Gy. In this report, although it was not statistically significant, there was an elevated risk of meningioma with an excess relative risk (ERR)/Sievert (Sv) of 0.64 (95% confidence interval; −0.01 to 1.8). In other data from both Nagasaki and Hiroshima bombs survivors, there was a correlation between the incidence of meningioma and the distance from the hypocenter of the atomic blast.[6] In Hiroshima, during the period between 1990 and 1992, the incidences of meningioma among the population within 1.0 km compared to the non-exposed group were 36.3 versus 5.6. The RR of radiation effect for meningioma was thus calculated as 6.48.[6]

Another seminal study that established association between ionizing radiation and meningiomas was the *Israel Tinea Capitis Cohort*. In its investigation, 10,834 individuals who were treated with cranial irradiation in the 1950s for a skin condition of the scalp were compared to nonexposed matched cohorts. The mean estimated radiation dose to the brain was 1.5 Gy. After 40 years, the ERR/Gy was found to be 4.63 (95% confidence interval; 2.43 to 9.12) for the development of benign meningiomas (data acquired through a national registry). This risk was positively associated with the radiation dose.[7]

In more recent evidence, even the low doses administered during dental X-rays, especially with older X-ray technology, were found to be associated with an increased risk of intracranial meningioma.[8]

Meningiomas associated with previous exposure to radiation differ from spontaneous meningiomas on many aspects, including age at presentation, multiplicity, clinical aggressiveness, and recurrence rate. In fact, multiplicity ranges from 4.6 to 18.7% in this particular subgroup of meningiomas (compared to 2.4% in spontaneous meningiomas in the *Israel Tinea Capitis Cohort*). In a series of 43 radiation-induced meningiomas, a 25.6% recurrence rate and an 11.6% rate of multiple recurrences were noted.[9] In our experience in treating these lesions, each patient often requires multiple operations and, during each surgical sitting, we do not hesitate to perform wide resection of the surrounding dura mater in the hope of reducing the recurrence rate.

4.3 Exogenous Hormones

The incidence of meningiomas is more than twofold higher in women than in men, an observation that has suggested very early on a role for sex hormones in the development and growth of meningiomas. The acceleration of meningioma growth during pregnancy, the subsequent shrinkage in size after delivery[10] and the association between breast cancer and meningiomas also supports this hypothesis.[11,12,13]

As a matter of fact, progesterone and estrogen receptors are very frequently expressed in meningiomas (progesterone in 61–95% of meningiomas and estrogens in 0–8.6% of cases).[14,15,16] Progesterone receptors have been shown to be associated with a more favorable prognosis, while the estrogen receptors are associated with an increased risk of tumor recurrence and progression. The meningioma's growth rate peaks during the reproductive life period.[10,17] In fact, molecular studies have shown that progesterone and estrogens together can stimulate cellular proliferation in meningiomas.[18] The precise mechanism involved in the hormonal induction and growth of meningiomas is not well understood but female hormones may modulate proliferation and cell cycle progression through transcriptional mechanisms involving the receptors.[18,19] In addition, estrogens have been postulated to affect genomic stability.[20,21] Lastly, estrogens interact with insulin-like growth factor, which stimulates tumor growth and prohibits cellular apoptosis.[22]

Consequently, several progesterone antagonist (mifepristone or onapristone) and antiestrogens (tamoxifen) have been proposed as potential therapeutic agents for unresectable meningiomas by blocking angiogenesis, although strong data is still lacking in this regard.[23,24,25]

4.3.1 Link between Cyproterone Acetate and Meningiomas

An important practical issue when managing intracranial meningiomas is the potential role of hormonal treatments.

Epidemiologic studies have shown either an absence or a weak relationship between meningiomas and hormone replacement therapy or oral contraception.[26] However, a definitive association between the prolonged use of high-dose progestational agents and meningiomas has been shown. More specifically, numerous patients treated with cyproterone acetate (CPA) for many years have been diagnosed with one or multiple meningiomas, mainly located on the anterior skull base and stabilizing or shrinking significantly after CPA withdrawal (cf. ▶ Fig. 4.1 and ▶ Fig. 4.2).[27,28,29,30]

CPA is prescribed mainly in Europe, predominantly in Spain and France, in Latin America and much less in some Asian countries. It is not available in the United States due to the risk of liver side effects. CPA's most common indications are signs of hyperandrogenism, such as those seen in polycystic ovary syndrome (PCOS), hirsutism, acne, and alopecia. It has also been used less commonly as an alternate contraceptive agent. In author's previously published series,[27] a link was reported between the duration of the exposure to CPA and the development of meningioma and an association between CPA and multiple meningiomas. It was also observed that the location of the meningiomas was more often found in the anterior skull base. Several authors subsequently reported similar findings.[30,31,32,33,34]

Pathophysiological mechanisms underlying this association between CPA and meningiomas, but also the significant tumor volume reductions seen after medication discontinuation are still unknown. Megestrol acetate and luteinizing hormone releasing hormone, both progesterone agonists have been reported to induce meningioma growth[35,36] but cases of spontaneous shrinkage after medication discontinuation are rare and have been reported with dramatic results only for CPA et chlormadinone acetate.[37] We also observed that peritumoral edema decreases after CPA withdrawal, which may be explained by the affinity of progesterone for glucocorticoid receptors of meningiomas.[38]

Meningiomas associated with CPA are located mainly in the anterior skull base. Genetic features related to meningiomas location have been studied previously and might also explain the behavior of these meningiomas induced on progestational agents. Clark et al reported that tumors with *NF2* mutations and/or chromosome 22 loss (*NF2/chr22loss*) were predominantly found in the hemispheres with nearly all posterior cerebral (parieto-occipital), cerebellar, or spinal meningiomas being *NF2/chr22loss* tumors.[39] They observed a difference between those originating from medial (*non-NF2*) versus lateral and posterior regions (*NF2/chr22loss*) of the skull base. Yuzawa et al also reviewed genetic patterns of 553 meningiomas and found a significant percentage of *NF2* mutation (55%).[40] They found several genes involved such as *TRAF7*, *AKT1*, *KLF4*, *PIK3CA*, and *SMO* and that 80% of cases harbored at least one of the genetic alterations in these

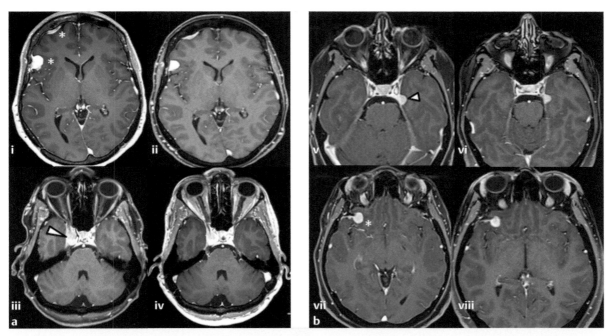

Fig. 4.1 Two (**a** and **b**) typical cases of multiple small meningiomas seen in association with cyproterone acetate. The preoperative T1-weighted axial images are seen in **i** and **iii** for the first case (**a**) and in **v** and **vii** for the second case (**b**). The same postoperative axial images are seen in **ii** and **iv** for the first case (**a**) and in **vii** and **viii** for the second case (**b**). The tumor's volume reduction was faster in both convexity meningiomas (*) than for the ones located in the anterior skull base (arrowhead).

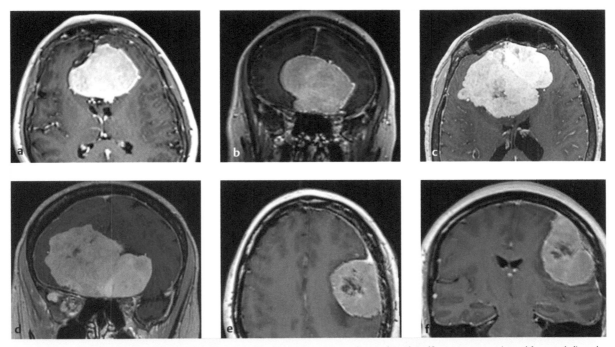

Fig. 4.2 Three cases of large solitary meningiomas on cyproterone acetate located in the olfactory groove (**a** and **b**, **c** and **d**) and convexity (**e** and **f**).

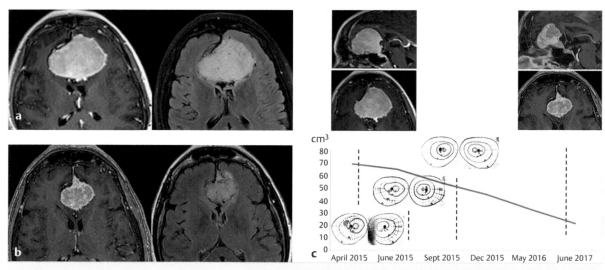

Fig. 4.3 A case of olfactory groove meningioma associated with cyproterone acetate [**a**, axial cuts in T1-weighted post-gadolinium and fluid attenuation inversion recovery (FLAIR) sequences] shrinking after hormone discontinuation (**b**, same sequences, 2 years after discontinuation). The signal changes seen on FLAIR suggest a modification of the tumor's vascularity. In **c**, the initial visual symptoms resolved over 2 months, neurobehavioral troubles over 8 months and there was a dramatic reduction in the tumor's volume over 26 months. Note that the rate of the tumor's volume reduction accelerated after December 2015, when the patient started losing weight following initiation of a strict diet.

genes. Tumors with the *TRAF7/AKT1* and *SMO* mutations shared specific features; they were located in the anterior fossa, median middle fossa, or anterior calvaria. Most of them were meningothelial or transitional meningiomas. Meningiomas associated with CPA might have similar genetic features, but this hypothesis warrants further investigation.

Additionally, in meningiomas associated with CPA, the duration of exposure to the medication has been shown to be a risk factor for the development of a meningioma and is proportional with the tumor's growth rate and volume.[27,30] We also observed that patients with multiple meningiomas had used CPA for a longer period of time (mean of 20.4 years) than patients with only one tumor (10 years) suggesting that longer exposure to CPA may induce the development of multiple tumors.[27] Another noteworthy observation made in our experience dealing with these cases is that the volume reduction rate in CPA-associated meningiomas may be slower in overweight patients (▶ Fig. 4.3). CPA is a lipophilic drug and it is possible that it is eliminated more slowly in overweight and obese patients.

4.4 Radiofrequency Electromagnetic Fields

The increasing use of mobile phones in our daily lives has led to concerns regarding potential adverse health effects, particularly development of tumors of the central nervous system (CNS) (including glioma, schwannomas, and meningiomas). In fact, studies have shown that the nonionizing radiofrequency emission of mobile phones can cause a small rise in the tissue temperature of the brain and adjacent organs.[41] However, large epidemiological studies have provided contrasted results and, as such, a clear causal relationship has not been established as of yet.

Among the earliest studies on this issue were conducted in Sweden that have provided some evidence for a possible association. One of the latest updates in this series of studies was a pooled analysis of two case-control studies of patients diagnosed with a meningioma between 1997 and 2003, and 2007 and 2009.[42] The investigators reported an increased risk of developing a meningioma among heavy users of mobile and cordless phones, especially in the highest quartile of cumulative use (wireless phones use > 1,486 hours), who had an odds ratio (OR) 1.3 (95% confidence interval; 1.1 to 1.6). The risk increased somewhat with latency, although this result was not statistically significant.

The *Danish Nationwide Study* followed up a cohort of 420,095 individuals who had signed a mobile phone contract from 1982 until 1995 and compared them to the rest of the adult Danish population. Follow-ups were then made in 1996, 2002, and 2007 through query of national registers. There was no overall increased risk of CNS tumors. Actually, the authors reported a 22% risk reduction for the development of meningiomas in men having a mobile phone subscription, while this risk was unchanged in women subscribers.[43]

The *INTERPHONE study*, an international population-based case-control study, had similar conclusions, although with some nuances. During this study, interviews were conducted with 2,425 patients with meningioma, 2,765 patients with glioma, and 7,658 control subjects. Overall, there was no compelling evidence that the risk of either glioma or meningioma was increased in association with the use of mobile phones. However, there were suggestions of an increased risk of glioma at the highest exposure levels, for ipsilateral exposures and gliomas of the temporal lobe. These suggestions were also documented for meningiomas, albeit with a much weaker statistical significance level.[44]

In a French multicentric case-control study (including 253 gliomas and 194 meningiomas), named the *CERENAT* study, there was no statistically significant difference in intracranial tumors between regular users of mobile phones and nonusers. In the heaviest mobile phone users (≥ 896 cumulative hours of use), an increased number of glioma were found, an association that was stronger after a 5-year latency period before the diagnosis. In meningiomas, an increased OR for more than 15 hours of calls/month was found (OR = 2.01, 95% confidence interval; 0.84 to 5.22). For cumulative duration of calls, a statistically significant association was observed in the last decile (OR = 2.57, 95% confidence interval; 1.02 to 6.44).[45]

Back in 2011, and in light of the available studies at the time, the International Agency for Research on Cancer (IARC) classified the radiofrequency electromagnetic fields as a "group 2B", or "possible", carcinogens. Some authors have more recently advocated reclassifying the REF as a "group 2A" ("probable") carcinogen.[46]

4.5 Metabolic Syndrome and Obesity

Obesity, and the metabolic syndrome more generally, have emerged as a major public health concern in the last decades. More recently, there has been accumulating evidence to the effect that obesity may be associated with the development of at least 13 types of cancer, including but not exclusive to postmenopausal breast cancer, endometrial cancer, colorectal adenomas, gallbladder cancer, pancreatic cancer, renal cancer, and liver cancer.[47,48]

Likewise, in a meta-analysis of the literature, obesity was found to be associated with an increased risk of having an intracranial meningioma (overall OR = 45, 95% confidence interval; 1.26 to 1.67).[47]

A British matched case-control study investigated the association of diabetes and intracranial meningiomas. In this study, 2,027 meningiomas were compared to 20,269 controls and an inverse relationship was found between diabetes and meningiomas (OR = 0.89, 95% confidence interval = 0.74 to 1.07). Interestingly, this association was driven by an inverse relation among women (OR = 0.78; 95% confidence interval = 0.62 to 0.98), in whom an inverse association with the duration of diabetes was also found (p = 0.071).[49] According to the authors, one possible explanation for such an association may be the reduced conversion of androgens into estrogens in the ovaries of female diabetic patients. Moreover, the authors suggested that exposure to different antidiabetic treatments may result in different outcomes in terms of meningioma development and growth. In the same study, sulfonylureas did not present any association with meningiomas and insulin was negatively associated with meningiomas. Conversely, metformin was found to be positively associated with meningioma, a finding that may indicate a possible role through modification of the hormonal balance in diabetic women using this medication (metformin may lead to reduction in the production of the luteinizing and follicle stimulating hormones).[49]

The metabolic syndrome is a cluster of metabolic risk factors that have been associated with an increased risk of cardiovascular diseases. Seliger et al have studied its potential association with meningiomas in a matched case-control study. Their findings suggest that only certain components of the metabolic syndrome are associated with meningiomas, namely obesity (OR = 1.33, 95% confidence interval; 1.17 to 1.52) and arterial hypertension (OR = 1.34, 95% confidence interval; 1.20 to 1.49). Dyslipidemia (low high density lipoprotein-cholesterol and high triglycerides) and impaired glucose tolerance, the other elements defining the metabolic syndrome, were not associated with meningioma. In addition to the hormonal hypothesis, the authors have suggested that chronic low grade inflammation, impaired immune function, increased oxidative stress, and decreased antioxidant mechanisms associated with the metabolic syndrome may also contribute to the development of meningiomas.[50]

4.6 Occupational Exposures

Occupational exposures and their possible carcinogenic effect in the development of meningiomas have also been the subject of intense interest. In the German subgroup from the *INTERPHONE* study, there was no association between six occupational categories (defined "a priori" as chemical, metal, agricultural, construction, electrical/electronic, and transport) and the risk of having a glioma, meningioma, or acoustic neuroma. However, data taken from the *INTEROCC* study group, a seven country population-based case-control study derived from the same *INTERPHONE* study, showed a positive association between exposure to iron (ever versus never exposed) and meningioma (OR = 1.26, 95% confidence interval; 1.00 to 1.58). An association that was stronger among women (OR = 1.70, 95% confidence interval; 1.00 to 2.89). Again, in the light of this gender-specific association, the authors of this study hypothesized that iron may interfere with meningioma development and growth through interaction with hormonal function.[51]

4.7 Smoking

Smoking is one of the most common and severe carcinogens which has been associated with numerous neoplastic processes. However, it has also been shown to be inversely associated with endometrial cancer, which like meningioma, has a hormonal etiology (Claus et al, 2013). In a meta-analysis of eight studies, and based on an ever versus never comparison, no statistical association was found between meningioma and smoking. More precisely, the same meta-analysis suggested that "ever" smoking was associated with an increased risk of meningioma in men but not in women.[52] Some studies have even shown a protective effect of smoking among women.[53] The hypothesis put forward by the authors of this study to explain this association is that cigarette smoking may reduce serum levels of estradiol through its inactivation into catechol estrogens, increased binding to the sex-hormone binding protein, and decreased adipose cell production of estradiol.

4.8 Immunity

Variations in the activity of the immune system has been implicated in various forms of tumoral and carcinogenic processes. More specifically, the association between allergy and/or eczema and meningioma has been the subject of many studies. A meta-analysis including case-control or cohort studies investigating this association between allergic conditions and meningioma found seven eligible studies.[54] In the pooled analysis of the results, there was a nonstatistically significant association of meningioma with overall allergic conditions, a category that included asthma, hay fever, and eczema, (OR = 0.91, 95% confidence interval; 0.79 to 1.04). However, a statistically significant inverse relationship was identified between eczema and meningioma (OR = 0.75, 95% confidence interval; 0.65 to 0.87). This finding provides clues as to a possible role for immunity in meningioma tumorigenesis, although the exact pathophysiological mechanisms behind this remain largely unknown.

4.9 Trauma

A causal relationship between head trauma and meningioma has long been suspected, although little evidence has been found in support of this claim. This possible interaction was even suggested by Harvey Cushing, who stated that "the conclusion that an etiological factor is involved is inescapable."[55] Among the strongest evidence against such an association comes from a Danish study that included 228,055 individuals hospitalized because of concussion, fractured skull, or other head injury between 1977 and 1992. These patients were tracked for an average of 8 years. In this cohort, the reported standardized incidence ratio for meningiomas after the first year was 1.2 (95% confidence interval; 0.8 to 1.7).[56]

4.10 Conclusion

In this overview of exogenous factors in meningioma tumorigenesis and growth, we have seen that the most clearly established risk factor is ionizing radiation. There is also accumulating evidence in support of a direct influence of female sex hormones on meningioma growth. As a matter of fact, exogenous hormone intake, especially progestational agents, has to be specifically inquired about when assessing a patient with a newly diagnosed meningioma. In such cases, hormonal therapy cessation may be the only required intervention in the management of these tumors.

Other probable or suspected risk factors for the development of meningioma discussed in this chapter are radiofrequency electromagnetic fields, such as those emitted by mobile phones, obesity, and exposure to iron. Interestingly, a few studies have shown that there are protective associations between smoking and diabetes, and meningioma. These gender-specific interactions also support the important role played by female sex hormone in meningioma. The interaction between some exogenous risk factors, hormonal balance, and meningiomas may be a promising way to better understand the evolution of these tumors.

In the future, a better understanding of the genetic and molecular profiles and subtypes of meningioma may provide additional clues as to the exact role played by these different environmental and potentially modifiable risk factors in the tumorigenesis of meningiomas.

References

[1] Ostrom QT, Gittleman H, Liao P, et al. CBTRUS statistical report: primary brain and central nervous system tumors diagnosed in the United States in 2007–2011. Neuro-oncol. 2014; 16 Suppl 4:iv1–iv63

[2] Couldwell WT, Cannon-Albright LA. A description of familial clustering of meningiomas in the Utah population. Neuro-oncol. 2017; 19(12):1683–1687

[3] Vijapura C, Saad Aldin E, Capizzano AA, Policeni B, Sato Y, Moritani T. Genetic syndromes associated with central nervous system tumors. Radiographics. 2017; 37(1):258–280

[4] Braganza MZ, Kitahara CM, Berrington de González A, Inskip PD, Johnson KJ, Rajaraman P. Ionizing radiation and the risk of brain and central nervous system tumors: a systematic review. Neuro-oncol. 2012; 14(11):1316–1324

[5] Taylor AJ, Little MP, Winter DL, et al. Population-based risks of CNS tumors in survivors of childhood cancer: the British Childhood Cancer Survivor Study. J Clin Oncol. 2010; 28(36):5287–5293

[6] Shintani T, Hayakawa N, Hoshi M, et al. High incidence of meningioma among Hiroshima atomic bomb survivors. J Radiat Res (Tokyo). 1999; 40(1):49–57

[7] Sadetzki S, Chetrit A, Freedman L, Stovall M, Modan B, Novikov I. Long-term follow-up for brain tumor development after childhood exposure to ionizing radiation for tinea capitis. Radiat Res. 2005; 163 (4):424–432

[8] Claus EB, Calvocoressi L, Bondy ML, Schildkraut JM, Wiemels JL, Wrensch M. Dental x-rays and risk of meningioma. Cancer. 2012; 118 (18):4530–4537

[9] Umansky F, Shoshan Y, Rosenthal G, Fraifeld S, Spektor S. Radiation-induced meningioma. Neurosurgical Focus. 2008; 24(5):E7

[10] Smith JS, Quiñones-Hinojosa A, Harmon-Smith M, Bollen AW, McDermott MW. Sex steroid and growth factor profile of a meningioma associated with pregnancy. Can J Neurol Sci. 2005; 32 (1):122–127

[11] Kubo M, Fukutomi T, Akashi-Tanaka S, Hasegawa T. Association of breast cancer with meningioma: report of a case and review of the literature. Jpn J Clin Oncol. 2001; 31(10):510–513

[12] Mehta D, Khatib R, Patel S. Carcinoma of the breast and meningioma. Association and management. Cancer. 1983; 51(10):1937–1940

[13] Custer B, Longstreth WT, Jr, Phillips LE, Koepsell TD, Van Belle G. Hormonal exposures and the risk of intracranial meningioma in women: a population-based case-control study. BMC Cancer. 2006; 6 (1):152

[14] Brandis A, Mirzai S, Tatagiba M, Walter GF, Samii M, Ostertag H. Immunohistochemical detection of female sex hormone receptors in meningiomas: correlation with clinical and histological features. Neurosurgery. 1993; 33(2):212–217, discussion 217–218

[15] Hsu DW, Efird JT, Hedley-Whyte ET. Progesterone and estrogen receptors in meningiomas: prognostic considerations. J Neurosurg. 1997; 86(1):113–120

[16] Rubinstein AB, Loven D, Geier A, Reichenthal E, Gadoth N. Hormone receptors in initially excised versus recurrent intracranial meningiomas. J Neurosurg. 1994; 81(2):184–187

[17] Hatiboglu MA, Cosar M, Iplikcioglu AC, Ozcan D. Sex steroid and epidermal growth factor profile of giant meningiomas associated with pregnancy. Surg Neurol. 2008; 69(4):356–362, discussion 362–363

[18] Jay JR, MacLaughlin DT, Riley KR, Martuza RL. Modulation of meningioma cell growth by sex steroid hormones in vitro. J Neurosurg. 1985; 62(5):757–762

[19] Wigertz A, Lönn S, Hall P, et al. Reproductive factors and risk of meningioma and glioma. Cancer Epidemiol Biomarkers Prev. 2008; 17(10):2663–2670

[20] Dickson RB, Stancel GM. Estrogen receptor-mediated processes in normal and cancer cells. Natl Cancer Inst Monogr. 2000; 27:135–145

[21] Henderson BE, Feigelson HS. Hormonal carcinogenesis. Carcinogenesis. 2000; 21(3):427–433

[22] Basen-Engquist K, Chang M. Obesity and cancer risk: recent review and evidence. Curr Oncol Rep. 2011; 13(1):71–76

[23] Elmaci İ, Altinoz MA, Sav A, Yazici Z, Ozpinar A. Giving another chance to mifepristone in pharmacotherapy for aggressive meningiomas-A likely synergism with hydroxyurea? Curr Probl Cancer. 2016; 40(5–)(6):229–243

[24] Miyai M, Takenaka K, Hayashi K, Kato M, Uematsu K, Murai H. [Effect of an oral anti-estrogen agent (mepitiostane) on the regression of intracranial meningiomas in the elderly]. Brain Nerve. 2014; 66(8):995–1000

[25] Ji J, Sundquist J, Sundquist K. Association of tamoxifen with meningioma: a population-based study in Sweden. Eur J Cancer Prev. 2016; 25(1):29–33

[26] Qi ZY, Shao C, Huang Y-L, Hui G-Z, Zhou Y-X, Wang Z. Reproductive and exogenous hormone factors in relation to risk of meningioma in women: a meta-analysis. PLoS ONE. 2013; 8(12):e83261

[27] Bernat AL, Oyama K, Hamdi S, et al. Growth stabilization and regression of meningiomas after discontinuation of cyproterone acetate: a case series of 12 patients. Acta Neurochir (Wien). 2015; 157(10):1741–1746

[28] Cebula H, Pham TQ, Boyer P, Froelich S. Regression of meningiomas after discontinuation of cyproterone acetate in a transsexual patient. Acta Neurochir (Wien). 2010; 152(11):1955–1956

[29] Gonçalves AMG, Page P, Domigo V, Méder JF, Oppenheim C. Abrupt regression of a meningioma after discontinuation of cyproterone treatment. AJNR Am J Neuroradiol. 2010; 31(8):1504–1505

[30] Kalamarides M, Peyre M. Dramatic shrinkage with reduced vascularization of large meningiomas after cessation of progestin treatment. World Neurosurg. 2017; 101:814.e7–814.e10

[31] Piper JG, Follett KA, Fantin A. Sphenoid wing meningioma progression after placement of a subcutaneous progesterone agonist contraceptive implant. Neurosurgery. 1994; 34(4):723–725, discussion 725

[32] Pozzati E, Zucchelli M, Schiavina M, Contini P, Foschini MP. Rapid growth and regression of intracranial meningiomas in lymphangioleiomyomatosis: case report. Surg Neurol. 2007; 68(6):671–674, discussion 674–675

[33] Zairi F, Aboukais R, LE Rhun E, Marinho P, Maurage CA, Lejeune JP. Close follow-up after discontinuation of cyproterone acetate: a possible option to defer surgery in patients with voluminous intracranial meningioma. J Neurosurg Sci. 2017; 61(1):98–101

[34] Alderman CP. Probable Drug-Related Meningioma Detected During the Course of Medication Review Services. Consult Pharm. 2016; 31 (9):500–504

[35] Konstantinidou AE, Korkolopoulou P, Mahera H, et al. Hormone receptors in non-malignant meningiomas correlate with apoptosis, cell proliferation and recurrence-free survival. Histopathology. 2003; 43(3):280–290

[36] Gruber T, Dare AO, Balos LL, Lele S, Fenstermaker RA. Multiple meningiomas arising during long-term therapy with the progesterone agonist megestrol acetate. Case report. J Neurosurg. 2004; 100(2):328–331

[37] Shimizu J, Matsumoto M, Yamazaki E, Yasue M. Spontaneous regression of an asymptomatic meningioma associated with discontinuation of progesterone agonist administration. Neurol Med Chir (Tokyo). 2008; 48(5):227–230

[38] Carroll RS, Zhang J, Dashner K, Black PM. Progesterone and glucocorticoid receptor activation in meningiomas. Neurosurgery. 1995; 37(1):92–97

[39] Clark VE, Erson-Omay EZ, Serin A, et al. Genomic analysis of non-NF2 meningiomas reveals mutations in TRAF7, KLF4, AKT1, and SMO. Science. 2013; 339(6123):1077–1080

[40] Yuzawa S, Nishihara H, Tanaka S. Genetic landscape of meningioma. Brain Tumor Pathol. 2016; 33(4):237–247

[41] Benson VS, Pirie K, Schuz J. Million Women Study Collaborators. Mobile phone use and risk of brain neoplasms and other cancers: prospective study. Int J Epidemiol. 2013; 42(3):792–802

[42] Carlberg M, Hardell L. Pooled analysis of Swedish case-control studies during 1997–2003 and 2007–2009 on meningioma risk associated with the use of mobile and cordless phones. Oncol Rep. 2015; 33(6):3093–3098

[43] Frei P, Poulsen AH, Johansen C, Olsen JH, Steding-Jessen M, Schüz J. Use of mobile phones and risk of brain tumours: update of Danish cohort study. BMJ. 2011; 343:d6387

[44] Cardis E, Armstrong BK, Bowman JD, et al. Risk of brain tumours in relation to estimated RF dose from mobile phones: results from five Interphone countries. Occup Environ Med. 2011; 68(9):631–640

[45] Coureau G, Bouvier G, Lebailly P, et al. Mobile phone use and brain tumours in the CERENAT case-control study. Occup Environ Med. 2014; 71(7):514–522

[46] Morgan LL. Miller AB, Sasco A, Davis DL. Mobile phone radiation causes brain tumors and should be classified as a probable human carcinogen (2A). Int J Oncol. 2015; 46(5):1865–1871

[47] Shao C, Bai LP, Qi ZY, Hui GZ, Wang Z. Overweight, obesity and meningioma risk: a meta-analysis. PLoS One. 2014; 9(2):e90167

[48] Steele CB, Thomas CC, Henley SJ, et al. Vital signs: trends in incidence of cancers associated with overweight and obesity—United States, 2005–2014. MMWR Morb Mortal Wkly Rep. 2017; 66(39):1052–1058

[49] Seliger C, Meier CR, Becker C, et al. Diabetes, use of metformin, and the risk of meningioma. PLoS ONE. 2017; 12(7):e0181089

[50] Seliger C, Meier CR, Becker C, et al. Metabolic syndrome in relation to risk of meningioma. Oncotarget. 2017; 8(2):2284–2292

[51] Sadetzki S, Chetrit A, Turner MC, et al. Occupational exposure to metals and risk of meningioma: a multinational case-control study. J Neurooncol. 2016; 130(3):505–515

[52] Fan Z, Ji T, Wan S, et al. Smoking and risk of meningioma: a meta-analysis. Cancer Epidemiol. 2013; 37(1):39–45

[53] Claus EB, Walsh KM, Calvocoressi L, et al. Cigarette smoking and risk of meningioma: the effect of gender. Cancer Epidemiol Biomarkers Prev. 2012; 21(6):943–950

[54] Wang M, Chen C, Qu J, et al. Inverse association between eczema and meningioma: a meta-analysis. Cancer Causes Control. 2011; 22(10): 1355–1363

[55] Jääskeläinen JE. Post-traumatic meningioma: three case reports of this rare condition and a review of the literature. Acta Neurochir (Wien). 2010; 152(10):1761–1761

[56] Inskip PD, Mellemkjaer L, Gridley G, Olsen JH. Incidence of intracranial tumors following hospitalization for head injuries (Denmark). Cancer Causes Control. 1998; 9(1):109–116

5 Instrumentation (Micro, Endo, IGS, MRI Application)

Oreste de Divitiis, Phillip A. Bonney, Teresa Somma, Federico Frio, Gabriel Zada

Abstract

Resection of skull base meningiomas represents a complex surgery in which the best surgical approach requires knowledge of all the possibility offered by modern neurosurgery. Traditional microneurosurgical approaches have taken advantages of technological evolution, for example, neuronavigation systems, to gain lesser bone removal and safer tumor debulking of such skull base lesions (minimally invasive surgery). On that way, the evolution of the extended endoscopic endonasal approaches, nowadays, offer minimal bone removal with safe debulking and dissection away from neurovascular structures. Besides, in selected procedures, the endoscope can be managed as an adjunct tool in traditional keyhole microsurgical approaches to obtain a detailed view of the structures in the shadow of the microscope beam, for inspection at the depth of a resection cavity (endoscope-assisted microneurosurgery).

Advances in technology have complemented the development of dedicated equipment and microinstruments designed for each approach. In an effort to lessen surgical trauma and to expand the mobility within such narrow corridors, low-profile shaft with well-established ergonomic features of newer micro-instruments have improved the surgical results and reduced brain damage.

In this chapter, we analyze the state-of-the-art of the instrumentation utilized in microscopic and endoscopic skull base surgery.

Keywords: skull base surgery, meningiomas, instrumentation, endoscope, operating microscope, imageguided surgery

5.1 Introduction

Meningiomas are common intracranial tumors often arising along the skull base or convexity regions.[1] The most challenging task confronting contemporary neurosurgeons remains the selection of the most appropriate surgical approach: multiple factors including surgeon's preference and experience, tumor size consistency and location, extent of dural attachment and relation with neurovascular structures should take in account for choosing the best corridor.

Traditional microsurgical approaches for resection of skull base meningiomas involve open microscopic craniotomy with fine tumor microdissection. Recently, extended endoscopic approaches have been utilized successfully to access and resect selected skull base meningiomas. Nowadays, the operating microscope, as well as the endoscope, are essential components of visual integration in the modern operating room (OR). The endoscope is the sole visualizing tool in pure extended endoscopic approaches and, in selected procedures, can be used in supporting the traditional microsurgical approaches, to simplify control of deep and hidden structures (endoscope-assisted microneurosurgery) (▶ Fig. 5.1).[2,3]

Preparation for complex skull base tumor surgery includes ensuring that the surgical team has access to all required equipment and instrumentation—the so-called "clock-gear mechanism" described by Cappabianca et al. A variety of optical equipment (e.g., microscopic or endoscopic), tumor resection devices, and microdissection instruments must be available to the surgeon to safely and efficiently perform complex meningioma resection procedures.

The growing technological developments brought the light on the concept of minimally invasive surgery. On that way, great attention has been focused on the idea of image-guided surgery (IGS), and it has been facilitated by the introduction of the neuronavigation systems (▶ Fig. 5.2). It allows the transfer of increasingly refined presurgical image information into the operating theater, to guide surgical procedures with a better knowledge of spatial orientation inside the skull base.

Future direction in skull base surgery, with improvements in technology, will led to robotic-assisted approaches that may become useful to enhance the surgeon expertise.[4,5,6]

5.2 The Role of the Microscopy in Skull Base Surgery

5.2.1 Positioning

The operative environment is an important "tool" for achieving a satisfactory operative result.[7,8]

Positioning the patient foresees methodic and consecutive steps, with the aim of achieving a comfortable working position for surgeon and the best working angle for reaching depth structures.

The head should be positioned using Sugita Head holder or three-pin Mayfield head holder, to get the best surgical operative angle, as regard to tissues and permitting gravity-assisted retraction.[9,10] Therefore, pin-fixation sites of the frames, as well as the arch and the counter arch of the Sugita frame, should allow total access to the operative field without hindering free movements of the neurosurgeon's hands or instruments or the operating microscope.[10]

The elevation of the head (20–30 cm over the level of the heart) facilitates venous drainage and the head should

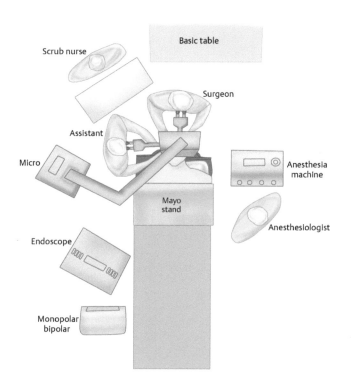

Fig. 5.1 Drawing representing a schematic disposition of the staff and equipment into the operating theater during endoscope-assisted microsurgical approach.

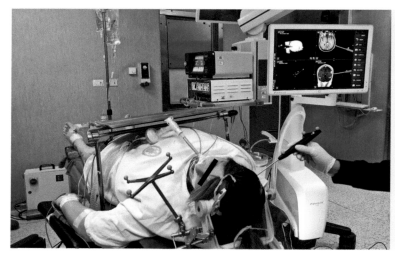

Fig. 5.2 Intraoperative photographs during a transcranial approach: the neuronavigation system guides the stereotactic centered craniotomy for a convexity meningioma.

not be turned too much, to avoid arterial and venous compression.

Most intracranial procedures are performed with the patient in the supine, three-quarters prone (lateral oblique or park-bench), or prone/concorde position, with the surgeon sitting at the head of the table.[11,12] Otherwise, modern operating tables offer easy and versatile adjustments, such as back elevation, lateral tilt, Trendelenburg, and anti-Trendelenburg position, which allow variations of working angle during surgery without moving the microscope.[13]

5.2.2 Operating Microscope

The operating microscope was first introduced in neurosurgical OR in 1957 by T. Kurze, which first removed a neurilemmoma of the eighth cranial nerve, and a crucial contribution provided by M.G. Yasargil, managed to overcome unwieldiness of the operating microscope, by permitting translational movements in the three planes.[14] It is the opening era of the modern neurosurgery.[15,16] Surgical procedures became more fluent and effective by the possibility of making fine adjustments to the position without repetitive use of the hands.[17,18]

Modern surgical microscopes provide the possibility of high magnification of the surgical field and stereoscopic perspective. Thanks to motorized zoom system, surgeon can suddenly change surgical field magnification to visualize small structures such as tumor vascular supplies. Equally important is also the possibility to visualize the depth of field by the stereoscopic perspective; this allows visualization of deep structures reducing brain retraction.

The light intensity is a fundamental aspect of gaining visual resolutions under the operating microscope: incandescent, fiber optic, halogen, and tungsten are available types of illumination.

Furthermore, the stability of the operating microscope permits movements during surgery and is guaranteed by a modern system of adjustable counterweights. This permits to reduce the operation time spent merely adjusting and moving the microscope, improving surgeon comfort. Finally, allows real-time observation and recording of operative details not otherwise visible by the integration with high-resolution 3CCD camera system.

This technical revolution changed the neurosurgery, permitting smaller cortical incisions and less brain retraction ("keyhole surgery"), but also safer and precise coagulation of bleeding points, less neural and vascular damage, and anastomosis of small vessels and nerves.[19]

Today's operating microscopes mount sophisticated imaging capabilities to better visualize malignant gliomas, such as blue light illumination and infrared technology, with administration of oral 5-aminolevulinic acid (5-ALA) and intravenous indocyanine green (ICG), respectively.

5.2.3 Microsurgical Instruments and Techniques

The instruments become extensions of the surgeon's own body. Every operation and even every technique for each type of operation requires a dedicated set of instruments (▶ Fig. 5.3).[20,21] Technological research permitted the realization of suitable handle microsurgical instruments, which are used, according to the "blind hand" technique, without direct visual control. Indeed, the straight bayoneted instruments are designed to avoid conflict between the surgeon's hands and the lens of the microscope. Bayonet forceps may be used to develop tissue planes, instead of straight scissors with fine blades or circular semisharp arachnoid blade, with a variety of tip sizes, is used for opening the most superficial arachnoid membrane, according to the "sharp dissection" (▶ Fig. 5.4).

The bipolar forceps provide accurate coagulation of bleeding areas in the scalp, muscles, dura, and intradural areas. Choosing the right lengths of bipolar forceps helps for delicate coagulation of brain tissue and tumor; furthermore, it permits arachnoid dissection and tumor manipulation, just adopting opening and closing maneuvers.

1- or 2-mm freer dissector or round-tip microdissector, are two important instruments. They are suitable for "blunt dissection"; indeed, they can be used for separating layers, vessels, and nerves, and surrounded tissue from tumor. In this scenario, the "water-jet" could be considered as one of the most elegant tool for dissection. Indeed, repeated injection of warm Ringer's solution in the subarachnoid space is currently used for separating arachnoid membranes or tumor from surrounding tissue.[22]

The suction is a multifunctional tool, in both neurosurgeon hands. Indeed, it could be used by right and left neurosurgeon hand for suction, retraction, and dissection. In particular, the modern suction tubes combine an ergonomic, surgeon-friendly design with the freedom

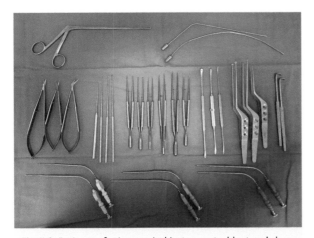

Fig. 5.3 Basic set of microsurgical instruments: blunt and sharp dissection instruments, different diameter wraparound tip aspirators, and different size Yasargil's tumor grasping forceps bayoneted shaped.

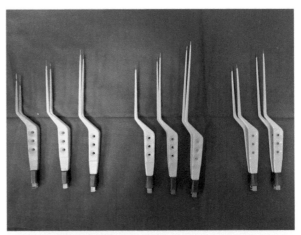

Fig. 5.4 Basic set of Yasargil's style stainless steel bipolar forceps.

and flexibility of many different lengths and diameters (from 3 to 7 French), with wraparound tip to minimize tissue injury. The slim, lightweight handpiece reduces fatigue during long procedures, while providing precise, intraoperative suction control with thumb or forefinger.

Brain retraction can increase the surgical working area but, several reports have claimed that "retractorless surgery" is superior for preserving neural function. Indeed, patient positioning, cerebrospinal fluid (CSF) drainage, neuroanesthesia, and suitable uses of bipolar forceps, suction tubes, cottonoids, and other instruments, provide to constantly move out the brain off the surgical working area. However, in some cases (e.g., subfrontal approach), with the aid of microcottonoids to protect the brain, the intermittent use of gentle brain spatulas or self-retaining retractors (Greenberg retractor, Fukushima holder system, or Sugita-type retractors) offers the necessary operative space in the depth.[7]

High-speed micro-drill with diamond-tipped burrs is fundamental to gently reduce the thickness of bones, such as the lesser and greater wing of the sphenoid in pterional or fronto-orbito-zygomatic approach, for increasing the surgical working area.

The Cavitron Ultrasonic Surgical Aspirator (CUSA) was introduced in neurosurgery approximately 30 years ago and, nowadays, it is a fundamental tool in modern OR (▶ Fig. 5.5). It is composed of an ultrasound generator, a sucker, and an irrigator that, together, combines aspiration, ultrasonic dissection, and irrigation in a single operation. The CUSA destroys selectively tissues with high water and low collagen content, so is used for fragmentation of solid tissues, such as meningioma, with relative sparing of vessels. Its widespread use is due to reduction of surgical time associated to respect of surrounding neural brain structures.[23]

5.3 Endoscopy

The endoscope can be a useful primary tool or surgical adjunct for a variety of meningiomas, when carefully selected. Skull base meningiomas in the region of the olfactory groove, planum sphenoidale, tuberculum sellae, or clivus can sometimes be approached via a pure extended endoscopic endonasal approach (EEA). Other times, keyhole access with endoscopic assistance can be utilized for skull base meningiomas (e.g., a supraorbital eyebrow craniotomy). For standard convexity meningiomas, the endoscope can be used as a surgical adjunct or exoscopic optic technology can be used for the entire operation. Finally, intraventricular meningiomas can be resected using surgical exoscopes via tubular retractor systems.

5.3.1 Introduction

Although early pioneers of neuroendoscopy introduced endoscopes into the ventricles in the early 1900s, the true era of the endoscopy in neurosurgery began in the 1970s when a confluence of technological advancements galvanized interest for third ventriculostomy and other intraventricular procedures.[24,25] Around the same time, neurosurgeons began using the endoscope as an adjunct to the microscope in several operations. In the mid-1990s, continued improvements in illumination and magnification led to purely EEAs to the sella, a development which has subsequently revolutionized the treatment of lesions accessible through the skull base.[26]

5.3.2 The Endoscope

The modern rigid endoscope consists of a rod lens system, a light source, and a camera system (▶ Fig. 5.6). The rod lens, developed by Hopkins in the late 1960s, utilizes glass rods in series interspersed between short segments of air over the length of the device to create a magnified image.[24] These glass rods make use of increasing indices of refraction moving inward radially, creating a sinusoidal path of light transmission.[27] This unique design allows for magnification across a long and narrow scope. The length of the instrument is commonly 15 to 30 cm, tailored to the depth of the surgical target, and the width ranges from 2 to 4 mm. The lens of the endoscope may be straight or angled. The 30-degree angled endoscope is the most commonly used angled endoscope and provides visualization off the long axis of the instrument. The light

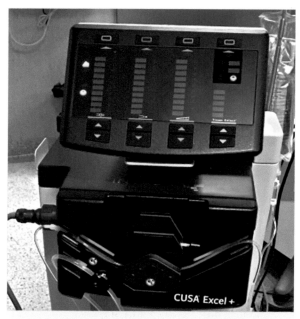

Fig. 5.5 CUSA Excel ultrasonic surgical aspirator system. It allows the selective dissection of target tissues while preserving vessels, ducts, and other delicate structures.

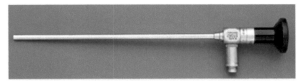

Fig. 5.6 The endoscope for endonasal transsphenoidal surgery: rigid, diagnostic rod lens telescopes (Hopkins scopes), 4-mm diameter, 18- or 30-cm long, with 0 30, or 45-degrees angled lenses. External sheath is connected to a manual or automated irrigation system. Recently, new generation of 3D endoscopes has been introduced for improved endoscopic depth perception. (This image is provided courtesy of Karl Storz Inc.)

source of the endoscope consists of fiber optic bundles which illuminate the surgical field from the working end of the instrument. A fiber optic cable attaches to the endoscope which provides illumination from an external source. The lens of the endoscope under direct illumination allows for excellent visualization at the depth of a surgical cavity. The image is relayed to a camera system that makes use of single or multiple charge coupled devices to transmit visual data onto a high-definition monitor to be viewed by the surgical team (▶ Fig. 5.7).

While capable solely of visualization, endoscopes are frequently incorporated into a system that allows for intervention as well. These systems include ports for suction/irrigation devices and working channels for endoscopy-tailored instruments. Such instruments include forceps, scissors, electrocautery (monopolar and bipolar), and numerous others, allowing the surgeon to perform the entirety of select procedures endoscopically. Accordingly, the endoscope may be employed either as the primary instrument of the operation or as an adjunct to the microscope.

5.3.3 Pure Endoscopic Approaches

Many skull base meningiomas can be targeted endonasally, particularly those arising along the midline anterior skull base. This minimally invasive approach provides relatively direct access to olfactory groove, tuberculum sellae, and planum sphenoidale meningiomas in a way that facilitates early identification and takedown of tumor vasculature as well as a complete bony and dural resection (true Simpson grade 1 resection). Using the endoscope, the tumor may be safely debulked and dissected away from critical neurovascular structures. For example, numerous groups have documented improved visual outcomes with an extended EEA to tuberculum and planum meningiomas compared with supraorbital approaches. Finally, angled endoscopes can be used to look around anatomical corners for residual tumor. Surgical instrumentation to augment these approaches and remove tumor that is visible using angled endoscopy is still evolving (▶ Fig. 5.8).

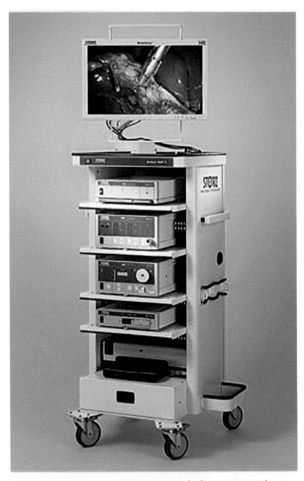

Fig. 5.7 Endoscopy tower is composed of a camera with 3 CCD technology, which can provide higher-quality images, a high-resolution monitor (HDTV or 3D endoscopic monitor), and a digital recording system that provides furthermore video editing and picture selection for didactic purposes.

The primary drawback relating to extended endonasal approaches is the increased difficulty of creating a watertight closure. As a result, postoperative CSF leak rates were historically as high as 25%, depending on the specific approach. However, closure techniques including autografts, synthetic materials, and vascular flaps (e.g., the pedicled nasal-septal flap) continue to improve, expanding the indications for these approaches.

In order to safely and seamlessly perform purely endoscopic endonasal skull base surgery, a variety of surgical instrumentation must be available. Cappabianca et al have referred to this paradigm as a "clock gear mechanism," in which all components must be properly functioning in order for the entire surgery to be successful.[28] Of course, any purely endoscopic approach relies on the availability of a functioning endoscope, light source, camera equipment, and high-resolution monitor. Surgical

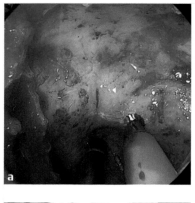
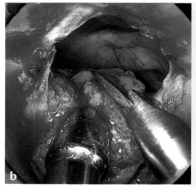
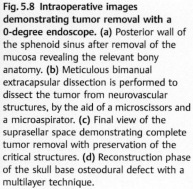
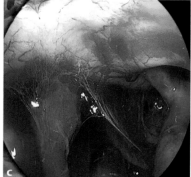
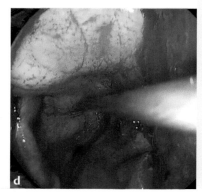

Fig. 5.8 Intraoperative images demonstrating tumor removal with a 0-degree endoscope. (a) Posterior wall of the sphenoid sinus after removal of the mucosa revealing the relevant bony anatomy. **(b)** Meticulous bimanual extracapsular dissection is performed to dissect the tumor from neurovascular structures, by the aid of a microscissors and a microaspirator. **(c)** Final view of the suprasellar space demonstrating complete tumor removal with preservation of the critical structures. **(d)** Reconstruction phase of the skull base osteodural defect with a multilayer technique.

adjuncts to extended endonasal endoscopic approaches may include neuronavigation (please see below), appropriate surgical instrumentation for sinus exposure (sinus tray and/or sinus microdebrider), bony removal (high-speed endoscopic drill or ultrasonic bone curette), tumor removal (including suction devices, grasping instruments, dissectors, microscissors, etc.), additional tumor resection devices (e.g., ultrasonic aspirators, side-cutting aspirators), autologous graft materials, dural sealants, and CSF diversion equipment.

5.3.4 Endoscope-Assisted Microneurosurgery

For meningioma cases in which a transcranial approach is used, the endoscope may play a role as an adjunct for visualization. In these cases, the magnification and illumination offered by the endoscope facilitates a particular aspect of the approach, such as inspection at the depth of a resection cavity which may be obstructed from view of the microscope. A common use is during supraorbital approaches, in which the 30-degree endoscope may be used to peer under and around structures of the anterior skull base to assess for the presence of tumor after the initial microscopic resection. For endoscopic-assisted keyhole operations, having access to low profile, long instruments is critical.

5.4 Image-Guided Surgery

The development of intraoperative navigation in neurosurgery has been instrumental in decreasing the morbidity and increasing the effectiveness of many skull base operations. Early frame-based navigation systems have now largely been replaced by frameless modalities.

Frameless neuronavigation systems relate the three-dimensional position of compatible instruments to the patient's anatomy represented on preoperative imaging (▶ Fig. 5.2). To do this, the exact position of the patient's head is determined and registered with the navigation software. Two common methods of registration include tracing skin landmarks with a pointer or other device and use of fiducials affixed to the patient's head. The former may be used in most cases of anterior pathology, while the latter may be necessary for posterior pathology. Most navigation systems make use of a rigid attachment to the Mayfield head clamp to ensure that the patient's head does not move in relation to the reference array.

Both MRI and CT are often relevant for the resection of skull base meningiomas, and many software packages enable toggling between the two or visualizing both simultaneously during neuronavigation. Neuronavigation is recommended for all extended endoscopic endonasal skull base approaches and for complex open approaches. For some open skull base craniotomies where the location of the tumor is easily identifiable (e.g., olfactory groove meningiomas), neuronavigation may be of limited benefit because the anatomy and location of pathology should be well known to the experienced surgeon.

5.5 Reconstruction Materials

The development of surgical approaches improved treatment of skull base lesions. However, CSF leaks represent a serious problem that could be controlled by a meticulous reconstruction of osteodural defects.[29]

5.5.1 Duraplasty and Hemostasis

Duraplasty is an important and complex step in tumor removal, especially in Simpson's grade I resection of skull base meningiomas, and it can be made using several dural substitutes (autologus materials, allografts, xenografts, and synthetic materials).[30]

The autologous materials (pericranium, fascia lata, temporalis fascia, fat, or muscles) offer different advantages: stability and facility of harvesting, immunologic activeness to potential contamination, faster healing process, and resistance to complementary radiation. The limitations are represented by small quantity availability (especially in minimally invasive approaches), and the eventual second skin incision.[31,32]

The xenograft materials, such as freeze-dried "lyophilized" dura and γ-rays sterilized bovine or equine pericardium, promote optimum fibroblastic proliferation and are not absorbable, acting as a guide for connective regeneration, but they are burdened by minimal risk of transmission of viral infection (e.g., Creutzfeldt–Jakob virus) and foreign body reactions.[33]

Plastic materials are represented by synthetic polymers that have the advantage of complete sterility. Absorbable Ethisorb Durapatch promotes fibroblastic reaction by replacing degraded graft by connective tissue, and demonstrated to show no tendency to local shrinkage.[34]

The concept of "watertight closure" of the dura is fundamental to prevent postoperative CSF leak. The first step is dural and/or graft suturing, which can be made by different suturing techniques (interrupted simple, running simple, or running locked), which should be performed always under microscopic technique. Application of surgical sealants directly on suture closure is useful to support dural reconstruction, ensuring rapid adhesion between human tissues and grafts and stimulating hemostasis and dural replacement.[35]

In selected case, "non-watertight closure" with collagen matrix represents an effective alternative, demonstrating to limit postoperative CSF leak: only application of matrix over the dura without dura suturing offers a rapid clot and fibrin formation, ensuring the holding of the graft in place, and promoting a rapid fibroblasts proliferation.[36]

Meticulous overview of the hemostasis is mandatory for controlling focal bleedings. Standard hemostatic techniques (pledge pressure, bipolar cautery, and oxidized cellulose) are usually effective in controlling bleeding, but in some cases, specific hemostatic agents and tissue sealant can come to surgeon's aid.[37] The available agents, such as gelatin sponges and thrombin-gelatin hemostatic materials, promote tissue adhesion and hemostasis either mechanically or by activating the coagulation cascade, demonstrated to be useful with ever- increasing employment in neurosurgery.[38]

References

[1] de Divitiis O, de Divitiis E. Anterior cranial fossa meningiomas: a new surgical perspective. World Neurosurg. 2012; 77(5–6):623–624

[2] de Divitiis E, de Divitiis O, Elefante A. Supraorbital craniotomy: pro and cons of endoscopic assistance. World Neurosurg. 2014; 82(1–2): e93–e96

[3] Cappabianca P, Cavallo LM, Esposito F, De Divitiis O, Messina A, De Divitiis E. Extended endoscopic endonasal approach to the midline skull base: the evolving role of transsphenoidal surgery. Adv Tech Stand Neurosurg. 2008; 33:151–199

[4] Apuzzo ML, Elder JB, Liu CY. The metamorphosis of neurological surgery and the reinvention of the neurosurgeon. Neurosurgery. 2009; 64(5):788–794, discussion 794–795

[5] Chauvet D, Hans S, Missistrano A, Rebours C, Bakkouri WE, Lot G. Transoral robotic surgery for sellar tumors: first clinical study. J Neurosurg. 2016:1–8

[6] Marcus HJ, Hughes-Hallett A, Cundy TP, Yang GZ, Darzi A, Nandi D. da Vinci robot-assisted keyhole neurosurgery: a cadaver study on feasibility and safety. Neurosurg Rev. 2015; 38(2):367–371, discussion 371

[7] Hernesniemi J, Niemelä M, Karatas A, et al. Some collected principles of microneurosurgery: simple and fast, while preserving normal anatomy: a review. Surg Neurol. 2005; 64(3):195–200

[8] Apuzzo ML, Weinberg RA. Architecture and functional design of advanced neurosurgical operating environments. Neurosurgery. 1993; 33(4):663–672, discussion 672–673

[9] Mayfield FH, Kees G, Jr. A brief history of the development of the Mayfield clip. Technical note. J Neurosurg. 1971; 35(1):97–100

[10] Zomorodi A, Fukushima T. Two surgeons four-hand microneurosurgery with universal holder system: technical note. Neurosurg Rev. 2017; 40(3):523–526

[11] Rhoton AL. Operative techniques and instrumentation for neurosurgery. In: Rothon AL, ed. Cranial Anatomy and Surgical Approaches, Chicago, IL: Lippincott William & Wilkins; 2003

[12] Clatterbuck R, Tamargo R. Surgical positioning and exposure for cranial procedures. In: Winn H, ed. Youmans Neurological Surgery. 5th ed., Philadelphia, PA: Saunders Elsevier Inc; 2004:623–645

[13] Mariniello G, de Divitiis O, Seneca V, Maiuri F. Classical pterional compared to the extended skull base approach for the removal of clinoidal meningiomas. J Clin Neurosci. 2012; 19(12):1646–1650

[14] de Divitiis O, de Divitiis E. The awe of the dura mater during the ages "Noli me tangere". World Neurosurg. 2015; 83(5):762–764

[15] Gelberman RH. Microsurgery and the development of the operating microscope. Contemp Surg. 1978; 13(6):43–46

[16] Kriss TC, Kriss VM. History of the operating microscope: from magnifying glass to microneurosurgery. Neurosurgery. 1998; 42(4): 899–907, discussion 907–908

[17] Uluç K, Kujoth GC, Başkaya MK. Operating microscopes: past, present, and future. Neurosurg Focus. 2009; 27(3):E4

[18] Yaşargil MG. Intracranial microsurgery. Clin Neurosurg. 1970; 17: 250–256

[19] de Divitiis E, Esposito F, Cappabianca P, Cavallo LM, de Divitiis O. Tuberculum sellae meningiomas: high route or low route? A series of 51 consecutive cases. Neurosurgery. 2008; 62(3):556–563, discussion 556–563

[20] Cappabianca P, de Divitiis O, Esposito F, Cavallo LM, de Divitiis E. Endoscopic skull base instrumentation. In: Schwartz TH, Anand VK, eds. Endoscopic Pituitary Surgery. New York, NY: Thieme; 2011:45–57

[21] Cappabianca P, Cavallo LM, Esposito F, de Divitiis E. Endoscopic endonasal transsphenoidal surgery: procedure, endoscopic equipment and instrumentation. Childs Nerv Syst. 2004; 20(11–12):796–801

[22] Nagy L, Ishii K, Karatas A, et al. Water dissection technique of Toth for opening neurosurgical cleavage planes. Surg Neurol. 2006; 65(1):38–41, discussion 41

[23] Tang H, Zhang H, Xie Q, et al. Application of CUSA Excel ultrasonic aspiration system in resection of skull base meningiomas. Chin J Cancer Res. 2014; 26(6):653–657

[24] Zada G, Liu C, Apuzzo ML. "Through the looking glass": optical physics, issues, and the evolution of neuroendoscopy. World Neurosurg. 2012; 77(1):92–102

[25] Apuzzo ML, Heifetz MD, Weiss MH, Kurze T. Neurosurgical endoscopy using the side-viewing telescope. J Neurosurg. 1977; 46(3):398–400

[26] Carrau RL, Jho HD, Ko Y. Transnasal-transsphenoidal endoscopic surgery of the pituitary gland. Laryngoscope. 1996; 106(7):914–918

[27] Esposito F, Cappabianca P. Neuroendoscopy: general aspects and principles. World Neurosurg. 2013; 79 s suppl 2:14.e7–14.e9

[28] Cavallo LM, Dal Fabbro M, Jalalod'din H, et al. Endoscopic endonasal transsphenoidal surgery. Before scrubbing in: tips and tricks. Surg Neurol. 2007; 67(4):342–347

[29] de Divitiis O, Di Somma A, Cavallo LM, Cappabianca P. Tips and tricks for anterior cranial base reconstruction. Acta Neurochir Suppl (Wien). 2017; 124:165–169

[30] Protasoni M, Sangiorgi S, Cividini A, et al. The collagenic architecture of human dura mater. J Neurosurg. 2011; 114(6):1723–1730

[31] Parízek J, Měricka P, Husek Z, et al. Detailed evaluation of 2959 allogeneic and xenogeneic dense connective tissue grafts (fascia lata, pericardium, and dura mater) used in the course of 20 years for duraplasty in neurosurgery. Acta Neurochir (Wien). 1997; 139(9):827–838

[32] Taha AN, Almefty R, Pravdenkova S, Al-Mefty O. Sequelae of autologous fat graft used for reconstruction in skull base surgery. World Neurosurg. 2011; 75(5–6):692–695

[33] Cavallo LM, Solari D, Somma T, Di Somma A, Chiaramonte C, Cappabianca P. Use of equine pericardium sheet (LYOMESH®) as dura mater substitute in endoscopic endonasal transsphenoidal surgery. Transl Med UniSa. 2013; 7:23–28

[34] Mello LR, Feltrin LT, Fontes Neto PT, Ferraz FA. Duraplasty with biosynthetic cellulose: an experimental study. J Neurosurg. 1997; 86(1):143–150

[35] Cappabianca P, Esposito F, Magro F, et al. Natura abhorret a vacuo—use of fibrin glue as a filler and sealant in neurosurgical "dead spaces". Technical note. Acta Neurochir (Wien). 2010; 152(5):897–904

[36] Sade B, Oya S, Lee JH. Non-watertight dural reconstruction in meningioma surgery: results in 439 consecutive patients and a review of the literature. Clinical article. J Neurosurg. 2011; 114(3):714–718

[37] Stendel R, Danne M, Fiss I, et al. Efficacy and safety of a collagen matrix for cranial and spinal dural reconstruction using different fixation techniques. J Neurosurg. 2008; 109(2):215–221

[38] Cappabianca P, Esposito F, Esposito I, Cavallo LM, Leone CA. Use of a thrombin-gelatin haemostatic matrix in endoscopic endonasal extended approaches: technical note. Acta Neurochir (Wien). 2009; 151(1):69–77, discussion 77

6 Intraoperative Neurophysiologic Monitoring during Surgery

Pietro Meneghelli, Francesco Sala

Abstract

Intraoperative neurophysiological monitoring (IONM) represents a valuable tool in the management of skull base meningiomas. First, through neurophysiological mapping techniques it is possible to identify, and spare, ambiguous neural structures that could be displaced or encased by the tumor. This is particularly valuable to identify cranial nerves when the anatomy is distorted. Second, the surgical manipulation of cranial nerves, perforating vessels, and brain or brainstem parenchyma may expose patients to substantial risk of neurological injury. In this perspective, IONM provides a continuous functional feedback on the functional integrity of motor, somatosensory, auditory, and visual pathways. Whenever warning criteria for changes in the evoked potentials are reached, the surgeon is informed of an impending injury and can adjust the surgical strategy in order to take corrective measures to reverse or minimize the risk of injury to the nervous system.

The combination of both mapping and monitoring techniques provides a multimodality approach, which offers the best chance to avoid neurological deficits. The application of different IONM strategies during skull base surgery must be tailored to the location of the tumor, according to the vascular and neural structures involved. This chapter will critically review the most common IONM techniques and their application during surgery for skull base meningiomas.

Keywords: somatosensory-evoked potential, motor-evoked potential, visual-evoked potentials, cranial nerve monitoring, intraoperative neurophysiologic monitoring, skull base meningiomas

6.1 Introduction

Surgical management of skull base meningiomas usually carries the risk of postoperative neurologic dysfunctions. The technique used for skull base surgery is based on microsurgical "navigation" inside the basal cisterns through the subarachnoid space in order to avoid or at least to reduce the manipulation of the brain as much as possible, which can cause contusions and/or hemorrhages. Brain arteries and cranial nerves run through the cisternal compartment and can be displaced, encased or even destroyed by skull base lesions. Thus, postoperative neurologic deficits are mainly related to arterial damage and/or injuries to one or more cranial nerves. Different locations and grow patterns of skull base tumors are related to different surgical risks. For example, the removal of an anterior clinoid meningioma that encases the carotid bifurcation and the proximal M1 segment is mainly related with the risk of damage to the perforating branches arising from the carotid bifurcation and/or the proximal part of the M1 segment; the removal of a cerebellopontine angle (CPA) tumor is mainly related with possible injury to the cranial nerves VII and VIII.

In the recent past, the standardization of skull base and cranial approaches as well as the wider use of endoscopic surgery has profoundly impacted on skull base surgery. The capability to approach a skull base tumor from its insertion on the dura, where the tumor receives its vascular supply, is a key factor for a successful surgery and, notably, this goal is nowadays reached through minimally invasive approaches. However, despite new technology and keyhole surgery, skull base tumors are still related with significant risk of postoperative morbidity and mortality.

IONM has increasingly gained value as a method to reduce the risk of neurologic injury. IONM evaluates the functional integrity of sensory, motor, auditory, and visual pathways; also, it permits to map ambiguous neural structures in order to define their functional role. Over the last two decades, IONM has become increasingly valuable during supratentorial brain tumor and cerebrovascular surgery.[1,2,3,4] IONM for infratentorial tumors relies on brainstem monitoring and, for skull base tumors, mainly on cranial nerve (CN) monitoring.[5,6,7] While monitoring techniques allow to assess the functional integrity of different neural pathways throughout the surgery, neurophysiologic mapping can assist in identifying peripheral CNs that may have been displaced, encircled, or encased by the tumor. The conjunction of both monitoring and mapping IONM techniques provides a valuable feedback to the surgeon during all the steps of the procedure (▶ Fig. 6.1).

The aim of this chapter is to provide a description of the IONM techniques that are useful during surgical removal of skull base meningiomas and to give a simple guide for their use in daily clinical practice.

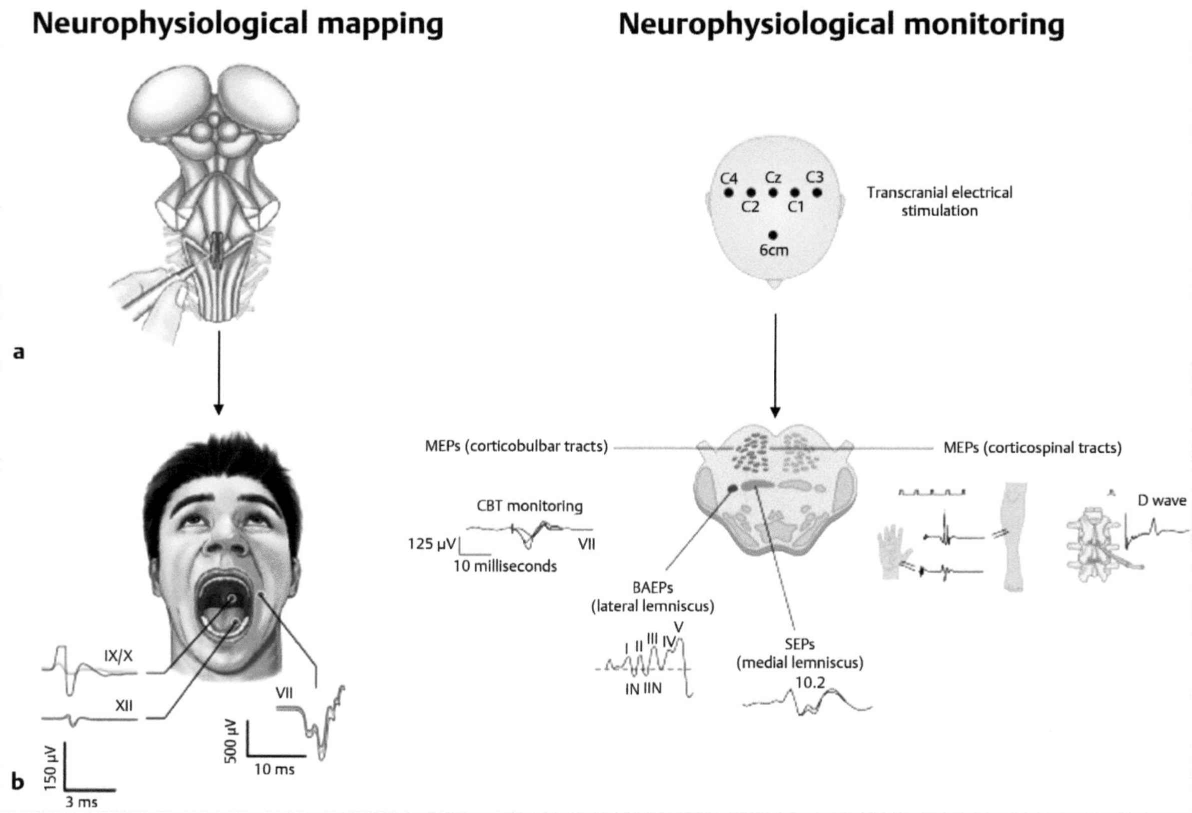

Neurophysiological mapping

Neurophysiological monitoring

Fig. 6.1 Schematic classification of intraoperative neurophysiology techniques in skull base surgery. *Left panel*: Neurophysiologic mapping allows to identify the functional landmarks in the brainstem as well as peripheral motor nerves. (a) A handheld monopolar probe is used to electrically stimulate the rhomboid fossa or the peripheral nerve. (b) Compound muscle action potentials are recorded from the muscles innervated by motor cranial nerves. *Right panel*: Neurophysiologic monitoring allows to keep under control the functional integrity of neural pathways (motor, sensory, auditory) throughout the surgery. See the text for further details on each monitoring technique. VII, recording from the orbicularis oris for the facial nerve; IX/X, recording from the posterior wall of the pharynx for the glossopharyngeal/vagus complex; XII, recording from the tongue muscles for the hypoglossal nerve. MEPs, motor-evoked potentials; *SSEPs*, somatosensory-evoked potentials; *BAERs*, brainstem auditory-evoked responses. CBT: corticobulbar tract (Modified from: F. Sala, P. Gallo, V. Tramontano. Intraoperative neurophysiological monitoring in posterior fossa surgery. In: M. Ozek, G. Cinalli, W. J. Maixner, C. Sainte-Rose, eds. Posterior Fossa Tumors in Children. Springer; 2015:239–262.)

6.2 Intraoperative Neurophysiologic Monitoring Techniques

6.2.1 Mapping Techniques to Identify Cranial Motor Nerves

A very useful technique in skull base surgery is the functional identification of oculomotor nerves by direct stimulation. Either a handheld monopolar probe or a bipolar concentric probe, which has the advantage of more focal stimulation, can be used to deliver low-intensity stimuli directly to the nerve. Rectangular pulses of 0.2-ms duration at 1 to 3 Hz and intensity up to 0.5 to 2 mA are generally used. The more focal is the stimulation, the more specific is the response, reducing the risk

of activation of nearby fibers due to current spreading. Recordings are obtained by inserting needle electrodes in the muscles innervated by the CNs. For small muscles such as the oculomotor muscles, wire Teflon-coated electrodes may be used as these are less traumatic. Typically, electrodes are inserted in the superior rectus, lateral rectus, and superior oblique muscles to record from the III, VI, and IV oculomotor nerve, respectively. The same technique can be used to localize oculomotor CN nuclei at the level of the midbrain (▶ Fig. 6.2).

When ambiguous tissue is encountered during surgery, the tip of the stimulator is placed on the tissue while the oscilloscope displays the recording muscles to determine whether this tissue is functional or, more simply, to confirm the visual identification of the nerve. For the oculomotor nerves one has to consider that compound muscle action potentials (CMAPs) from extraocular muscles are of low

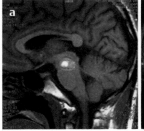
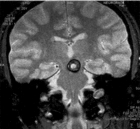
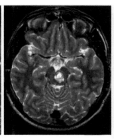

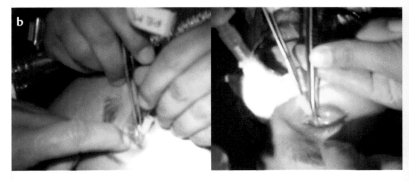

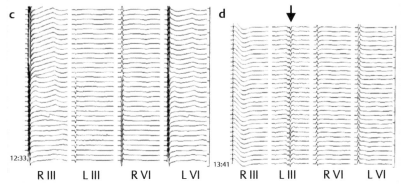

Fig. 6.2 Identification of the oculomotor nerve nuclei at the level of the tectal plate. (a) Sagittal (*left*), coronal (*middle*), and axial (*right*) magnetic resonance images of a midbrain cavernoma. (b) One pair of wire electrodes is inserted in the upper and lateral rectus muscles, bilaterally, to record compound action muscle potentials. (c) Initially (time 12.33), direct stimulation of the superior colliculus (*left panel*) does not elicit any response from the oculomotor muscles innervated by the cranial nerves III and VI. (d) Later on (time 13.41), stimulation from inside the surgical cavity, during removal of the cavernoma, elicits a consistent response (*arrow*) from the left upper rectus muscles (L III), indicating stimulation of the nearby nuclei. R III, right upper rectus muscle; L III, left upper rectus muscle; R VI, right lateral rectus muscle; L V, left lateral rectus muscle. (Modified from: F. Sala, P. Gallo, V. Tramontano. Intraoperative neurophysiological monitoring in posterior fossa surgery. In: M. Ozek, G. Cinalli, W. J. Maixner, C. Sainte-Rose, eds. Posterior Fossa Tumors in Children. Springer; 2015:239–262.)

amplitude due to the small number of fibers innervated by each axon, when compared to peripheral muscle units. The latency of the response depends on the point of stimulation along the peripheral nerve, being shorter and shorter as the nerve is stimulated more distally, and it ranges between 2 and 5 ms.[8,9] This technique is often indicated during surgery for meningiomas involving the cisternal, cavernous, or intra-orbital segment of the oculomotor nerves.

When meningiomas involve the posterior fossa and CPA, mapping of motor CNs V to XII may be valuable. The same stimulation parameters indicated for oculomotor nerve mapping apply. As a general rule, it should be considered that direct stimulation of an intact peripheral cranial motor nerve should elicit a CMAP with as little as 0.1 to 0.3 mA of intensity (▶ Fig. 6.3). Higher intensities may be required either if the nerve is injured or if the nerve fibers are encased in tumoral tissue. For recording, needle or wire electrodes are inserted in the following muscles innervated by motor CNs: the masseter (CN V), orbicularis oculi and oris (CN VII), posterior wall of the

pharynx (CN IX), vocal cords (CN X), trapezius (CN XI), and tongue (CN XII). There is some debate whether a threshold difference between proximal (close to the brainstem) and distal stimulation of the nerve retains a prognostic value for postoperative nerve function. For example, during CPA surgery, some authors suggest that a low proximal stimulating threshold is indicative of good prognosis of the facial nerve (FN).[10] However, others[11] have shown that a proximal stimulation threshold less than 0.05 mA is highly specific (90%) but little sensitive (29%), and therefore does not exclude postoperative facial palsy.

6.2.2 Monitoring Techniques

Somatosensory-Evoked Potentials Monitoring

Somatosensory-evoked potentials (SSEPs) are used to monitor the dorsal column pathway, from the periphery

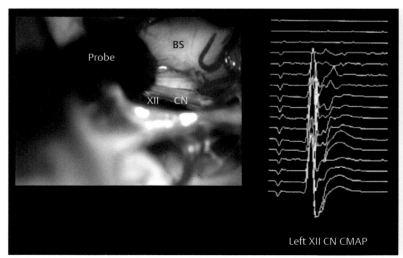

Fig. 6.3 Identification of cranial motor nerves through direct stimulation of the peripheral nerve. Left panel: Direct stimulation (monopolar handheld probe, intensity 0.2 mA, single stimulus of 0.5-ms duration) of the left hypoglossal nerve (CN XII) at its exit zone from the brainstem (BS). **Right panel:** Compound muscle action potentials recorded from the left hypoglossal muscles.

Left XII CN CMAP

to cerebral cortex. SSEPs monitoring is obtained through the stimulation of the median nerve for the upper extremities and of the posterior tibial nerve for the lower extremities. Because of the different somatotopy at the cord and at the cortex and to the different vascular territories involved in the cortical generators of these potentials, upper and lower SSEPs should be monitored separately. More specifically, the median nerve SSEP would better assess the middle cerebral artery territory and tibial nerve SSEP the anterior cerebral artery territory.

The electrical stimulation of the median nerve induces the depolarization that will generate the upper limb SSEPs; the action potential volley travels through the sensory fibers of the dorsal root and reach the fasciculus cuneatus (above T6); beyond the nucleus cuneatus, the action potential decussates (internal arcuate fibers), reaches the contralateral medial lemniscus, and terminates in the ventral posterolateral (VPL) nucleus of the thalamus. Finally, third-order neurons reach the somatosensory cortex and parietal association fields and are processed by cortical scalp leads. The electrical stimulation of the posterior tibial nerve induces the lower extremity SSEPs; the action potential travels through the fasciculus gracilis to the nucleus gracilis; second-order neurons decussate, travel through the contralateral medial lemniscus, and terminate in the VPL nucleus of thalamus. Third-order neurons project to the somatosensory area and parietal association fields and are processed by scalp leads. Scalp leads are placed at CP3 and CP4 with a forehead reference (Fpz or Fz). Parameters monitored are the SSEP amplitude, latency, and central conduction time (CCT), which refers to the transit time from the dorsal column nuclei to the cortex.

Baseline values are recorded prior to any significant patient positioning (this will help to detect and correct pressure or traction on the brachial plexus or peripheral nervous system), prior to incision, at the craniotomy and at the beginning of the intracranial manipulation. A standard protocol is then used for decision making in case of SSEP changes; the following warning criteria are usually adopted: decrease of SSEP amplitude greater than 50%, latency delay greater than 10%, and CCT prolongation of greater than 1 ms.

Motor-Evoked Potentials Monitoring

Motor-evoked potentials (MEPs) monitoring is used to assess the integrity of the corticospinal tracts (CTs). Two different techniques are available according to the site of the craniotomy: transcranial electrical stimulation (TES), which is used when the motor strip is not exposed and direct cortical stimulation (DCS), which is applied in case of surgical exposure of the motor strip. The former (TES) is by far the most common technique used for skull base surgery, as the motor strip is almost never directly exposed. TES of the motor cortex is usually applied using corkscrew electrodes, which guarantee low impedance.[12] Our routine MEP protocol is based on six electrodes (C1, C2, C3, C4, Cz–1 cm, and Cz + 6 cm) according to the 10/20 International Electroencephalography system. Using different montages of stimulating electrodes provides flexibility to optimize elicitation of mMEPs without muscle twitching, which can interfere with surgery. In most cases, C1/C2 is a better electrode montage for eliciting mMEPs in all contralateral limbs. Occasionally, the montage Cz–1 cm versus Cz + 6 cm can better elicit mMEPs from lower extremities, offering also the advantage of less intense muscle twitching than other montages. MEP recording is obtained from muscle of the upper and lower extremities using pairs of needle electrodes.

TES is considered a safe method, and there are no major contraindications to its use in the clinical setting.[13] However, there is a potential risk of distal activation of the CT as far as the brainstem, if too high intensity is used.[14] In such a situation, this may produce a false-negative result (meaning, the patient wakes up hemiparetic in spite of present mMEPs) because the point of CT activation can be distal to the level of a subcortical injury (e.g., due to an ischemic event). For this reason, stimulation intensity immediately above threshold is chosen in order to avoid unnecessary charge load and also to minimize the risk of distal activation of the descending motor pathways.

MEP amplitude and latency should be evaluated in comparison with baseline values and through a standard step-by-step protocol in order to exclude anesthesiologic or technical abnormalities as possible causes of changes in the evoked potentials. Although there is still an ongoing debate on what is considered a "significant" MEP change, modifications in amplitude are more relevant than those affecting latency and any amplitude drop, which exceeds 50% of baseline values, should be reported to the surgeon as it may predict an impending injury to motor pathways.[15,16,17,18] In brain surgery, complete loss of MEPs correlate with a permanent paresis and postoperative evidence, at the neuroimaging, of subcortical ischemia.[18] No changes in MEPs usually predict a good motor outcome from early after surgery. However, robust criteria to interpret MEP changes in intracranial surgery are still not well defined and reports referring specifically to skull base surgery are scarce.

MEPs are generally more suitable to monitor subcortical areas while SSEPs are more sensitive to ischemic derangements at the cortical level. Therefore, SSEP recording seems inadequate to monitor function in vascular territories supplied by the perforators while it is certainly indicated when cortical ischemia represents the main risk of surgery. From a methodological standpoint, it should be kept in mind that evoked potentials' recording should be tailored to the location of the tumor and, therefore, to the territory at risk for ischemia. For example, a tumor which encases the anterior communicating artery, anterior cerebral artery, or basilar artery branch would be better monitored using a bilateral tibial nerve SSEPs and bilateral MEP recordings, while for tumors which encase the internal carotid artery bifurcation and M1 segment, contralateral recordings may suffice.

Visual-Evoked Potentials Monitoring

Visual-evoked potentials (VEPs) monitoring is used to assess the integrity of the visual pathway in order to prevent postoperative visual deterioration. A light-stimulating device, or goggles, is placed on closed eyelids; flashing light intensity can be adjusted with an electric current ranging from 0 to 20 mA. Each eye is stimulated separately in order to obtain averaged VEP waveforms. Overall, 40 to 100 flashes are recorded to obtain each averaged VEP waveform, with a stimulus average of one flash (40 ms) per second. Recording montage requires five channels, with electrodes placed on the bilateral earlobes and the left occiput, occipital midline, and the right occiput. A small negative potential and a large positive potential at around 100 ms of latency are recorded, and the amplitude of the VEP is defined as the voltage difference between these two potentials. In order to verify the arrival of the light at the retina, needle electrodes are inserted subcutaneously at the lateral canthi for electroretinogram (ERG) recording. It is useful to record at least two consecutive ERG and VEP in order to confirm the reproducibility of the ERG and VEP waveforms after setup and before surgery.[19] Although many attempt have been made in order to improve the reproducibility of VEPs, stable recordings are difficult to obtain and consequently a clear clinical usefulness remains unclear. However, the use of ERG permits the distinction between clinical and technical problems, such as light goggles displacement or inappropriate visual stimulus delivery. Moreover, the improvement in neuroanesthesia, with the widespread use of total intravenous anesthesia (TIVA), has contributed to improve the reproducibility of VEPs.

Brainstem Auditory-Evoked Responses Monitoring

Brainstem auditory-evoked responses (BAERs) monitoring provides data on the auditory pathway.[20] Bilateral ear transducers create alternate compression and rarefaction square wave clicks with duration of 100 to 200 ms and intensity of 70 dB. The stimulation produces a 7-peak wave and each peak is related to a specific sequence of synapsis along the auditory pathway: cochlear nerve (1-degree peak), cochlear nuclei (2-degrees peak), contralateral superior olivary complex (3-degrees peak), lateral lemniscus (4-degrees peak), inferior colliculi (5-degrees peak), medial geniculate body (6-degrees peak), and acoustic radiation (7-degrees peak). BAERs provide information on the general status of the brainstem, especially when manipulation and dissection around it occur during skull base tumor removal. The interpretation of BAERs can be summarized as follows: dysfunction of the eighth nerve proximal to its cochlear end will cause a prolongation of the I to III interpeak interval, attenuation of waves III and V, or both; the latencies of waves III and V increase in parallel, while the III to V interpeak interval remains almost unchanged as long as the auditory pathways within the brainstem are not affected. A disappearance of wave I only may also be indicative of cochlear ischemia secondary to the compromise of the internal auditory artery. Vice versa, if the cochlea is not injured and the damage to the eighth nerve occurs in the CPA, wave I may persist even if the eighth nerve is completely transected. Damage to the lower pons, around the area of the cochlear nucleus or the superior olivary complex, will also affect waves III and V with delay in latency and drop in amplitude. Damage to the brainstem at the level of the midbrain will affect waves IV or V, but not waves I or III.

Cranial Nerve Monitoring

Free-Running Electromyography

The standard technique for cranial motor nerve monitoring is the evaluation of the spontaneous electromyography (EMG) activity in the muscles innervated by motor CNs.[21] The criteria proposed to identify EMG activity patterns related with nerve injury have been modified through the years. During manipulation of the nerve irritative activity may appear, but it usually stops shortly after the manipulation has stopped. This pattern is generally related with good prognosis for postoperative nerve function. Conversely, neurotonic discharges and especially high-frequency trains usually last longer than surgical manipulation and are related with possible nerve injury. The clinical interpretation of EMG modification has been studied especially for FN during vestibular schwannoma surgery.[22] However, the reliability of free-running EMG for other motor CNs remains controversial; it should be kept in mind that the same electrical silence (no EMG activity) suggesting that no changes are occurring can be observed even after the section of the peripheral nerve; conversely, the irrigation of the surgical field with cold saline can produce some irritative EMG activity. So, although several criteria have been proposed to identify EMG activity patterns indicative of nerve injury, the terminology remains somehow confusing, and convincing data regarding a clinical correlation between EMG activity and clinical outcome are still lacking.[8] This has been particularly disappointing for lower cranial motor nerves in skull base surgery,[23] while the results are more convincing for monitoring the FN in vestibular schwannoma surgery, especially when considering A-train analysis.[24,25]

Monitoring of Corticobulbar MEPs

In recent years, in the attempt to introduce a more reliable technique than free-running EMG for monitoring motor CNs, the principle of MEP monitoring used in monitoring limb muscles has been extended to the muscles innervated by motor CNs. The first reported application for this technique was focused on facial nerve monitoring during vestibular schwannoma surgery.[26] We used a similar technique to monitor CNs VII, IX/X complex, and XII in brainstem surgery.[27] These so-called "corticobulbar" MEPs permit to assess the functional integrity of the entire corticobulbar pathway, from the cortex to the muscle. Corticobulbar MEPs are recorded after TES with a train of four stimuli of 0.5-ms duration at a rate of 1 to 2 Hz and intensity ranging between 60 and 140 mA. The montage used for the electrode is usually C3/Cz for right-side muscles and C4/Cz for left-side muscles (▶ Fig. 6.4).

For recording, electrodes are placed in the following muscles bilaterally: orbicularis oculi and oris (CN VII), the posterior wall of the pharynx or vocal cords (CN IX/X complex), trapezius (CN XI), and tongue (CN XII). The major drawbacks reported for this technique are (1) high-intensity TES stimulation with a C3/C4 montage increases the risk of distal activation of the corticobulbar pathways deep in the brain or even at the level of the brainstem or peripheral nerve, therefore, exposing to false-negative results. A single versus train of stimuli protocol can be used to distinguish between centrally conducted and peripherally activated muscle response.[27] (2) The lateral montage (C3/Cz and C4/Cz) can produce muscle twitches in some patients, especially at higher stimulation intensities and these twitches can interfere with surgery thus forcing the surgeon to transiently stop the procedure. By increasing the number of stimuli and reducing stimulation intensity, muscle twitches sometimes can be reduced, while still obtaining a muscle response. (3) Spontaneous EMG activities, which is common during manipulation of CNs, can hinder the recordings of reliable MEPs from the same muscles, therefore compromising the correct interpretation of electrophysiologic signals. If so, to transiently halt surgery may facilitate the disappearance of the firing activity.

6.2.3 Anesthetic Considerations

The anesthesiological management of the surgical procedure can deeply influence the value of IONM. The inhalational agents such as isoflurane, sevoflurane, and desflurane may affect the reliability of IONM by blocking neural transmission at the synaptic level. Halogenated anesthetics elevate muscle MEP stimulus thresholds and block muscle MEPs in a dose-dependent fashion, and therefore should be avoided.

TIVA is the preferable choice during INM. Anesthesia is therefore maintained with a constant infusion of propofol (100–150 µg/kg/min) and fentanyl (usually around 1 µg/kg/h). Nitrous oxide not exceeding 50% can be used. Bolus injections of both intravenous agents should be avoided because this temporarily disrupts SSEPs and MEPs recordings. For anesthesia, short-acting muscle relaxants are given for intubation but not thereafter because with full relaxation muscle MEP monitoring and cortical/subcortical mapping are unfeasible. We try also to avoid any partial relaxation because a physiologic variability in the mMEP amplitude across repetitive trials and in the compound muscle action potential response already exists, so that any muscle relaxation would add another variable to the interpretation of motor responses.

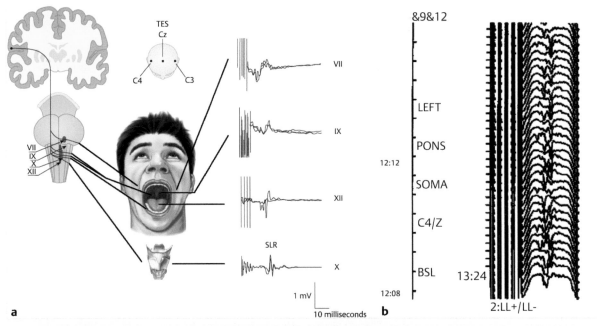

Fig. 6.4 Continuous monitoring of corticobulbar motor-evoked potentials. (a, *left panel*) Schematic illustration of corticobulbar motor-evoked potentials elicited after transcranial electrical stimulations at C4/Cz (left-side muscles) and C3/Cz (right-side muscles). Responses are recorded directly from the muscles innervated by motor cranial nerves VII, IX/X, and XII. The entire corticobulbar pathway, from the motor cortex to the muscles, is monitored with this technique (see text for details). **(b,** *right panel*) Continuous monitoring of the corticobulbar tracts from the right IX/X and XII cranial nerves following transcranial electrical stimulation delivered at C3(anode)/Cz(cathode) with a train of 4 stimuli, 0.2-ms duration each, at 95 mA. Modified from: F. Sala, G. Squintani, V. Tramontano. Intraoperative neurophysiologic monitoring during brainstem surgery. In: C.M. Loftus, J. Biller, E.M. Baron, eds. Intraoperative Neuromonitoring. McGraw-Hill; 2014:285–297.

6.3 Clinical Application in Skull Base Surgery

6.3.1 IONM for Sellar and Cavernous Sinus Surgery

Approaches directed to the sellar and parasellar region are complicated by the intimate relationship between skull base vessels and CNs. Direct mechanical injury to the III to VI CNs as well as subcortical ischemia due to vascular injury may occur. For example, during endoscopic surgery, the oculomotor nerve is vulnerable in the interpeduncular cistern via the transsphenoidal and transplanum routes, with potential vascular injury to the inferolateral trunk of the cavernous carotid or its branches. Both direct identification of the peripheral nerve through neurophysiologic mapping and/or monitoring of neural pathways may assist the surgeon.

The utility of SSEPs monitoring during skull base surgery has been proven useful during both transcranial[28] and endoscopic endonasal surgery (EES).[29] Bejjani et al[28]

reported a positive predictive value of 100%, and a negative predictive value of 90% in a series of 244 skull base procedures. Furthermore, the author evaluated the risk factors potentially related to true positive and true negative results in order to highlight the characteristics of the tumor that can augment the predictive value of SSEPs monitoring. On univariate analysis, the factors were pathologic abnormality, vessel encasement, vessel narrowing, degree of cavernous sinus involvement, brainstem edema, middle fossa location, final amount of resection, age, and tumor size. SSEPs have a high positive predictive value for postoperative deficit; they are therefore mainly helpful in predicting the occurrence of postoperative deficits and not their absence. According to the authors, SSEPs will predict outcome better if a patient has a high risk of postoperative deficits than if he or she has a small risk. This explains why the aforementioned factors are associated with a high predictive value of SSEPs. Thirumala et al[29,30] investigated the role of SSEP in endoscopic surgery to the sellar region; in one retrospective review of 976 patients submitted to skull base surgery, SSEPs changes were reported in 20 cases (2%) with subsequent evidence of 5 cases (0.5%) of new postoperative deficit; in this study there were 2 false negative (0.2%) and 4 false positive (0.4%) results reported. In a second study by the same group, 138 patients underwent endoscopic surgery for skull base tumors and SSEP changes were detected in five patients, three of which were true positive findings. Intraoperative changes of SSEPs emerged in both of these studies and were usually resolved after raising the mean arterial blood pressure. However, while SSEPs provide information regarding an impending cortical ischemia, they are not fully sensitive to subcortical ischemia and do not provide any information specific to the motor pathways. These limitations can lead to false-negative neurophysiologic findings and may need to be supplemented by additional modalities, such as MEPs.

The utility of VEPs for intraoperative monitoring of the optic tract is still under debate in both endoscopic[31] and transcranial surgery.[19] As the technology for stimulation devices advances, VEPs may play a larger role in monitoring. At the moment, setup for monitoring is time consuming because skin flaps sometimes disturb goggle placement. Even if the warning signs are vague and influenced by many factors, a decrease of more than 50% in amplitude is accepted as a warning threshold.[32] The TIVA anesthetic protocol helps stabilize the trial-by-trial variability that is present in the VEP responses. Further research is needed to assess if VEPs can be reliably used as an adjunct to monitor procedures where the visual tracts are affected. Nowadays, there is still little evidence from any intracranial procedure that VEPs are reliable predictors of postoperative function and their role remains controversial also in the case of transsphenoidal surgery.[31,33] For that reason, they are not recommended as part of a comprehensive IONM plan during skull base surgeries.

Cavernous sinus surgery is related with high risk for CN damage. However, the use of IONM during cavernous sinus surgery for the identification of ocular motor nerves and the assessment of their functional integrity is rarely reported. Weisz et al[34] questioned the benefits of IONM for ocular motor nerves; CNs in the cavernous sinus can be dislocated, infiltrated, or invaded by the tumor or, conversely, can be completely independent from the mass. Therefore, the authors argued that while the nerves that are invaded or infiltrated by the tumor cannot be spared, those being visible to the surgeon do not require any neurophysiologic monitoring. Conversely, Sekiya et al[35] described IONM for motor ocular CN as very useful and comparable to facial nerve monitoring for vestibular schwannomas. Recently, Kaspera et al[36] prospectively described the use of IONM for CNs III and VI during surgery for cavernous sinus meningiomas; the authors analyzed the reliability of IONM during the stages of identification and sparing of the CNs. The percentage of CNs identified with IONM was higher than that of CNs identified with visual inspection only, and this was true

for both CNs III and VI; notably, IONM particularly helped in the identification of CNs III and VI during the resection of intra-extracavernous and intracavernous component of the tumor. The authors conclude that the quality of postresection recordings correlated to the clinical status of the nerves on long-term follow-up.

Overall, in spite of the fact that the value of oculomotor nerve monitoring remains to some extent controversial, still it may represent a valuable adjunct in skull base surgery, especially when functional identification of anatomically ambiguous structure is needed.

6.3.2 IONM for Cerebellopontine Angle Surgery

Meningiomas of the CPA can be divided into five groups according to their relationships with the internal auditory canal (IAC)[37]: the tumors may arise anterior to IAC (group 1), involve the IAC (group 2), grow superior to the IAC (group 3), inferior to the IAC (group 4), or posterior to the IAC (group 5). The preservation of facial nerve function is possible in the majority of patients, ranging from 76.3% in group 1 tumors to 90% in group 5 tumors (lying posterior to the IAC). In tumors involving the IAC (group 2), normal facial nerve function could be maintained in 79% of patients. Tumor location also strongly affected the auditory outcome; the best rate of hearing preservation was obtained in groups 3 and 5 (81.3 and 81%, respectively) and the worse rate was reported in group 4 (54.5%).

Facial nerve monitoring during CPA surgery is mainly related to three techniques: direct electrical stimulation, free-running EMG, and corticobulbar MEPs. The evaluation of the CMAP triggered by direct electrical stimulation can be used intermittently and after the identification of the nerve. This can be particularly difficult during surgery for large tumors in which the proximal FN can be inaccessible for the most part of the procedure. Furthermore, it has been demonstrated that FN identification and the recording of the brainstem-to-distal IAC CMAP ratio cannot be performed in 30 to 35% of monitored patients due to technical reasons, distorted anatomy, or surgical approach. Thus, it may not be possible to assess continuously the FN function, even if the method is available in all cases.[26]

Free-running EMG relies on neurotonic discharges in response to surgical maneuvers that can indicate injury to the facial nerve. Irritation of the FN produces two specific patterns: burst and trains. Burst patterns are paroxysmal simple or polyphasic EMG activities of short duration and have been associated with direct mechanical trauma, irrigation, and electrocautery.[38] Trains are of longer duration (seconds to minutes) and are constituted by groups of repetitive high-frequency discharges. They have been associated with nerve traction, contusion, heat, or saline irrigation. According to their EMG characteristics, trains can be divided in three types: types A, B, and C. The "A-train" is composed of sinusoidal symmetric elements with high interpeak frequency and it has a sudden onset and sudden termination. It has been reported as pathognomonic for postoperative FN paresis.[22] However, no standardization of terminology exists between different IONM labs and trains classification has not been widely accepted. Furthermore, it necessitates special software for real-time and postprocessing analysis and it provides only an approximate correlation between the frequency of the discharges and the degree of the nerve injury.[22]

The introduction of corticobulbar MEPs monitoring during CPA surgery has been considered a promising method in FN monitoring because it permits to overcome the disadvantages of standard techniques. A corticobulbar MEPs reduction of 50% at the end of surgery has been identified as a good predictor for postoperative FN outcome after CPA surgeries.[26,39,40,41] Fukuda et al[41] examined the correlation between the final-to-baseline FN MEP ratio and postoperative facial nerve function. They concluded that an FN MEP ratio of less than 50% consistently predicted immediate postoperative facial palsy, while all patients had satisfactory facial nerve function (House and Brackmann grades I and II) postoperatively if the FN MEP ratio remained at greater than 50%.

Acioly et al[39] thoroughly investigated different MEP threshold among these two muscles; by using the receiver operating characteristic (ROC) curves, the authors found a statistical correlation at different cutoff values for both monitored muscles. For orbicularis oculi muscle, an 80% ratio (20% amplitude decrease) was calculated and for orbicularis oris muscle, a 35% ratio (65% amplitude decrease) significantly correlated with the postoperative FN motor function. Nevertheless, monitoring orbicularis oris muscle FN MEP was more consistent leading to stronger statistical results.

BAEPs monitoring is regularly applied during CPA surgery. Standard criteria adopted for the interpretation of BAEPs are usually based on the examination of the amplitude and latency of peaks and waves I, III, and V[42]; a 50% decrease in the amplitude and/or 1-ms prolongation in the absolute latency of wave V or the I to V interpeak interval are considered warning criteria. Another sensitive criterion for changes in latency is a delay more than 10% of the baseline peak V latency.[42] BAEPs dysfunction can be caused by various surgical maneuvers: compression and traction of CN VIII, thermal injury to the nerve, vascular derangements at the level of the cochlea, the auditory nerve, and the brainstem. However, with the exception of vascular injury to the internal auditory artery, the majority of these changes occurs in a stepwise fashion, giving us time for adopting corrective measures and reverse impending injuries.

6.3.3 IONM for Jugular Foramen—Clival and Foramen Magnum Surgery

During surgery for tumors around the jugular foramen and from the clival region to the foramen magnum, CNs are constantly at risk of injury. Furthermore, surgical manipulation and traction of the surrounding structures in order to dissect the tumors can cause damage of the brainstem and of the CTs. Therefore, during these surgical procedures a multimodality IONM approach should be applied; BAEPs monitoring is routinely used due to its capability to detect impending injury of the brainstem; FN monitoring can be introduced according to the extension of the tumor at the level of the CPA; SEP and MEP monitoring are used in order to detect impending injuries to the brainstem and the CT. During endoscopic surgery, the abducens nerve, being the longest and most ventrally located CN at the level of the clivus and cavernous sinus, is particularly at risk during approaches to petroclival lesions via the midline transclival, paramedian suprapetrous, and medial petrous apex approaches. As endoscopic approaches are extended to the inferior clivus, as well as through the transcondylar, and transjugular corridors, attention must be placed on lower CN monitoring, including the glossopharyngeal, vagus, accessory, and hypoglossal nerves.

As for facial nerve MEP monitoring described during CPA surgery, our group described a similar methodology for MEP monitoring of IX/X complex, CNs XI and XII for intrinsic brainstem tumors.[27] Keeping in mind the theoretical and practical drawbacks described in the previous section, even if data supporting the prognostic value of corticobulbar MEPs are still lacking, our experience suggests that the warning criteria used for limb muscle MEPs can be applied also in this setting; a complete disappearance of the corticobulbar MEP is indicative of significant and long-lasting deficits of that specific nerve (▶ Fig. 6.5), whereas transient and/or permanent drop in amplitude are of lesser concern but can still indicate some degree of worsening. The stability of the potentials during surgery generally correlates with good functional outcome. However, complex reflexes such as coughing and swallowing cannot be completely investigated in their functional integrity because only the efferent pathway mediated by lower CNs can be monitored. Very recently, however, a novel method has been proposed to monitor the laryngeal adductor response and this may well open a new perspective in the intraoperative neurophysiology of the lower brainstem.[43,44]

Kodama et al[45] had recently reviewed the intraoperative course of long-tract monitoring during infratentorial surgery to evaluate MEP and SEP relationship with clinical outcome; the authors pointed out that long-tract MEPs and SEPs behavior mostly follows the "all or nothing" criteria applied for spine procedures and is

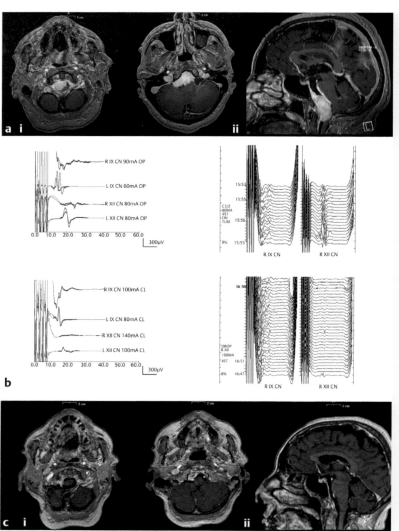

Fig. 6.5 **(a)** A 67-year-old woman with 3-month history of paresthesia on both hands, mainly on the right side, headache, and neck pain. Preoperative MRI showed a large right anterolateral foramen magnum meningioma with upward expansion along the lower segment of the clivus. The patient underwent surgical removal of the tumor through a right far lateral approach in semisitting position. **(b)** IONM included corticobulbar MEPs for the cranial nerves IX and XII. **(a-i)** Opening (OP) baseline MEPs for the right and left CNs IX and XII. **(a-ii, c-ii)** During surgery, the right XII CN MEPs were still present at 15.55 **(a)** but it disappeared progressively and was lost at 16.50 **(c)**; the left XII CN MEPs showed a decrease in amplitude but were still present at closure. The IX CN MEPs remained stable on both sides. After surgery, the patient showed right XII CN palsy, dysphonia, and dysphagia. The latter two symptoms disappeared during rehabilitation within 1 month from surgery. **(c-i)** At closing (CL), the right CN MEPs are lost, in spite of the increased stimulation intensity (140 vs. 80 mA). **(c)** MRI scan 1 year after surgery showed the near radical resection of the tumor (*lower panels*); at that time the right XII CN palsy was still present.

therefore different than in supratentorial surgery in which minor changes such as increase of motor threshold or amplitude decrement can be followed by long-lasting neurologic sequelae. In fact, in infratentorial surgery, permanent losses are related with long-lasting deficits. The negative predictive value in their series was very high (0.989), and this demonstrates the efficacy of long-tract monitoring to predict postoperative outcome. On the contrary, the positive predictive value was only 0.467; the authors states that this can be explained by the fact that they did not distinguish between permanent and transient alterations in monitoring. In the same study, the authors report a 35% incidence of MEP and SEP deterioration during posterior fossa surgery and they pointed out that the risk for MEP and SEP deterioration is mainly at the final stage of the tumor removal; at this point the higher risk is due to the maneuvers around the brainstem and to the manipulation of the perforating vessels.

6.4 IONM Changes and Surgical Strategy

During surgery for skull base meningiomas, the strategy for tumor removal relies on a careful judgment of the preoperative neuroimaging, the clinical examination of the patient, the selection of the most appropriate surgical approach, and the surgeon's experience. While all these aspects remain essential, IONM may offer an additional information that the surgeon can use to tailor the intraoperative decision-making process. For a valuable IONM, it is of outmost importance to tailor the selection of the IONM techniques to the characteristics of the tumor (site, involvement of CN, vessels) (▶ Table 6.1). A multimodality IONM strategy is indicated when different neural pathways are at risk. By combining mapping and monitoring techniques, we can improve the reliability of IONM as a valid diagnostic test and, above all, increase the

Table 6.1 Anatomical regions combined with surgical approaches (microsurgical and endoscopic) and recommended IONM modalities

Anatomical region and approaches	IONM montage
Sellar/suprasellar region	
• Transcranial microsurgical approach	
○ To suprasellar region	EEG, SSEPs, MEPs, VEPs (?)
• Endoscopic transsphenoidal	None
○ To sella	EEG, SSEPs, MEPs
○ To suprasellar (transplanum, transtuberculum)	
Cavernous sinus	
• Transcranial and endoscopic	EEG, SSEPs, MEPs, EMG (CNs III, IV, VI) (?)
CP angle	
• Transcranial microsurgical	EEG, SSEPs, MEPs, CB-MEP
• Endoscopic transclival/ transpetrous to posterior fossa	(CN VII) EMG (CNs VI, VII), BAERs
Jugular foramen, clival region, foramen magnum	
• Transcranial and endoscopic (transcondylar, transjugular)	EEG, SSEPs, MEPs, CB-MEP (CNs VII, IX–X, XI, XII) EMG (CNs VI, VII, IX–X, XI, XII), BAERs

Abbreviations: BAERs, brainstem auditory-evoked responses; CB-MEP, CNs, cranial nerves; EEG, electroencephalogram; EMG, electromyography; MEPs, motor-evoked potentials; SSEPs, somatosensory-evoked potentials; VEPs, visual-evoked potentials.

chance to detect an impending injury to the nervous system in time to be reverted.

Changes in IONM parameters do occur during skull base surgery and should be taken seriously into account. When warning criteria are reached, the strategy that we adopt is summarized by the acronym TIP: time, irrigation, and papaverine.[27] Time is a crucial variable. Our experience showed that if surgery is transiently stopped after MEPs disappearance or deterioration, these potentials often spontaneously recover. Conversely, to sustain a surgical maneuver that has induced MEP changes will likely transform a reversible injury into an irreversible one. It must be kept in mind that during skull base surgery if evoked potentials suddenly disappear without recover even after rescue maneuvers, it is usually due to a vascular injury to perforators. The use of warm irrigation accelerates the rate of recovery of evoked potentials; this technique is adopted during brain and spinal cord surgery in order to correct the relative hypothermia of the exposed surgical field, which possibly lead to a further deterioration of the potentials. While there is virtually no data on the efficacy of this method specifically during skull base surgery, there is no specific reason why the same principles should not apply. Finally, correction of any hypotension, as well as improving local perfusion by

the instillation of papaverine directly on the vessels exposed in the surgical field, may help to counteract any incipient ischemia.

6.5 Conclusions

IONM has exponentially grown over the last two decades as a valuable discipline that can assist neurosurgeons when facing challenging surgical procedures where the risk of injury to the central or peripheral nervous system is substantial. Although the vast majority of the literature has addressed IONM mainly with regard to brain tumor, brainstem, and spinal cord surgery, there is a growing interest also for the role of IONM in skull base surgery. Interestingly, the use of free-running EMG of the facial nerve during CPA surgery was, historically, the first IONM technique which was recommended by the NIH as standard of care in 1991.[46] Almost 30 years later the field of IONM has gained new interest; thanks also to the improvement in terms of reliability of mapping and monitoring techniques. Although the value of IONM in skull base surgery remains controversial when referring to the standards of evidence-based medicine, yet there is no less evidence for the benefit of IONM than the evidence we can offer for most of our skull base surgeries, many of those being well accepted as standard of care for their respective conditions. More refined IONM mapping techniques will be likely needed in the years to come to allow their intraoperative use during endoscopic approaches, and larger studies will hopefully provide more evidence for the benefit as well as the limitations of IONM in skull base surgery.

References

[1] Kombos T, Suess O, Ciklatekerlio O, Brock M. Monitoring of intraoperative motor evoked potentials to increase the safety of surgery in and around the motor cortex. J Neurosurg. 2001; 95(4): 608–614

[2] Neuloh G, Pechstein U, Schramm J. Motor tract monitoring during insular glioma surgery. J Neurosurg. 2007; 106(4):582–592

[3] Szelényi A, Kothbauer K, de Camargo AB, Langer D, Flamm ES, Deletis V. Motor evoked potential monitoring during cerebral aneurysm surgery: technical aspects and comparison of transcranial and direct cortical stimulation. Neurosurgery. 2005; 57 s uppl 4: 331–338, discussion 331–338

[4] Sala F, Lanteri P. Brain surgery in motor areas: the invaluable assistance of intraoperative neurophysiological monitoring. J Neurosurg Sci. 2003; 47(2):79–88

[5] Broggi G, Scaioli V, Brock S, Dones I. Neurophysiological monitoring of cranial nerves during posterior fossa surgery. Acta Neurochir Suppl (Wien). 1995; 64:35–39

[6] Acioly MA, Gharabaghi A, Liebsch M, Carvalho CH, Aguiar PH, Tatagiba M. Quantitative parameters of facial motor evoked potential during vestibular schwannoma surgery predict postoperative facial nerve function. Acta Neurochir (Wien). 2011; 153(6):1169–1179

[7] Jackson LE, Roberson JB, Jr. Vagal nerve monitoring in surgery of the skull base: a comparison of efficacy of three techniques. Am J Otol. 1999; 20(5):649–656

[8] Schlake HP, Goldbrunner R, Siebert M, Behr R, Roosen K. Intra-operative electromyographic monitoring of extra-ocular motor

nerves (Nn. III, VI) in skull base surgery. Acta Neurochir (Wien). 2001; 143(3):251–261

[9] Sekiya T, Hatayama T, Shimamura N, Suzuki S. Intraoperative electrophysiological monitoring of oculomotor nuclei and their intramedullary tracts during midbrain tumor surgery. Neurosurgery. 2000; 47(5):1170–1176, –discussion 1176–1177

[10] Lalwani AK, Butt FY, Jackler RK, Pitts LH, Yingling CD. Facial nerve outcome after acoustic neuroma surgery: a study from the era of cranial nerve monitoring. Otolaryngol Head Neck Surg. 1994; 111(5): 561–570

[11] Sughrue ME, Kaur R, Kane AJ, et al. The value of intraoperative facial nerve electromyography in predicting facial nerve function after vestibular schwannoma surgery. J Clin Neurosci. 2010; 17(7):849–852

[12] Journée HL, Polak HE, de Kleuver M. Influence of electrode impedance on threshold voltage for transcranial electrical stimulation in motor evoked potential monitoring. Med Biol Eng Comput. 2004; 42(4):557–561

[13] MacDonald DB. Safety of intraoperative transcranial electrical stimulation motor evoked potential monitoring. J Clin Neurophysiol. 2002; 19(5):416–429

[14] Rothwell JC, Thompson PD, Day BL, Boyd S, Marsden CD. Stimulation of the human motor cortex through the scalp. Exp Physiol. 1991; 76 (2):159–200

[15] Nossek E, Korn A, Shahar T, et al. Intraoperative mapping and monitoring of the corticospinal tracts with neurophysiological assessment and 3-dimensional ultrasonography-based navigation. Clinical article. J Neurosurg. 2011; 114(3):738–746

[16] Krieg SM, Schäffner M, Shiban E, et al. Reliability of intraoperative neurophysiological monitoring using motor evoked potentials during resection of metastases in motor-eloquent brain regions: clinical article. J Neurosurg. 2013; 118(6):1269–1278

[17] Neuloh G, Pechstein U, Cedzich C, Schramm J. Motor evoked potential monitoring with supratentorial surgery. Neurosurgery. 2004; 54(5): 1061–1070, discussion 1070–1072

[18] Szelényi A, Hattingen E, Weidauer S, Seifert V, Ziemann U. Intraoperative motor evoked potential alteration in intracranial tumor surgery and its relation to signal alteration in postoperative magnetic resonance imaging. Neurosurgery. 2010; 67(2):302–313

[19] Kodama K, Goto T, Sato A, Sakai K, Tanaka Y, Hongo K. Standard and limitation of intraoperative monitoring of the visual evoked potential. Acta Neurochir (Wien). 2010; 152(4):643–648

[20] Legatt AD, Arezzo JC, Vaughan HG, Jr. The anatomic and physiologic bases of brain stem auditory evoked potentials. Neurol Clin. 1988; 6 (4):681–704

[21] Grabb PA, Albright AL, Sclabassi RJ, Pollack IF. Continuous intraoperative electromyographic monitoring of cranial nerves during resection of fourth ventricular tumors in children. J Neurosurg. 1997; 86(1):1–4

[22] Prell J, Rachinger J, Scheller C, Alfieri A, Strauss C, Rampp S. A real-time monitoring system for the facial nerve. Neurosurgery. 2010; 66 (6):1064–1073, discussion 1073

[23] Schlake HP, Goldbrunner RH, Milewski C, et al. Intra-operative electromyographic monitoring of the lower cranial motor nerves (LCN IX-XII) in skull base surgery. Clin Neurol Neurosurg. 2001; 103(2):72–82

[24] Prell J, Rampp S, Romstöck J, Fahlbusch R, Strauss C. Train time as a quantitative electromyographic parameter for facial nerve function in patients undergoing surgery for vestibular schwannoma. J Neurosurg. 2007; 106(5):826–832

[25] Romstöck J, Strauss C, Fahlbusch R. Continuous electromyography monitoring of motor cranial nerves during cerebellopontine angle surgery. J Neurosurg. 2000; 93(4):586–593

[26] Dong CC, Macdonald DB, Akagami R, et al. Intraoperative facial motor evoked potential monitoring with transcranial electrical stimulation during skull base surgery. Clin Neurophysiol. 2005; 116(3):588–596

[27] Sala F, Lanteri P, Bricolo A. Motor evoked potential monitoring for spinal cord and brain stem surgery. Adv Tech Stand Neurosurg. 2004; 29:133–169

[28] Bejjani GK, Nora PC, Vera PL, Broemling L, Sekhar LN. The predictive value of intraoperative somatosensory evoked potential monitoring: review of 244 procedures. Neurosurgery. 1998; 43(3):491–498, discussion 498–500

[29] Thirumala PD, Kassasm AB, Habeych M, et al. Somatosensory evoked potential monitoring during endoscopic endonasal approach to skull base surgery: analysis of observed changes. Neurosurgery. 2011; 69 s uppl o perative 1:ons64–ons76, discussion ons76

[30] Thirumala PD, Kodavatiganti HS, Habeych M, et al. Value of multimodality monitoring using brainstem auditory evoked potentials and somatosensory evoked potentials in endoscopic endonasal surgery. Neurol Res. 2013; 35(6):622–630

[31] Chung SB, Park CW, Seo DW, Kong DS, Park SK. Intraoperative visual evoked potential has no association with postoperative visual outcomes in transsphenoidal surgery. Acta Neurochir (Wien). 2012; 154(8):1505–1510

[32] Sasaki T, Itakura T, Suzuki K, et al. Intraoperative monitoring of visual evoked potential: introduction of a clinically useful method. J Neurosurg. 2010; 112(2):273–284

[33] Kamio Y, Sakai N, Sameshima T, et al. Usefulness of intraoperative monitoring of visual evoked potentials in transsphenoidal surgery. Neurol Med Chir (Tokyo). 2014; 54:606–611

[34] Weisz DJ, Sen C, Yang B. Neurophysiological monitoring during cavernous sinus surgery. In: Eisenberg MB, Al-Mefty O, eds. The Cavernous Sinus—A Comprehensive Text. Philadelphia, PA: Lippincott Williams & Wilkins; 2000:123–13

[35] Sekiya T, Hatayama T, Iwabuchi T, Maeda S. Intraoperative recordings of evoked extraocular muscle activities to monitor ocular motor nerve function. Neurosurgery. 1993; 32(2):227–235, discussion 235

[36] Kaspera W, Adamczyk P, Ślaska-Kaspera A, Ładziński P. Usefulness of intraoperative monitoring of oculomotor and abducens nerves during surgical treatment of the cavernous sinus meningiomas. Adv Med Sci. 2015; 60(1):25–30

[37] Nakamura M, Roser F, Dormiani M, Matthies C, Vorkapic P, Samii M. Facial and cochlear nerve function after surgery of cerebellopontine angle meningiomas. Neurosurgery. 2005; 57(1):77–90, discussion 77–90

[38] Baldwin M, McCoyd M. Intraoperative facial nerve monitoring. In: Loftus CM, Biller J, Baron EM, eds. Intraoperative Monitoring. New York, NY: McGraw-Hill; 2014:261–272

[39] Acioly MA, Liebsch M, Carvalho CH, Gharabaghi A, Tatagiba M. Transcranial electrocortical stimulation to monitor the facial nerve motor function during cerebellopontine angle surgery. Neurosurgery. 2010; 66 s uppl o perative 6:354–361, discussion 362

[40] Akagami R, Dong CC, Westerberg BD. Localized transcranial electrical motor evoked potentials for monitoring cranial nerves in cranial base surgery. Neurosurgery. 2005; 57 suppl 1:78–85, discussion 78–85

[41] Fukuda M, Oishi M, Takao T, Saito A, Fujii Y. Facial nerve motor-evoked potential monitoring during skull base surgery predicts facial nerve outcome. J Neurol Neurosurg Psychiatry. 2008; 79(9): 1066–1070

[42] Mullatti N, Coakham HB, Maw AR, Butler SR, Morgan MH, American Clinical Neurophysiology Society. Guideline 9C: guidelines on short-latency auditory evoked potentials. J Clin Neurophysiol. 2006; 23(2): 157–167

[43] Sinclair CF, Téllez MJ, Tapia OR, Ulkatan S, Deletis V. A novel methodology for assessing laryngeal and vagus nerve integrity in patients under general anesthesia. Clin Neurophysiol. 2017; 128(7): 1399–1405

[44] Sala F. A spotlight on intraoperative neurophysiological monitoring of the lower brainstem. Clin Neurophysiol. 2017; 128(7):1369–1371

[45] Kodama K, Javadi M, Seifert V, Szelényi A. Conjunct SEP and MEP monitoring in resection of infratentorial lesions: lessons learned in a cohort of 210 patients. J Neurosurg. 2014; 121(6):1453–1461

[46] Acoustic neuroma. Consensus Statement National Institutes of Health Consensus Development Conference. 1991;9(4):1–24

7 Role of Stereotactic Radiosurgery

Gautam U. Mehta, Jeyan Kumar, Mohana Rao Patibandla, Jason P. Sheehan

Abstract

Stereotactic radiosurgery (SRS) is an important component of a multimodality approach to primary and metastatic tumors of the brain. In this chapter, we will discuss the role of SRS in the treatment of skull base meningiomas. To date, clinical studies have largely demonstrated durable tumor control for meningiomas treated with SRS. Compared to convexity meningiomas, radiosurgical management of meningiomas at the skull base requires specific pretreatment considerations, given the proximity to critical neurovasculature and the potential for cerebrospinal fluid outlet obstruction with posterior fossa lesions. As surgical treatment of skull base lesions may also carry increased risk, careful patient selection is essential, and factors such as patient age, tumor location, tumor size, distance from cranial nerves, and medical comorbidities must be considered. Further research is necessary to better understand the long-term outcomes of SRS in order to define optimal management of skull base meningiomas.

Keywords: meningioma, radiation, skull base, stereotactic radiosurgery

7.1 Introduction

SRS is a neurosurgical procedure that delivers radiation that is highly conformal, allowing high treatment doses to selected targets. Unlike fractionated radiotherapy or fractionated stereotactic radiotherapy, SRS is most frequently performed in a single session. The first clinical applications of SRS for meningioma were performed by Lars Leksell in the 1970s and with modern applications in the 1980s, with the advent of postcontrast MRI.[1,2] Because meningiomas of the skull base can be challenging to resect, these tumors are more frequently referred for radiation than those at other locations. Although convexity meningiomas have similar biology to those of the skull base, similar to skull base resection, SRS of skull base meningiomas presents with unique challenges. Despite steep radiation dose falloff with SRS, minimizing radiation doses to neurovascular structures at the base of the brain becomes critical. Furthermore, management and patient selection require special considerations, which will be discussed in this chapter.

7.2 Radiobiology of Skull Base Meningiomas

Initial understanding of the radiobiology of intracranial meningiomas was largely based on initial clinical results with nonstereotactic radiation therapy reported in the 1970s. Despite lack of modern neuroimaging to assess tumor response, patients with subtotal resection of meningiomas and postoperative irradiation were found to have prolonged survival in these early studies.[3] Unlike these clinical results, in vitro study of radiation for meningiomas has demonstrated modest to equivocal results, likely due to the slow proliferative rate of these tumors in culture.[4] More sophisticated recent models have shown that radiation inhibits angiogenesis in murine models of these tumors.[5]

Large series of SRS for meningiomas over the past two decades have helped further elucidate the radiobiology of these tumors. Initial results with the first large series published at the University of Pittsburgh in 1991.[6] Kondziolka and colleagues demonstrated that Gamma Knife radiosurgery could result in a 96% actuarial control at 2 years, with reduction in tumor volume in 17 of 50 patients (34%).[6] Margin doses in this initial study were relatively high, with 96% of patient receiving 12 Gy or higher and 48% of patients receiving 18 Gy or higher. Later studies analyzing the effect of margin dose found that a margin dose greater than or equal to 12 Gy was effective in tumor control of these patients.[7] Of 10 patients treated with 10 Gy or less, 4 tumors increased in size and 6 tumors were stable. Of 11 tumors treated with 12 Gy or more, 7 tumors were stable and 4 decreased in size. The largest study to date of meningiomas treated by SRS was performed by the European Gamma Knife Society.[8] This included 4,565 patients treated with SRS using a median margin dose of 14 Gy. The authors found that SRS resulted in a 5- and 10-year progression-free survival of 95.2 and 88.6%, respectively.

7.3 Outcomes of Stereotactic Radiosurgery for Skull Base Meningiomas

7.3.1 Radiological Response

Over the past two decades, several studies on the treatment outcomes for SRS of skull base meningiomas have been reported. In 1996, Nicolato and colleagues reported the results of Gamma Knife radiosurgery for 50 patients with skull base meningiomas.[9] This included 26 patients with cavernous sinus meningiomas. Mean tumor volume was 8.6 cm³ and mean margin dose was 18 Gy. 49 patients had tumor control at last follow-up, however, only 3 patients had follow-up of at least 2 years in this study. Two modern, single-center studies with more than 200 patients using a mean and/or median margin dose of 14 Gy, resulted in a 5-year progression-free survival of 96 to 98.5%.[10,11] Median tumor volume was 6.5 cm³ in one study and mean tumor volume was 5 cm³ in another. Another study of SRS for foramen magnum meningiomas, demonstrated a 5-year progression-free survival of 97% (▶ Fig. 7.1). Because increased tumor volume has been associated with worse SRS outcomes for skull base meningioma, separate studies have looked at the outcomes of SRS for larger skull base meningiomas.[12] We previously analyzed the results of SRS for skull base meningiomas greater than 8 cm³ (which corresponds to a diameter of approximately 2.5 cm).[13] Among 75 patients, we found 5- and 10-year progression-free survivals of 88.6 and 77.2%, respectively. Patients with tumors greater than 14 cm³

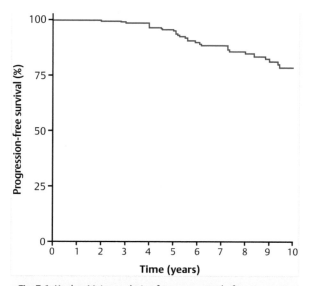

Fig. 7.1 Kaplan-Meier analysis of tumor control after stereotactic radiosurgery in 57 foramen magnum meningiomas demonstrates 5- and 10-year progression free survival of 97 and 92%, respectively. Dashed lines represent 95% confidence intervals. (Reproduced from Mehta G. U., Zenonos G., Patibandla M. R., et al. Outcomes of stereotactic radiosurgery for foramen magnum meningiomas: an international multicenter study. 2017; in press.)

were more likely to progress (hazard ratio 6.86, 95% confidence interval [CI] 0.88–53.36).

7.3.2 Cranial Neuropathy

Cranial neuropathies associated with SRS of skull base meningiomas are largely dependent on the location of the meningioma treated. Regardless, studies that have combined the results of all skull base meningiomas have demonstrated a rate of new or progressive cranial neuropathy in 1.5 to 8.6% of patients.[10] The risks of cranial neuropathies based on tumor location are detailed in ▶ Table 7.1. The cranial neuropathy risks associated with SRS for larger meningiomas may be greater than for small- to medium-volume tumors. Bledsoe and colleagues, who analyzed large (> 10 cm³) meningiomas at all sites, reported a 23% complication rate, with an 8% rate of cranial neuropathy.[12] Looking at only skull base meningiomas, we previously found that new or worsened cranial neuropathy occurred in 14% of patients who had SRS for tumors greater than 8 cm³. Hypofractionated SRS may be an option for patients with larger skull base meningiomas and help to mitigate complications associated with single-session SRS for large targets.

7.3.3 Brainstem Toxicity

As skull base meningiomas may be directly adjacent to or compressing the brainstem, radiation exposure with SRS is often unavoidable. Because of the steep radiation falloff with SRS and shielding strategies, this radiation burden can be significantly minimized.[17] The American Society for Radiation Oncology (ASTRO) funded a review of the maximum tolerated dosages of radiation on normal tissue called Quantitative Analysis of Normal Tissue Effects in the Clinic (QUANTEC).[18] The brainstem-specific study for this initiative reviewed prior reports of radiation therapy and radiosurgery for lesions adjacent to the brainstem.[19] This review found that brainstem doses of less than or equal to 12.5 Gy were associated with less than 5% risk of complications. Clinical evidence of brainstem toxicity is rare. A multicenter study of SRS for 675 posterior fossa

Table 7.1 Outcomes of some large series of skull base meningiomas by location

Author/date	Location	Patients	Mean/median volume	Mean/median margin dose	Progression-free survival (PFS)	Adverse radiation effects
Skeike et al/ 2010[14]	Cavernous	100	7.39 cm³	12.4 Gy	5 year: 94% 10 year: 92%	Optic neuropathy (2%)
Sheehan et al/ 2014[15]	Sellar/parasellar	763	8.8/6.7 cm³	13.2/13 Gy	5 year: 95% 10 year: 82%	New/worsening CN deficits (9.6%)
Starke et al/ 2014[16]	Petroclival	254	7.8 ± 6.6 cm³	13.4 ± 2.4 Gy	5 year: 93% 10 year: 84%	Hydrocephalus (2.8%)
Mehta et al/ in press[37]	Foramen magnum	57	Median: 2.9 cm³	Median: 12.5 Gy	5 year: 97% 10 year: 92%	Hearing loss/ numbness in one patient (2%)

meningiomas did not demonstrate any cases with apparent brainstem toxicity.[20]

7.3.4 Other Complications

Vascular injury is a potential complication of SRS, particularly at the skull base, but the risk of major injury to a cerebrovascular structure from radiosurgery for a skull base meningioma is quite rare. Bledsoe and colleagues noted vascular infarct in 2 of 91 patients with skull base meningiomas who were treated with Gamma Knife radiosurgery.[12] After SRS, tumor swelling may result in ventricular outlet obstruction and hydrocephalus. In the previously described study of 675 patients treated with SRS for posterior fossa meningiomas, 2.1% developed hydrocephalus on imaging and 1.7% required surgery for cerebrospinal fluid diversion.[20]

7.4 Management of Skull Base Meningiomas and Indications for Stereotactic Radiosurgery

7.4.1 General Indications

Patient selection is critical for effective utilization of SRS for skull base meningiomas. As many such tumors are found incidentally, observation is an important option for these patients, particularly with older patients or those with nongrowing, asymptomatic tumors. For growing and symptomatic tumors, most patients should consider treatment. In general, the procedural morbidity of SRS is significantly less than open surgical resection. This includes risks associated with general anesthesia, as well as surgery. This is particularly important in the management of meningiomas of the skull base as open surgical resection may require lengthy surgery with dissection around or manipulation of cranial nerves, the brainstem, and major arteries and veins. Therefore, patients who are older, and who carry greater medical comorbidities may be better suited for SRS (► Table 7.1). With young patients, and with tumors that are amenable to complete resection, open surgical options provide the possibility of histological confirmation of the tumor and grade and long-lasting, curative therapy. Regardless, even in the modern, microsurgical era, Simpson's grade I resections are associated with some small risk of recurrence.[21,22] Several studies have suggested that gross total tumor

resection at the expense of subtotal resection with neurologic preservation, followed by radiosurgery, may be a more valid approach in the contemporary era.[23] Others have concluded that tumor control and recurrence-free survival are comparable for Simpson's grade I resected patients and those treated with radiosurgery for a World Health Organization (WHO) grade I meningioma.[24]

The risks and benefits of radiosurgery compared with observation are largely dependent on the natural history of meningiomas. Several natural history studies of asymptomatic meningiomas have been reported, demonstrating growth in only 11 to 37% of patients over more than 5 years follow-up.[25,26,27] These rates of quiescence may be comparable to the rates of tumor stability seen with some studies of SRS. However, the natural history of meningiomas is rarely tumor regression while tumor regression is seen frequently after SRS. In a recent survey in the United Kingdom, SRS was found to be the preferred approach for incidental but progressive meningiomas of the skull base.[28] To more clearly understand the tumor control benefits of SRS, future observational studies will be required with matched untreated controls.

7.4.2 Specific Tumor Locations

Although meningiomas of the skull base share a common proximity to critical neurovascular structures, the benefits and risks of radiosurgery may be unique to specific locations. The risks of cranial neuropathy documented in the previous section are clearly related to tumor location. In particular, proximity to the optic apparatus may be particular to certain meningiomas of the anterior cranial base. Likewise, the risk of brainstem toxicity is an important consideration for tumors of the posterior fossa. Therefore, it is critical to analyze the results of SRS, specific to these tumor locations to more clearly understand risk–benefit profile compared with observation or surgery (► Table 7.2). Furthermore, within various locations, some skull base meningiomas may be more amenable to surgery than others (lateral vs. middle or medial sphenoid wing, posterior vs. anterior or anterolateral foramen magnum). These factors should be considered in a patient-based and lesion-specific approach to management.

Despite these considerations, the radiobiology of tumors of different locations may be similar. Based on large, retrospective cohort data, several authors have suggested that meningiomas may be less likely to be atypical or anaplastic in skull base locations than over the convexity.[29,30,31] These

Table 7.2 Factors favoring stereotactic radiosurgery and surgical resection of skull base meningiomas

Treatment modality	Stereotactic radiosurgery	Surgical resection
Preoperative factors	Older age Greater medical comorbidities Smaller tumor size Distant from optic apparatus	Younger age Few medical comorbidities Larger tumor size Compressing optic apparatus Symptomatic mass effect

data from retrospective studies may be limited by factors related to symptom development as small, slow-growing convexity meningiomas may go undetected due to their location. Specific tumor locations within the skull base, however, have not been reported to predispose to more aggressive phenotypes.

7.4.3 Primary, Residual, and Recurrent Disease

SRS for meningioma can be performed either for previously untreated tumors with radiological findings consistent with meningioma, with no histological confirmation, or for residual or recurrent disease. The comparative results of SRS for these different indications may be difficult to determine as most studies combine these groups in their analysis. However, in the European Gamma Knife Society, report on SRS for benign meningiomas, multivariate analyses found that radiological tumor control was better for those patients who had not undergone prior surgery ($p < 0.001$).[8] For some patients with tumor adherent to critical neurovascular structures, gross total resection may not be possible. In such instances, a paradigm of maximal operative resection followed by SRS of residual disease may be reasonable. Recurrent disease after resection of meningiomas may occur even after Simpson's grade I resection.[22] In select cases of recurrence, without significant mass effect, SRS may be a viable alternate treatment option.

7.4.4 Atypical and Anaplastic Meningiomas

Atypical and anaplastic meningiomas likely represent a larger proportion of all meningiomas (> 20%) than previously recognized.[32] In a study of 140 meningiomas, 117

of the benign tumors had 5-year overall survival of 85% compared to 23 atypical or anaplastic tumors with 58%.[33] Aichholzer and colleagues studied 46 patients with skull base meningiomas with mean follow-up of 40 months found survival rates of 97.5% in benign tumors and 83% for malignant tumors.[34] SRS for these tumors is performed after resection and histological identification of a high-grade tumor. Milker-Zabel and colleagues found local tumor failure after SRS was significantly greater in WHO grade II tumors versus grade I ($p < 0.002$).[35] In this study, they also demonstrated that patients treated with SRS at recurrence had worse progression-free survival than patients treated with SRS immediately following resection or biopsy. Also, higher radiosurgical doses are certainly required to treat grade II and III meningiomas. In our review of 647 cases of grades II and III meningiomas, margin doses were typically 16 to 20 Gy for grade II and 18 to 22 Gy for grade III meningiomas.[36] Despite these higher doses, the median 5-year progression-free survival rates for grades II and III meningiomas were 59 and 13%, respectively. While SRS affords low rates of tumor control for WHO grades II and III meningiomas, radiosurgery does appear to represent a valuable tool in the multimodality management often required for patients harboring such tumors. Future prospective study will be required to compare the natural history of higher-grade meningiomas to those treated with SRS.

7.4.5 Case Example

A 63 year-old woman presented with gradually progressive changes in taste, decreased sensation on the left side of her face, and diminished hearing in the left ear. MRI showed a well-defined, extra-axial mass in the left cerebellopontine angle consistent with a meningioma. The tumor was 1.2 cm³ upon presentation in November 2008 (▶ Fig. 7.2a).

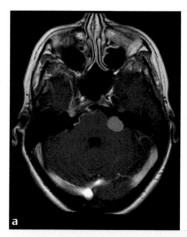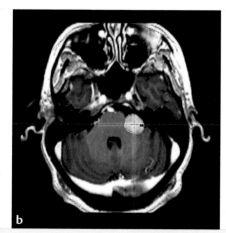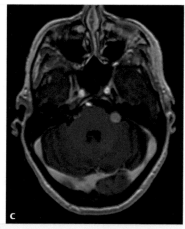

Fig. 7.2 MRI of a cerebellopontine angle meningioma treated with Gamma Knife stereotactic radiosurgery. (a) Axial postcontrast T1-weighted MRI at presentation in November 2008 revealed a tumor volume of 1.2 cm³. **(b)** By July 2010, the tumor had grown to 3.8 cm³, at which point it was treated with Gamma Knife SRS (treatment isodose line denoted in yellow). **(c)** At last follow-up in April 2016, the tumor had diminished in size to 0.95 cm³.

The patient initially chose conservative management, however, serial imaging, over the next 2 years, demonstrated interval growth to 3.8 cm^3 in July 2010 (▶ Fig. 7.2b). At this point, the patient elected to have Gamma Knife SRS. She was treated with a prescription dose of 13 Gy to the tumor margin. Clinical and radiological follow-up were performed at approximately 6-month intervals for the first 2 years after SRS and then annually thereafter. Her facial sensation improved over the first 6 months, whereas her hearing had declined slightly by last follow-up. At 6 years post-SRS, her tumor had diminished in sized to 0.95 cm^3 (▶ Fig. 7.2c).

7.5 Conclusions

Overall, SRS can play an important role in the management of skull base meningiomas. SRS can provide durable tumor control in the majority of patients with small to medium skull base meningiomas. SRS for larger-volume tumors can be effective in controlling tumor growth, but it carries a higher risk of adverse radiation effects. Additionally, tumor location, preexisting deficits, and volume, largely dictate the relative morbidity and risks of SRS. Finally, careful patient selection is crucial to the success of this treatment.

References

[1] Leksell L. Stereotactic radiosurgery. J Neurol Neurosurg Psychiatry. 1983; 46(9):797–803

[2] Lunsford LD, Flickinger J, Lindner G, Maitz A. Stereotactic radiosurgery of the brain using the first United States 201 cobalt-60 source gamma knife. Neurosurgery. 1989; 24(2):151–159

[3] Wara WM, Sheline GE, Newman H, Townsend JJ, Boldrey EB. Radiation therapy of meningiomas. Am J Roentgenol Radium Ther Nucl Med. 1975; 123(3):453–458

[4] Fischer H, Hartmann GH, Sturm V, et al. In vitro model for the response to irradiation of different types of human intracranial tumours. Acta Neurochir (Wien). 1987; 85(1–2):46–49

[5] Kılıç K, Avsar T, Akgün E, et al. Gamma Knife radiosurgery inhibits angiogenesis of meningiomas: in vivo rat corneal assay. World Neurosurg. 2013; 80(5):598–604

[6] Kondziolka D, Lunsford LD, Coffey RJ, Flickinger JC. Stereotactic radiosurgery of meningiomas. J Neurosurg. 1991; 74(4):552–559

[7] Ganz JC, Backlund EO, Thorsen FA. The results of Gamma Knife surgery of meningiomas, related to size of tumor and dose. Stereotact Funct Neurosurg. 1993; 61 suppl 1:23–29

[8] Santacroce A, Walier M, Régis J, et al. Long-term tumor control of benign intracranial meningiomas after radiosurgery in a series of 4565 patients. Neurosurgery. 2012; 70(1):32–39, discussion 39

[9] Nicolato A, Ferraresi P, Foroni R, et al. Gamma Knife radiosurgery in skull base meningiomas. Preliminary experience with 50 cases. Stereotact Funct Neurosurg. 1996; 66 suppl 1:112–120

[10] Starke RM, Williams BJ, Hiles C, Nguyen JH, Elsharkawy MY, Sheehan JP. Gamma knife surgery for skull base meningiomas. J Neurosurg. 2012; 116(3):588–597

[11] Kreil W, Luggin J, Fuchs I, Weigl V, Eustacchio S, Papaefthymiou G. Long term experience of gamma knife radiosurgery for benign skull base meningiomas. J Neurol Neurosurg Psychiatry. 2005; 76(10):1425–1430

[12] Bledsoe JM, Link MJ, Stafford SL, Park PJ, Pollock BE. Radiosurgery for large-volume (> 10 cm3) benign meningiomas. J Neurosurg. 2010; 112(5):951–956

[13] Starke RM, Przybylowski CJ, Sugoto M, et al. Gamma Knife radiosurgery of large skull base meningiomas. J Neurosurg. 2015; 122(2):363–372

[14] Skeie BS, Enger PO, Skeie GO, Thorsen F, Pedersen PH. Gamma knife surgery of meningiomas involving the cavernous sinus: long-term follow-up of 100 patients. Neurosurgery. 2010; 66(4):661–668, discussion 668–669

[15] Sheehan JP, Starke RM, Kano H, et al. Gamma Knife radiosurgery for sellar and parasellar meningiomas: a multicenter study. J Neurosurg. 2014; 120(6):1268–1277

[16] Starke R, Kano H, Ding D, et al. Stereotactic radiosurgery of petroclival meningiomas: a multicenter study. J Neurooncol. 2014; 119(1):169–176

[17] Schlesinger D, Snell J, Sheehan J. Shielding strategies for Gamma Knife surgery of pituitary adenomas. J Neurosurg. 2006; 105 suppl: 241–248

[18] Marks LB, Yorke ED, Jackson A, et al. Use of normal tissue complication probability models in the clinic. Int J Radiat Oncol Biol Phys. 2010; 76 suppl 3:S10–S19

[19] Mayo C, Yorke E, Merchant TE. Radiation associated brainstem injury. Int J Radiat Oncol Biol Phys. 2010; 76 s suppl 3:S36–S41

[20] Sheehan JP, Starke RM, Kano H, et al. Gamma Knife radiosurgery for posterior fossa meningiomas: a multicenter study. J Neurosurg. 2015; 122(6):1479–1489

[21] Gousias K, Schramm J, Simon M. The Simpson grading revisited: aggressive surgery and its place in modern meningioma management. J Neurosurg. 2016; 125(3):551–560

[22] Nanda A, Bir SC, Maiti TK, Konar SK, Missios S, Guthikonda B. Relevance of Simpson grading system and recurrence-free survival after surgery for World Health Organization Grade I meningioma. J Neurosurg. 2017; 126(1):201–211

[23] Heald JB, Carroll TA, Mair RJ. Simpson grade: an opportunity to reassess the need for complete resection of meningiomas. Acta Neurochir (Wien). 2014; 156(2):383–388

[24] Bir SC, Patra DP, Maitl TK, Bollam P, Minagar A, Nanda A. Direct comparison of gamma knife radiosurgery and microsurgery for small size meningiomas. World Neurosurg. 2017; 101:170–179

[25] Go RS, Taylor BV, Kimmel DW. The natural history of asymptomatic meningiomas in Olmsted County, Minnesota. Neurology. 1998; 51 (6):1718–1720

[26] Olivero WC, Lister JR, Elwood PW. The natural history and growth rate of asymptomatic meningiomas: a review of 60 patients. J Neurosurg. 1995; 83(2):222–224

[27] Yano S, Kuratsu J, Kumamoto Brain Tumor Research Group. Indications for surgery in patients with asymptomatic meningiomas based on an extensive experience. J Neurosurg. 2006; 105(4): 538–543

[28] Mohammad MH, Chavredakis E, Zakaria R, Brodbelt A, Jenkinson MD. A national survey of the management of patients with incidental meningioma in the United Kingdom. Br J Neurosurg. 2017; 31(4): 459–463

[29] Sade B, Chahlavi A, Krishnaney A, Nagel S, Choi E, Lee JH. World Health Organization Grades II and III meningiomas are rare in the cranial base and spine. Neurosurgery. 2007; 61(6):1194–1198, discussion 1198

[30] Cornelius JF, Slotty PJ, Steiger HJ, Hänggi D, Polivka M, George B. Malignant potential of skull base versus non-skull base meningiomas: clinical series of 1,663 cases. Acta Neurochir (Wien). 2013; 155(3):407–413

[31] Kane AJ, Sughrue ME, Rutkowski MJ, et al. Anatomic location is a risk factor for atypical and malignant meningiomas. Cancer. 2011; 117 (6):1272–1278

[32] Willis J, Smith C, Ironside JW, Erridge S, Whittle IR, Everington D. The accuracy of meningioma grading: a 10-year retrospective audit. Neuropathol Appl Neurobiol. 2005; 31(2):141–149

[33] Goldsmith BJ, Wara WM, Wilson CB, Larson DA. Postoperative irradiation for subtotally resected meningiomas. A retrospective analysis of 140 patients treated from 1967 to 1990. J Neurosurg. 1994; 80(2):195–201

[34] Aichholzer M, Bertalanffy A, Dietrich W, et al. Gamma knife radiosurgery of skull base meningiomas. Acta Neurochir (Wien). 2000; 142(6):647–652, discussion 652–653

[35] Milker-Zabel S, Zabel A, Schulz-Ertner D, Schlegel W, Wannenmacher M, Debus J. Fractionated stereotactic radiotherapy in patients with benign or atypical intracranial meningioma: long-term experience and prognostic factors. Int J Radiat Oncol Biol Phys. 2005; 61(3): 809–816

[36] Ding D, Starke RM, Hantzmon J, Yen CP, Williams BJ, Sheehan JP. The role of radiosurgery in the management of WHO Grade II and III intracranial meningiomas. Neurosurg Focus. 2013; 35(6):E16

[37] Mehta GU, Zenonos G, Patibandla MR, Lin CJ, Wolf A, Grills I, et al. Outcomes of stereotactic radiosurgery for foramen magnum meningiomas: an international multicenter study. 2017; in press

8 Sphenoid Wing Meningiomas

Francesco Tomasello, Domenico La Torre, Filippo Flavio Angileri, Alfredo Conti, Salvatore Massimiliano Cardali, Antonino F. Germanò

Abstract

Sphenoid wing meningiomas (SWMs) are the most common tumors in the anterior skull base, accounting for approximately 20% of supratentorial meningiomas and represent a great surgical challenge due to their invasion of the bone and, especially, to their close relationship to main arteries and cranial nerves. Lateral or pterional meningiomas usually grow into the sylvian fissure, are fed by middle meningeal artery and its branches, and reach clear relationship with middle cerebral artery (MCA), distal carotid artery, and carotid bifurcation. Medial SWMs grow compressing the proximal internal carotid artery (ICA) and its branches, are fed by dural branches of the ICA, and compress the optic nerve, the third cranial nerve; in some cases, they can invade the cavernous sinus and the optical canal. Surgical excision remains the preferred treatment. Stereotactic radiosurgery and external-beam radiotherapy are being used increasingly for surgically inaccessible, recurrent, or subtotally excised tumors, particularly if they are atypical or anaplastic. We present our experience in the surgical management of SWMs.

Keywords: meningioma, sphenoid wing, skull base, surgery

8.1 General Considerations and Definition

Meningiomas are the most common benign intracranial tumors, accounting for 13 to 26% of all primary intracranial tumors.[1,2] Meningiomas are generally slow-growing tumors composed of neoplastic arachnoidal (meningothelial) cells. Occasional tumors, particularly those lying next to the sphenoid ridge, grow in a more diffuse pattern over the dura; in these cases, they are termed meningiomas *en plaque*.

They can be classified according to their dural site of origin, the involvement of adjacent tissues (e.g., venous sinuses, bone, brain, and neurovascular structures), and their histological grading. Histological grading of meningiomas is based on the current WHO classification. Most of them (about 90%) are WHO grade I, reflecting their benign nature. However, atypical meningiomas (WHO grade II), which make up 5 to 7%, and anaplastic variants (WHO grade III), 1 to 3%, are recognized by several histological characteristics.

Typical genetic features of meningiomas are monosomy 22 and inactivating mutations of neurofibromatosis type 2 (NF2). More recently, mutations in TRAF7, AKT1, KLF4, SMO, and PIK3CA were identified. More than 80% of meningiomas harbored at least one of the above genetic alterations. NF2 alterations and mutations of the other genes were mutually exclusive with a few exceptions. Clinicopathologically, tumors with mutations in TRAF7/AKT1 and SMO shared specific features; they were located in the anterior fossa, median middle fossa, or anterior calvarium, and most of them were meningothelial or transitional meningiomas. TRAF7/KLF4 type meningiomas occurred in the lateral middle fossa and median posterior fossa as well as anterior fossa and median middle fossa, and contained a secretory meningioma component.[3]

Meningiomas present clinically with focal or generalized seizure disorders, focal neurologic deficits, or neuropsychological decline. However, an estimated 2 to 3% of the population has an incidental asymptomatic meningioma.[4] Asymptomatic meningiomas can be treated conservatively because they usually show minimal growth. Nevertheless, close clinical and radiological follow-up is necessary in order to exclude a rapidly growing tumor, particularly in young patients because of the higher growth potential.[5] Serial volumetric measurements are useful for determining the natural history of meningioma. Furthermore, meningiomas with the evidence of calcification on CT scans and low signal intensity on T2-weighted MRI have been associated with slower growth rate. Nevertheless, even if growth has been confirmed, the decision to operate depends on patient's age, symptomatology, and comorbidities. Furthermore, in series with surgically treated asymptomatic meningiomas the morbidity rate was not negligible especially for patients older than 70 years of age. For symptomatic patients, resection is usually necessary to relieve neurologic symptoms. Complete resection is often curative even if recurrences may develop after many years. Thus, the length of follow-up is the main aspect dealing with recurrence rate in meningioma series. In elderly patients, although complications are more frequent, after detailed preoperative evaluation and appropriate postoperative care, an operation is justified. Recently, a grading system has been proposed to standardize the surgical indication of intracranial meningiomas in the elderly.[6] For the majority of incompletely resected or recurrent tumors, a "wait and see" strategy or for those not previously irradiated, radiotherapy, conventional or stereotactic, is a viable alternative. Furthermore, when the meningioma is considered unresectable or all other treatments (surgery and radiotherapy) have failed, hormonal therapy or chemotherapy may be considered.

Surgical excision remains the preferred treatment. Stereotactic radiosurgery and external-beam radiotherapy are being used increasingly for surgically inaccessible, recurrent, or subtotally excised tumors, particularly if they are atypical or anaplastic. Recent advances in clarification of the genetics, molecular biology, and neuropathology of meningiomas, are becoming useful in prediction of prognosis after various treatments.[3]

SWMs are the most common tumors in the anterior skull base, accounting for approximately 20% of supratentorial meningiomas and represent a great surgical challenge due to their invasion of the bone and, especially, to their close relationship to main arteries and cranial nerves.[7] Anatomically, the sphenoid wing extends from the anterior clinoid process to the pterion with the greater wing constituting the outer third and the lesser wing the inner two-thirds. The greater wing and the lateral half of the lesser wing represent the lateral and middle portions of the sphenoid wing. The lateral/pterional SWMs are usually accompanied by epilepsy, focal weakness, and trouble with language function when present on the dominant side. The tumors of the medial (inner) sphenoid ridge usually present with early unilateral visual impairment due to compression of the optic nerve. Those tumors may also involve the cavernous sinus and oculomotor nerves and cause double vision and numbness of the face.

SWMs were first described in detail by Drs. Cushing and Eisenhardt, who distinguished between globoid SWMs and en plaque SWMs.[7,8] Globoid meningiomas were subdivided into three groups, namely, deep, inner/medial, or clinoidal, middle or alar, and outer or pterional.[7] In this classification scheme, the lesser sphenoid wing is divided into thirds: a medial third, which represents the segment most adjacent to the anterior clinoid process; a middle third, which runs medial to lateral; and a lateral third, which runs anterior to posterior, eventually joining with the temporal squama. Later on, Bonnal and Brotchi divided SWMs in into five groups that raised specific surgical problems: (A) deep or clinoidal or sphenocavernous; (B) invading en plaque the sphenoid wings; (C) invading en mass the sphenoid wings; (D) middle ridge meningiomas; and (E) pterional or sylvian point meningiomas.[9] According to Yasargil, we prefer to distinguish medial and lateral SWMs.[10] Middle or alar meningiomas have clinical, radiological, and surgical characteristics similar to lateral or pterional meningiomas. Moreover, even during surgical excision, the exact site of attachment of these two groups cannot be distinguished and thus, they could be considered in a unique group. Lateral or pterional meningiomas usually grow into the sylvian fissure, are fed by middle meningeal artery and its branches, and reach clear relationship with MCA, distal carotid artery, and carotid bifurcation. These arteries may be compressed, engulfed, and rarely invaded by the tumor. On the other hand, medial SWMs grow compressing the proximal ICA and its branches, are fed by dural branches of the ICA and compress the optic nerve, the third cranial nerve; in some cases, they can invade the cavernous

sinus and the optical canal. More frequently, these tumors may compress, engulf, or invade the arterial wall. Medial SWMs may be classified according to their origin around the anterior clinoid process and the lateral wall of the cavernous sinus. Accordingly, Al-Mefty made a subdivision of clinoidal meningiomas into three groups. Group 1 included all tumors that have an attachment on the lower part of the clinoid and that develop in the carotid cistern and encase the artery, adhering directly to the adventitia in the absence of an arachnoidal membrane; group II lesions originate from the superior or lateral aspect of the anterior clinoid process and, as they grow, come into contact with the carotid artery, with interposition of an arachnoid membrane deriving from carotid and sylvian cisterns; group III included tumors that originate from the optic foramen in which the arachnoid membrane is present between vessels and tumor, but may be lacking between tumor and optic nerve.[11]

Therefore, it is quite clear that meningiomas originating from the medial region of the sphenoid wing are more challenging for neurosurgeons, given their proximity to the optic nerve, to the cranial nerves entering the superior orbital fissure, and to the cavernous sinus (▶ Fig. 8.1). On the contrary, lateral SWMs push the sylvian fissure medially, and for this reason the optic nerve is less at risk.

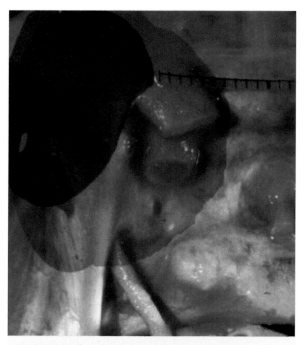

Fig. 8.1 Growth pattern of medial sphenoid wing meningiomas. The dark area is the site of origin while the shadowed area represents the area involved when the tumor progressively grows.

8.2 Lateral or Pterional Sphenoid Wing Meningiomas

8.2.1 General Aspects and Clinical Presentation

Pterional or lateral SWMs arise from the dura covering the outer sphenoid wing. Headache and psychological deficit represent the most common clinical presentation due to the fact that they are slowly growing tumors and their diagnosis is often delayed until they reach quite a large size. Seizures and other symptoms suggestive of increased intracranial pressure such as blurring of vision and vomiting were also common symptoms. Less frequent symptoms are gradual progressive diminution of vision, usually affecting the same side of the tumor, motor weakness, and altered consciousness. This group includes both globular and hyperostotic en plaque tumors (also called "spheno-orbital" meningiomas). Large tumors with middle cranial fossa extension compressing the temporal lobe or brainstem result in seizures or hemiparesis, respectively. Such tumors may also cause cognitive and memory deficits, personality changes, and dysphasia. Tumor-induced hyperostosis of the sphenoid wing and lateral orbit may present with proptosis, diplopia, and orbital pain. *En plaque* meningiomas of the sphenoid wing, also called spheno-orbital meningiomas, present with such ocular manifestations (▶ Fig. 8.2). These tumors can invade the lateral wall of the cavernous sinus, superior orbital fissure, floor of the middle cranial fossa, and the extracranial infratemporal fossa. These tumors carry a high rate of recurrence, due to frequent bone involvement, cavernous sinus, or infratemporal fossa invasion. Also for these reasons, the most appropriate surgical treatment should be total removal, including the dural attachment and bone that is involved with the tumor.[12] For this reason, bone reconstruction, orbital repair, soft tissue repair, and esthetic, represent fundamental steps of surgical techniques. Moreover, large tumors may have considerable surgical difficulties because of their possible close relationship with MCA and its branches. Usually an arachnoidal plane may be recognized and sharply dissected. In some cases, the arachnoidal plane between the tumor and artery is not clearly present; in these cases, a small fragment might be left in place, whereas needed to avoid direct damage to the main arterial trunk or even to small branches.

8.2.2 Evaluation

A thorough history and physical examination with particular attention to the symptoms and signs mentioned above are required. Thin-cut or high-resolution MRI, while including fat suppression sequences through the orbits, can assess orbital involvement. Angiographic evaluation with MR angiography or CT angiography determines the meningioma's relationship to the surrounding vasculature and their degree of encasement. However, these studies are rarely necessary as the T2-weighted MR images are adequate for identification of relevant vasculature. The bone windows on CT angiography also determine the extent of tumor-infiltrated hyperostosis. Digital subtraction angiography (DSA) may be helpful in identifying feeding vessels from the middle meningeal artery and the relationship with sylvian fissure vessels (mainly the MCA, its branches, and sylvian veins). Preoperative embolization is rarely necessary because feeding arteries can be identified, coagulated, and transected early during operation by extending to the base of the craniotomy and drilling the sphenoid wing. These maneuvers, usually, devascularize the tumor before the intradural procedure.

8.2.3 Indications for Procedure

Surgical resection is the mainstay of treatment for lateral SWMs. These tumors can be safely excised relieving the mass effect and the related clinical syndrome. Stereotactic radiosurgery is an option for recurrent small tumors in high-risk patients. Rarely, this option should be proposed for asymptomatic small tumors without mass effect. Observation is also a reasonable treatment plan for small incidental tumors.

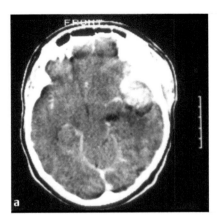
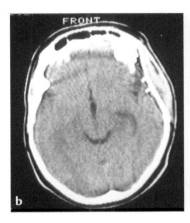

Fig. 8.2 En plaque lateral sphenoid wing meningioma. (a) Preoperative CT scan demonstrating bone involvement and invasion. **(b)** Postoperative CT scan demonstrating surgical removal including the involved bone and reconstruction with a titanium plate.

8.2.4 Surgical Approach

The choice of surgical approach for these meningiomas depends on the location of the tumor and extent of its dural attachment. Pterional and fronto-orbitozygomatic are the most commonly used surgical approaches. However, a pterional craniotomy offers several unique advantages, mainly a direct approach to the dural attachment along the sphenoid ridge, which allows an early devascularization of the tumors. This step converts a skull base meningioma in a convexity one as suggested by a fundamental mandate of skull base surgery. Even in large or giant lateral sphenoid wing tumors, an orbital or orbitozygomatic osteotomy is rarely necessary. Hyperostosis of the greater sphenoid wing with involvement of the posterolateral orbit and floor of the middle fossa should suggest an orbitozygomatic approach (▶ Fig. 8.3) facilitating removal of the involved bone in the posterolateral orbit above and below the superior orbital fissure and medially to the foramen rotundum and foramen ovale.[11,13,14] We believe that lumbar drainage is not necessary because early cerebrospinal fluid (CSF) release and brain relaxation can be obtained intraoperatively even in large tumors.

A standard pterional craniotomy is performed. A temporal craniectomy and a wide sphenoid wing drilling is mandatory to identify the meningeal branches feeding the tumor. These can be coagulated extradurally obtaining a wide devascularization that will help during the intradural steps of tumor debulking. The dura is opened circumferentially from the posterior pole to the middle cranial fossa floor and anteriorly toward the removed sphenoid wing. At this step, tumor debulking starts with the aim of reaching the dural implant to complete devascularization. As soon as the tumor is partially debulked, the relationship with the sylvian fissure vessels should be identified. Usually distal MCA branches are early identified and dissected, while in other cases, a proximal control is better obtained. Distal or proximal control should be obtained before attempting final vessel dissection. This step is better achieved with sharp instruments avoiding unnecessary traction on vessels and its small perforators. Traction may lead to spasm and cerebral infarction even

if the vessel is preserved. Identification and preservation of an arachnoidal plane is mandatory. Identification of an arachnoidal plane should guide the choice of starting vessel dissection either distally or proximally. As soon as the tumor is dissected free from the vessel, it can be removed. The dural attachment is removed and the involved bone drilled away. During this step, use of abundant rinsing with saline is suggested to avoid heat damage to surrounding cranial nerves especially at the superior orbital fissure and in the middle cranial base. Duraplasty is usually needed. A galeal-pericranial flap is ideal. In case this is not available (previous surgery or radiotherapy), an allograft with dural substitute is needed.

8.3 Medial Sphenoid Wing Meningioma

8.3.1 General Aspects and Clinical Presentation

The most common clinical presentation of medial SWMs includes headache and visual disturbances. The latter is usually a combination of visual acuity and visual field defects. Tumors that invade the cavernous sinus or superior orbital fissure may cause additional cranial neuropathies. In these cases, diplopia (usually from cranial nerve VI impairment) and facial hypoesthesia (from trigeminal involvement) are the most common symptoms. Medial SWMs are an heterogeneous group of tumor with the common feature to originate from the dura covering the lesser sphenoid wing. Many different nomenclatures have been proposed although not always justified by the real different pattern of growth or clinical picture. Yasargil proposed to differentiate medial sphenoid wing in four groups according to the site of origin and growth pattern: clinoidal, sphenocavernous, spheno-orbital, and sphenopetrosal. In general terms, we believe that clinoidal meningiomas, as described by Al-Mefty, should be differentiated from tumors arising from the dura covering the medial portion of the sphenoid bone, occupying the region of the anterior clinoid and adjacent medial

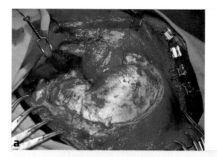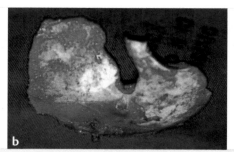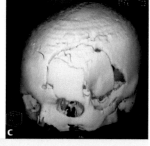

Fig. 8.3 Orbitopterional approach. (a) The bone flap including orbital osteotomy has been elevated. **(b)** One-piece orbitopterional flap and **(c)** 3D CT scan demonstrating repositioning of the bone flap after surgical removal.

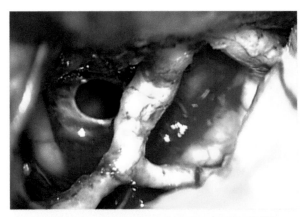

Fig. 8.4 Main neurovascular structures involved in medial sphenoid wing meningiomas. After radical tumor removal, the proximal internal carotid artery, carotid bifurcation, and the optic nerve are medialized by tumor growth. The third cranial nerve is preserved. The Lilicquist membrane is recognized and preserved during resection.

sphenoid wing and involving the pericavernous or cavernous sinus structures. We prefer to differentiate these tumor as sphenocavernous meningiomas.[15] They have a different pattern of growth involving a more distal portion of the ICA (▶ Fig. 8.4). Moreover, they compress the optic nerve later on in comparison with clinoidal meningiomas. This differentiation has many clinical and surgical implications. Sphenocavernous · meningiomas usually become symptomatic with a less specific clinical picture (chronic headache, seizures, altered mental status, and personality changes), while visual acuity and visual field impairment are present in only about 20% of patients. Moreover, in sphenocavernous meningioma surgery, the carotid artery proximal control may be obtained in the early steps of the surgical procedure.

8.3.2 Evaluation

CT scan may be used as emergency evaluation in case of seizure for an initial presumptive diagnosis. It can detect the presence of intratumoral calcifications, predicting a more firm and fibrous appearance at surgery. In some cases, CT scan may show cerebral edema. This is usually due to vein compression and/or pial penetrations. The latter aspect is very important because it may predict the absence of an arachnoidal plane between the tumor and the parenchyma. There is no direct relationship between the grade of edema and the size of the tumor. CT angiography may be helpful in studying vessel dislocation and encasement.

MRI is the ideal study for medial SWMs. It better defines tumor extension and characteristics in terms of perilesional edema, mass effect, and presumptive consistency. Brainstem compression may be clearly evaluated on MRI. Gadolinium enhancement is usually intense and

uniform. T2-weighted images may sometimes predict tumor consistency. Hyperintense tumor on T2-weighted images may predict a soft tumor, while hypointense signal is more frequently associated to a firm tumor. These correlations are not so strong to allow a reliable presurgical plan. MRI is fundamental in evaluating tumor extension to the cavernous sinus and optic canal. MR angiography may be helpful in studying arterial dislocation and compression, even if it is not possible to predict the absence of an arachnoidal plane that is a contraindication to aggressively attempt a radical removal.

DSA is rarely indicated in the standard preoperative work-up of a medial SWM. It may clearly elucidate the pattern of feeding arteries. In medial SWM, it usually comes from dural branches of the ICA. Moreover, even medial SWMs may be early devascularized during surgical exposure by aggressive resection of the sphenoid wing and anterior clinoid as well as cauterization of the involved dura. For these reasons, preoperative embolization is not usually suggested. Information about vessel dislocation and encasement, as mentioned before, may be obtained even with less invasive studies such as MR angiography and CT angiography. In cases when an ICA sacrifice is planned or is at high risk during surgery, DSA may be helpful to obtain a preoperative carotid occlusion test. However, in such cases, we strongly advocate a more conservative approach preserving ICA and its branches. Small residual tumor may be followed up and treated with radiosurgery in case of progression.

Finally, a complete neuro-opthalmologic and endocrinologic assessment should be performed in all patients harboring symptomatic parasellar tumors, including meningiomas.

8.3.3 Indications for Procedure

Surgical management is the first therapeutic option for medial SWMs. The treatment decisions may be sometimes difficult because symptoms may be mild; the natural history is variable with some tumors having a very indolent course. However, some general guidelines for the treatment of these tumors can be outlined. Factors determining the choice of surgical excision should be clinical picture, size of the lesion, patient's clinical conditions and risk factors, and presence of and amount of cerebral edema. Differently from lateral SWM, surgery should be preferred even for asymptomatic medial SWM in young patients due to the risk of early visual deterioration even in case of small tumors. In this case, preventing visual deficits and safe radical excision should be the goal of surgery. In elderly patients or in case of significant medical contraindication, close follow-up and radiosurgical treatment may be another option. As general rule, in meningioma surgery "the first shot is the best shot," thus complete removal should be attempted at first surgery. An experienced neurosurgeon knows when this can be safely accomplished keeping well in mind that functional integrity and quality of life are the main and indispensable goals of surgery.

8.3.4 Surgical Procedure

In the experience of the senior author, a pterional craniotomy is the approach of choice for most medial SWM. It is a standard, simple, and widely used approach that allows exposure and resection of these tumors (▶ Fig. 8.5). Other more extensive skull base approach, such as fronto-temporo-orbitozygomatic, have been proposed with the main purpose to reduce brain manipulation, widening the bone window offering a wide angle of attack to the tumor.[16] As a general consideration, we believe that, even if these approaches should be part of the armamentarium to deal with different skull base tumor, they are infrequently necessary to resect medial SWM. A strict microsurgical technique aimed at early relieving CSF, obtaining brain relaxation, tumor debulking, and early devascularization is the mainstay in medial SWM surgery. Neurovascular decompression and a safe radical removal may be obtained in most cases.

The patient is positioned supine with the head fixed in a three-pin headrest, extended and slightly turned toward the contralateral side. I suggest no more than a 30-degree rotation to allow a better exposition and control of the proximal ICA.

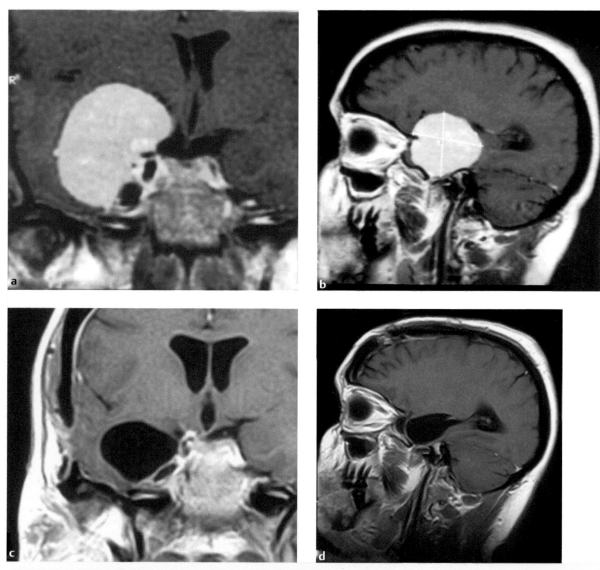

Fig. 8.5 Medial sphenoid wing meningioma. (a) Coronal and **(b)** sagittal preoperative contrast-enhanced T1-weighted images. **(c)** Coronal and **(d)** sagittal postoperative contrast-enhanced T1-weighted images demonstrating radical surgical removal.

The skin incision, the temporalis muscle preparation, and the bony steps are performed for a standard pterional craniotomy, including extensive drilling of the sphenoid wing and temporobasal craniectomy. In this step, care must be taken to identify and coagulate the deep branches of the middle meningeal artery (e.g., orbitomeningeal artery and its branches) allowing partial devascularization of the tumor. After opening the dura, the sylvian fissure is dissected and widely opened. This maneuver is mandatory because it allows elevation of the basal posterior aspect of the frontal lobe with minimal retraction pressure, also as a consequence of the upward dislocation of the frontal lobe exerted by the tumor itself.

The tumor capsule is coagulated and incised. Central tumor enucleation is alternated to coagulation of the feeding vessels at the base of the tumor along the sphenoid ridge, as well as control and coagulation of leptomeningeal feeding arteries. Tumor devascularization results in reduction in turgor and consistency and facilitates its debulking. It is important to underline that tumor debulking creates enough space to proceed in the dissection. Gradually, the MCA branches are identified and the artery is followed proximally to establish a dissection plane. This maneuver allows a better spatial identification of the seeming "intratumoral" position of the encased vessels. The tumor is removed in a piecemeal fashion under strict visual control of the MCA and its branches, which can be shifted, stretched, or encased. An arachnoidal plane should strictly be recognized and followed. Dissection should be conducted either with sharp instruments or blunt dissecting instruments. When possible, sharp dissection should be preferred avoiding any stretching on small vessels. During this phase small arterial branches from the ICA nourishing the tumor are coagulated and divided. Although vascular encasement is common on imaging in these tumors, most often, the arachnoidal plane remains intact allowing to dissect the vessel free from the tumor. If the tumor is too adherent for this maneuver, a small sheet of tumor must be left on the vessels for prevention of vasospasm or even direct injury. As soon as sufficient tumor volume reduction has been achieved, the proximal (paraclinoid segment) carotid artery, the optic nerve, and the cisternal portion of the third cranial nerve are recognized and dissected free from the tumor. After control of the paraclinoid ICA is gained, dissection of the MCA and its perforating branches, and the posterior communicating and anterior choroidal arteries can be completed. The base of the tumor is finally fully exposed and devascularization completed. The invaded dura is coagulated and resected. At this point, the falciform ligament is opened and the optic canal explored to allow decompresssion of the optic nerve, if needed. The dissection is finally carried out on the lateral wall of the cavernous sinus, peeling the walls with sharp instruments and completing tumor removal with cautious bipolar coagulation. In case of frank cavernous sinus invasion, we do not suggest to attempt resection of the intracavernous portion of the tumor to avoid oculomotor nerves and intracavernous carotid injury. The intracavernous residual tumor can be postoperatively followed up and treated with radiosurgery in case of progression. Dissection of fibrous or firm tumors can be more challenging and more caution should be reserved in these cases. Use of high-voltage bipolar coagulation or even ultrasonic aspirator may lead to heat injury to neurovascular structures.

After obtaining accurate hemostasis, the dura is closed and the bone flap repositioned.

8.4 Final Considerations

- Surgical excision is the first option in the great majority of patients harboring a sphenoid wing meningioma.
- Gross total removal is the best option for patients. First shot (first surgery) is the best chance to pursue this goal.
- Look for an arachnoidal layer. This is your best ally during dissection from neurovascular structure.
- Use sharp dissection. It avoids undue tractions and stretching on small vessels and cranial nerves.
- If an arachnoidal layer is not recognized, do not force dissection. A small remnant may be followed up and treated at progression. This strategy guides in preserving quality of life of your patients without compromising long-term tumor control.
- Large tumors produce large "birth channels." Do not manipulate brain to obtain more room for dissection. As soon as tumor debulking is obtained, you will obtain the space for further dissection.
- In case of intracavernous meningioma extension, radical removal is seldom possible. Resection of intracavernous portion often results in significant adjunctive morbidity.

References

[1] Bondy M, Ligon BL. Epidemiology and etiology of intracranial meningiomas: a review. J Neurooncol. 19 96; 29(3):197–205

[2] Longstreth WT, Jr, Dennis LK, McGuire VM, Drangsholt MT, Koepsell TD. Epidemiology of intracranial meningioma. Cancer. 1993; 72(3): 639–648

[3] Yuzawa S, Nishihara H, Tanaka S. Genetic landscape of meningioma. Brain Tumor Pathol. 2016; 33(4):237–247

[4] Whittle IR, Smith C, Navoo P, Collie D. Meningiomas. Lancet. 2004; 363(9420):1535–1543

[5] Ojemann R. Meningiomas: clinical features and surgical management. In: Wilkins RH RS, ed. Neurosurgery. New York, NY: McGraw-Hill; 1985:635–654

[6] Sacko O, Haegelen C, Mendes V, et al. Spinal meningioma surgery in elderly patients with paraplegia or severe paraparesis: a multicenter study. Neurosurgery. 2009; 64(3):503–509, discussion 509–510

[7] Nakamura M, Roser F, Jacobs C, Vorkapic P, Samii M. Medial sphenoid wing meningiomas: clinical outcome and recurrence rate. Neurosurgery. 2006; 58(4):626–639, discussion 626–639

[8] Cushing H, Eisenhardt L. Meningiomas, their classification, regional behaviour, life history, and surgical end results. Springfield, IL: Charles C Thomas; 1938

[9] Bonnal J, Thibaut A, Brotchi J, Born J. Invading meningiomas of the sphenoid ridge. J Neurosurg. 1980; 53(5):587–599

[10] Yasargil M. Microneurosurgery of CNS tumours. In: Yasargil M, ed. Microneurosurgery. Vol IV B. New York, NY: Georg Thieme Verlag; 1986:136

[11] Al-Mefty O. Clinoidal meningiomas. J Neurosurg. 1990; 73(6): 840–849

[12] Krisht A. Clinoidal meningiomas. In: Al-Mefty O, ed. Al-Mefty's Meningiomas. New York, NY: Georg Thieme Verlag; 2011

[13] Bikmaz K, Mrak R, Al-Mefty O. Management of bone-invasive, hyperostotic sphenoid wing meningiomas. J Neurosurg. 2007; 107 (5):905–912

[14] Leake D, Gunnlaugsson C, Urban J, Marentette L. Reconstruction after resection of sphenoid wing meningiomas. Arch Facial Plast Surg. 2005; 7(2):99–103

[15] Tomasello F, de Divitiis O, Angileri FF, Salpietro FM, d'Avella D. Large sphenocavernous meningiomas: is there still a role for the intradural approach via the pterional-transsylvian route? Acta Neurochir (Wien). 2003; 145(4):273–282, discussion 282

[16] McDermott MW, Durity FA, Rootman J, Woodhurst WB. Combined frontotemporal-orbitozygomatic approach for tumors of the sphenoid wing and orbit. Neurosurgery. 1990; 26(1):107–116

9 Clival Meningiomas

Rami O. Almefty, Ossama Al-Mefty

Abstract

True "clival meningiomas" arise from a broad attachment to the central upper two-thirds of the clivus, distinct from the more lateral petroclival or more inferior foramen magnum meningiomas. Because of their midline origin, clival meningiomas grow to compress the brainstem and encase the basilar artery and multiple cranial nerves bilaterally. They are often large in size at the time of diagnosis and represent a considerable therapeutic challenge. Because of their proximity to the brainstem and often large size, surgical resection is the optimal treatment. Complete resection should be pursued to reduce the risk of recurrence. This chapter describes the preoperative assessment, techniques, potential complications and advise for their avoidance, and management in pursuing resection of clival meningiomas.

Keywords: meningioma, clivus, petrosal, petrosectomy, tumor

9.1 Preoperative Definition of Lesion Features

9.1.1 Definition

The classification of meningiomas involving the posterior fossa has evolved with time and is a nontrivial task, as proper classification of these tumors allows for a useful comparison of treatment outcomes and allows the surgeon to better predict the pathologic anatomy in planning surgery.[1] Cushing and Eisenhardt classified posterior fossa meningiomas into four groups based on the location of the tumor mass.[2] Castellano and Ruggiero revised the classification based on the site of tumor origin using postmortem analysis[3] and Yasargil et al refined the classification based on intraoperative microsurgical findings. They differentiated basal posterior fossa meningiomas into clival, petroclival, sphenopetroclival, lower clival, and cerebellopontine angle tumors.[4] Clival meningiomas are defined as those arising from a broad attachment to the central upper two-thirds of the clivus. These are distinct from the more lateral petroclival subtype and more inferior lower clival (or foramen magnum) meningiomas.

9.1.2 Anatomical Considerations

Because of their origin in the midline on the clivus, these tumors grow to involve and typically encase the basilar artery, its perforators, and a multitude of cranial nerves bilaterally. The tumor is obscured by the petrous temporal bone, and the brainstem is typically compressed and deflected in a posterior direction (▶ Fig. 9.1). This is in contrast to petroclival meningiomas which originate slightly more laterally and deflect the basilar artery rather than encasing it and compress the brainstem laterally. Clival meningiomas are typically large in size at the time of diagnosis and can extend to involve Meckel's cave, the cavernous sinus, the internal auditory canal, and jugular foramen to either side.

9.2 Surgical Indications

With rare exception, clival meningiomas' typical large size, brainstem compression, and relentless natural progression necessitate surgical resection.[4,5,6] Small, asymptomatic tumors in elderly or medically ill patients may best be observed. Rarely radiation is the primary treatment and only in those patients who are poor surgical candidates due to advanced age or medical comorbidities with proven growing tumors.

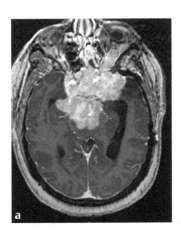
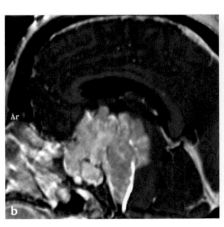

Fig. 9.1 Contrast-enhanced (a) axial and **(b)** sagittal MRI showing the potentially extensive nature of clival meningiomas with spread throughout the skull base, encasement of the basilar artery, and compression and posterior displacement of the brainstem.

9.3 Surgical Techniques

9.3.1 Preoperative Assessment

A critical component of the surgical management of clival meningiomas is the preoperative work-up and planning. All patients should be studied with contrast-enhanced magnetic resonance imaging (MRI), computed tomography (CT), angiography, venography, and audiogram. These studies play a critical role in planning the approach and anticipating the pathologic anatomy. MRI provides unparalleled detail of the tumor's soft tissue extension and relationship to the brainstem as well as vascular encasement. CT scan delineates the patient's skull base anatomy and the tumor's involved bone. Typically, noninvasive angiography and venography is sufficient. We have found dynamic CT angiography (CTA) to be particularly useful.[7] Angiography details the relationship of the major arteries to the tumor as well as the tumor's vascularity. Study of the venous anatomy is critical in approach selection and should include bilateral demonstration of the transverse and sigmoid sinuses, their connection at the torcula, the venous drainage of the temporal lobe and its relationship to the superior petrosal sinus, tentorium, and sigmoid sinus, and the location of the jugular bulb.[8] The audiogram aids in determining whether a hearing preserving approach is worthwhile.

9.3.2 Approach Selection

The ideal approach offers direct visualization and illumination of the tumor, brainstem, and critical neurovascular structures with a short operating distance, avoidance of brain retraction, multiple trajectories, freedom of movement, and early devascularization of the tumor. In approaching clival meningiomas, the temporal bone is obstructive and lateral skull base approaches are needed to optimize the approach. Since these tumors lie anterior to the brainstem and typically extend below the level of the internal auditory canal, they require either a combined petrosal approach[9] or a total petrosectomy with the patient's hearing status being the determinant. However, midclival tumors represent a formidable challenge and even patients with intact hearing may warrant total petrosectomy. The venous anatomy, although important to understand prior to surgery and may necessitate adaption of the approach, rarely prohibits an approach.[1,8,10]

Anesthesia and Intraoperative Neuromonitoring

The anesthetic care of the patient is a critical component in a successful operation and the surgeon must work closely with the anesthesiologist with an open line of communication. Total intravenous anesthesia is used to optimize brain relaxation and neuromonitoring. Mild hypothermia is induced, normotension is maintained throughout induction, and the duration of the case and hypervolemia is avoided. We avoid the use of mannitol to preserve the arachnoid dissection plane and avoid its anticoagulant effect. We also avoid the use of lumbar drains because of their potential catastrophic complications.[11] Skull base approaches allowing access to cerebrospinal fluid (CSF) egress without brain retraction obviate their need. In the event of a tumor that extends down to crowd the foramen magnum, awake fiberoptic intubation may be necessary.

Intraoperative neuromonitoring is a critical adjunct and is used in all cases. Somatosensory-evoked potentials, brainstem auditory-evoked responses, and cranial nerve monitoring, which may include any cranial nerve III to XII, are performed in all cases.

Combined Petrosal Approach

Patient Positioning

The patient is placed supine with an ipsilateral shoulder roll. The trunk is elevated to place the head above the heart and facilitate venous drainage. The head is turned slightly to the opposite side and the vertex dropped to allow the temporal lobe to fall away. Excessive turning or flexion of the head will compromise venous drainage and must be avoided. The abdomen is prepped for harvesting fat.

Soft Tissue Dissection

The scalp incision begins 1 cm in front of the tragus, curves anteriorly along the hairline, behind the frontalis branch of the facial nerve, gently curves posteriorly two fingerbreadths above the pinna of the ear, and finally turns down, two fingerbreadths behind the pinna to below the level of the mastoid tip. During the scalp incision, the superficial temporal artery is preserved and the scalp incision is reflected inferiorly separately from the underlying muscle and fascia. The temporalis muscle is incised along its inferior, anterior, and superior aspect and elevated off of the temporalis muscle in continuity with the sternocleidomastoid muscle which is incised posteriorly and reflected inferiorly. This creates a long, wide, thick vascularized combined myofascial flap for reconstruction. The zygoma is then sectioned allowing the temporalis muscle to reflect well inferiorly. The temporalis muscle can also be used as a vascularized flap.

Bone Work

Four burr holes are placed bridging the sinus anteriorly and posteriorly and additional burr holes are placed as needed to safely dissect the dura. A combined posterior fossa, occipital, temporal craniotomy is then performed. The burr holes bridging the sinus are connected with the drill rather than crossing the sinus with the footplate. Following the craniotomy, a piece of the mastoid cortex is harvested for later reconstruction. A mastoidectomy is then completed, skeletonizing the sigmoid sinus from its junction with the transverse sinus down to the jugular bulb and exposing the presigmoid dura. A middle fossa dissection is then performed to expose the petrous apex. The middle meningeal artery is identified in the foramen spinosum, coagulated, cut, and waxed. Posterior and medial to it, the greater superficial petrosal nerve is identified and preserved. The dissection is carried medial up to the posterior fossa dura and posteriorly to the internal auditory canal. Care must be taken during the dissection as there may be a dehiscence of the bone overlying the petrous carotid or the genu of the facial nerve. The area of bone to be drilled is bounded by the trigeminal ganglion anteriorly, the petrous carotid laterally, the internal auditory canal posteriorly, and the posterior fossa dura medially. The drilling is carried inferiorly to the level of the inferior petrosal sinus and can be extended medially into the clivus.

Dural Opening and Sectioning of the Superior Petrosal Sinus

The dura is incised both along the inferior temporal lobe and in the presigmoid dura. Separating the two incisions is the superior petrosal sinus and the tentorium. Prior to connecting the cuts by sectioning the superior petrosal sinus, it is critical that the venous drainage of the temporal lobe is identified. The sinus must be sectioned and the tentorium cut anterior to where the temporal lobe venous drainage enters. Once the sinus is ligated and cut, the incision is extended on the tentorium in an anterior and medial direction to the incisura. Prior to completing the cut, the fourth nerve must be identified and the final cut made posterior to where the fourth nerve enters the tentorium. Completing this cut releases the sigmoid sinus allowing it to mobilize posteriorly, opening up the presigmoid exposure, and connecting the posterior and middle fossa.

Intradural Dissection and Tumor Removal

Once the dura is opened, the first objective is to open the cisternal arachnoid to allow for CSF egress. Once CSF has been released and the brain relaxed, a wide and shallow exposure to the tumor without the need for retraction is obtained. The tumor is then devascularized from its attachment along the clivus. Once the tumor has been devascularized, the arachnoid membrane is dissected off of a safe portion of the tumor, allowing it to be entered and intracapsular debulking to be performed. Debulking must be done with caution as the basilar artery, its perforators, and branches can be encased by the tumor. Once the tumor is debulked, using high magnification and meticulous technique the critical neurovascular structures are dissected free utilizing the arachnoidal plan. Maintaining the dissection within the proper arachnoid plane is the key to the safe and total removal. In cases where an arachnoidal plane is not present, total removal

is not possible and it is better to leave a small residual than risk injury to the critical neurovascular structures.

Closure

Primary closure of the dura is not typically possible and it must be grafted. Following a good dural grafting, the cavities created in the petrous apex and mastoid are obliterated with fat. The vascularized myofascial flap is reflected to cover the defect. The bone is replaced along with the mastoid cortex using standard cranial fixation techniques and the wound is closed in layers.[1]

Total Petrosectomy

The soft tissue dissection for the total petrosectomy is similar to that for the combined petrosal approach; however, it includes the sectioning and blind sac closure of the external canal. The bone work also begins similarly but following the mastoidectomy, the drilling is continued to include translabyrinthine and transcochlear exposures. Although the facial nerve can be completely liberalized from its bony canal and reflected posteriorly, we prefer to leave it protected in a thin bony canal which has allowed for good facial nerve outcomes when using this approach.[8] The middle ear is emptied and the eustachian tube obliterated prior to completion of the drilling including the cochlea and internal auditory canal[1,12] (▶ Fig. 9.2).

9.4 Complications

Dr. Harvey Cushing is credited as saying "All said and done, it is the final result that counts, and having been brought up to believe that convalescence is shortened by attention to the technical details while the patient is on the operating table, I have no dread of a long session." This idiom is never more pertinent than when embarking on the resection of a clival meningioma. Clival meningiomas are located deep in the skull base, obscured by the clivus and temporal bones, often large in size, and encasing the basilar artery and its perforators. A myriad of complications is possible; however, modern skull base approaches and microsurgical technique have made their resection safe and effective. Meticulousness in technique must be constantly maintained to best avoid complications.

9.4.1 Vascular

Appropriate care involving the transverse and sigmoid sinus as well as the venous drainage of the temporal lobe must be ensured. The sinuses must be crossed carefully, separated meticulously, and the temporal venous drainage identified and preserved. The basilar artery, as well as its perforators and branches can be encased by the tumor. Their preservation is critical and must be done with meticulous dissection within the arachnoid plane under high magnification after careful debulking. If the arachnoid plane is not present, residual tumor must be accepted.

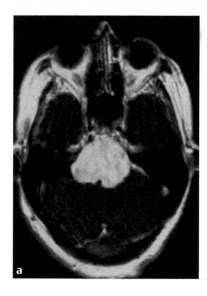 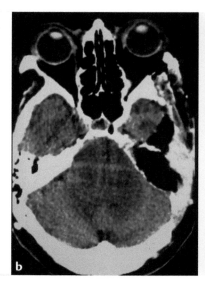

Fig. 9.2 **(a)** Axial contrast-enhanced MRI showing a midclival meningioma extending bilaterally, encasing the basilar artery, and compressing the brainstem posteriorly. **(b)** Postoperative CT scan demonstrating the bony removal and fat packing following a total petrosectomy and the complete resection of the tumor.

9.4.2 Cranial Nerve

Lower cranial nerve paralysis can lead to significant morbidity and mortality. Every effort is made to preserve them intraoperatively and their adequate function must be ensured postoperatively with a formal swallow evaluation. This may necessitate tube feeding in the interim. As the function often improves in the short term, we avoid early placement of gastrostomy–jejunostomy tubes and their associated complications. In the event of a persistent deficit, vocal cord injections can be helpful. The seventh and eight cranial nerves are best preserved by avoiding lateral to medial traction and preserving their blood supply from the labyrinthine artery. In the event of seventh nerve dysfunction, if the patient is unable to close the eye, it must be protected. This is particularly troublesome if concomitant fifth nerve palsy is present rendering the cornea insensate. Placement of a lid weight allows for eye closure and its protection while the nerve recovers. Patients with unilateral hearing loss, desiring better sound localization can be aided by contralateral routing devices. The rootlets of the fifth nerve may be sharply displaced as they enter Meckel's cave in the middle fossa and careful attention is needed in elevating the outer wall of Meckel's cave to follow the tumor. After the sixth nerve travels superiorly intradurally and enters Dorello's canal, it runs under the dura and is susceptible to injury when the involved bone of the clivus and petrous apex is removed. In clival meningiomas, bilateral sixth nerves are frequently at risk. Deficits of cranial nerves III, IV, and VI are initially treated with patching to alleviate double vision and are given a chance to recover. In the event of a fixed deficit, diplopia can be improved with prism glasses or strabismus surgery.

9.4.3 Brainstem

Injury to the brainstem from subpial transgression or vascular injury can lead to devastating consequences and mandates the utmost care and attention. The tumor at the brainstem interface is only dissected after considerable debulking has left only a thin shell of tumor allowing intra-arachnoidal dissection, preserving a layer of arachnoid over the brainstem. If an arachnoid plane is not present, then it is better to leave a small remnant of tumor than risking neurologic injury.

9.4.4 CSF Leak

CSF leak is a potentially fatal complication and requires careful planning and execution to avoid when removing skull base meningiomas. The most important factor in preventing CSF leak is planning the approach to provide vascularized flaps for reconstruction. The petrosal approaches described earlier provide a vascularized myofascial flap as well as a temporalis flap. Next, the dura can rarely be closed primarily and good grafting is essential, particularly at the sinodural angle. The petrous apex and mastoid defects are packed with fat to obliterate dead space. When performing a total petrosectomy, the eustachian tube must be packed closed with fat and fascia. Dural sealants can be used to reinforce closure and hold the fat packing in place but are no substitute for a vascularized reconstruction.

In the event of a suspected CSF leak, it must be dealt with urgently. First, the presence of hydrocephalus is excluded with cranial imaging. The diagnosis and site of the defect is then confirmed with CT cisternography. Once the site and extent of the defect is identified, the optimal strategy can be planned. In the event of small, low flow defects, early in the course, temporary CSF diversion may suffice. Otherwise, a more robust vascularized repair must be performed.

9.4.5 Cholesteatoma

During a total petrosectomy and the obliteration of the external canal, the potential for an iatrogenic cholesteatoma is created. In order to avoid this complication, the remnant of the ear with the eardrum must be removed.

9.5 Early and Long-term Postoperative Management

The fact that meningioma recurrence is directly related to the extent of resection has been well established.[13,14,15] Therefore, every effort should be made at the outset to optimize the resection, and total removal should be pursued with zeal. A premeditated strategy of planned debulking and radiation therapy subjects the patient to all the risks of surgery, all the risks of radiation, and eliminates the opportunity for curative removal. Having said that, despite the surgeon's best attempt, total removal is not always safely possible and one must accept a subtotal resection. Many advocate for upfront radiation therapy at this time[16,17,18,19]; however, we believe a small residual is best observed. In the event of further growth, the decision can be made at that time to continue observation, reoperate, or radiate depending on the extent of recurrence and patient circumstances.

References

[1] Al-Mefty O. Operative atlas of meningiomas. Philadelphia, PA: Lippincott-Raven; 1998

[2] Cushing H, Eisenhardt L. Meningiomas: their classification, regional behavior, life history, and surgical end results. Springfield, ILs: Charles C Thomas; 1938

[3] Castellano F, Ruggiero G. Meningiomas of the posterior fossa. Acta Radiol Suppl. 1953; 104:1–177

[4] Yasargil M. Meningiomas of basal posterior cranial fossa. Vol 7. Vienna, VA: Springer-Verlag; 1980

[5] Cherington M, Schneck SA. Clivus meningiomas. Neurology. 1966; 16 (1):86–92

[6] Mayberg MR, Symon L. Meningiomas of the clivus and apical petrous bone. Report of 35 cases. J Neurosurg. 1986; 65(2):160–167

[7] Bi WL, Brown PA, Abolfotoh M, Al-Mefty O, Mukundan S, Jr, Dunn IF. Utility of dynamic computed tomography angiography in the preoperative evaluation of skull base tumors. J Neurosurg. 2015; 123(1):1–8

[8] Erkmen K, Pravdenkova S, Al-Mefty O. Surgical management of petroclival meningiomas: factors determining the choice of approach. Neurosurg Focus. 2005; 19(2):E7

[9] Cho CW, Al-Mefty O. Combined petrosal approach to petroclival meningiomas. Neurosurgery. 2002; 51(3):708–716, discussion 716–718

[10] Haddad GF, Al-Mefty O. The road less traveled: transtemporal access to the CPA. Clin Neurosurg. 1994; 41:150–167

[11] Snow RB, Kuhel W, Martin SB. Prolonged lumbar spinal drainage after the resection of tumors of the skull base: a cautionary note. Neurosurgery. 1991; 28(6):880–882, discussion 882–883

[12] Pieper DR, Al-Mefty O. Total Petrosectomy Approach for Lesions of the Skull Base. Oper Techn Neurosurg. 1999; 2(2):62–68

[13] Simpson D. The recurrence of intracranial meningiomas after surgical treatment. J Neurol Neurosurg Psychiatry. 1957; 20(1):22–39

[14] Gousias K, Schramm J, Simon M. The Simpson grading revisited: aggressive surgery and its place in modern meningioma management. J Neurosurg. 2016; 125(3):551–560

[15] Almefty R, Dunn IF, Pravdenkova S, Abolfotoh M, Al-Mefty O. True petroclival meningiomas: results of surgical management. J Neurosurg. 2014; 120(1):40–51

[16] Mathiesen T, Gerlich A, Kihlström L, Svensson M, Bagger-Sjöbäck D. Effects of using combined transpetrosal surgical approaches to treat petroclival meningiomas. Neurosurgery. 2007; 60(6):982–991, discussion 991–992

[17] Frostell A, Hakim R, Dodoo E, et al. Adjuvant stereotactic radiosurgery reduces need for retreatments in patients with meningioma residuals. World Neurosurg. 2016; 88:475–482

[18] Przybylowski CJ, Raper DM, Starke RM, Xu Z, Liu KC, Sheehan JP. Stereotactic radiosurgery of meningiomas following resection: predictors of progression. J Clin Neurosci. 2015; 22(1):161–165

[19] Aboukais R, Zairi F, Reyns N, et al. Surgery followed by radiosurgery: a deliberate valuable strategy in the treatment of intracranial meningioma. Clin Neurol Neurosurg. 2014; 124:123–126

10 Petroclival Meningiomas

Danica Grujicic, Rosanda Ilic, Teresa Somma, Rosa Maria Gerardi, Luigi Maria Cavallo, Dragan Savic, Mihailo Milicevic

Abstract

Petroclival meningiomas are one of the most challenging pathology because of their deep-seated locations and intimate relationship with important neurovascular structures. Patients could be asymptomatic or affected by symptoms due to raised intracranial pressure or due to cranial nerves, cerebellum, or brainstem compression. The choice of the approach should be tailored on the patient and tumor characteristics, while the goal of the surgical treatment should be the radical resection, without neurological damage.

Stereotaxic radiosurgery is an effective and safe tool that gives good control of small residual tumor. We considered the retrosigmoid approach for tumors localized in posterior fossa, and the pterional, subtemporal, and orbitozygomatic for tumors with middle cranial fossa extension. Follow-up should be carried out according to neuro-oncological principles.

Keywords: petroclival meningioma, retrosigmoid approach, stereotaxic radiosurgery, transpetrous approach

10.1 Introduction

Petroclival meningiomas are defined as those originating at the upper two-thirds of the clivus, lateral to the midline, at the level of the petroclival junction and medial to the trigeminal nerve.[1,2,3,4] These lesions represent a permanent challenge for neurosurgeons because of their deep-seated locations and intimate relationship with important neurovascular structures. Petroclival meningiomas are a rare entity accounting for 0 to 15% of all intracranial tumors and comprising only 3 to 10% of the posterior fossa meningiomas. Nevertheless, these lesions are still one of the "hottest" topics for debate in neurosurgical community, mostly with regards to the choice of the surgical approach as well as to the growing application of stereotactic radiosurgery.

Because of slow growth rate, and relatively scarce symptoms, sometimes they can reach extensive dimensions at the time of diagnosis, extending into posterior portion of the cavernous sinus and middle cranial fossa, with involvement of the petrous apex and cave of Meckel. Spheno-petroclival meningiomas involve the entire cavernous sinus (including its anterior portion), sella turcica, with wide middle cranial fossa extension. Sometimes cavernous sinus is infiltrated bilaterally, with clivus and sphenoid sinus involvement.[2,3] Treatment of these tumors will also be considered in this chapter. Other meningiomas of posterior fossa, including clival meningiomas (midline clivus), foramen magnum meningiomas (lower third of clivus) and anterior and posterior petrosal meningiomas (lateral to trigeminal nerve) do not share anatomic relations with true petroclival meningiomas and will not be addressed further.[1]

10.2 Anatomical Considerations

Petroclival meningiomas grow at the posterior cranial fossa, where they occupy the space between brainstem and cerebellar hemispheres posteriorly, pyramid laterally, and clivus anteriorly. Usually, neurovascular structures are displaced in the typical pattern, III and IV nerves above the tumor, V and VII nerves laterally and posteriorly, VI nerve medially,[5] and lower group (IX–XI) on the caudal pole of the tumor. These structures might also be encased by the tumor as it gradually enlarges, although seldom there is any apparent cranial nerve palsy. As this is the most frequent cause of morbidity related to petroclival meningioma surgery, it is of great importance to accurately predict their localization preoperatively and high definition magnetic resonance tractography seems a promising tool to identify displaced and/or encased cranial nerves.[6,7]

One of the most important features is the relationship with the brainstem; usually it is displaced by the tumor posteriorly and contralaterally, along with vertebral and basilar arteries and their branches.[1] MRI T2 sequences are useful to identify the arachnoidal layer of the brainstem, which appears as a space between the tumor and the brainstem, predicting a more favorable tumor resection; absence of this radiological sign indicates that this border is disturbed, thus probability of brainstem and perforating blood vessels damage during the resection is higher.[8,9]

Spheno-petroclival lesions are the most extensive of these lesions involving one or both cavernous sinuses or establishing a close relationship with optical nerves, chiasm, intradural portion of carotid artery, and their branches.

10.3 Clinical Presentation

Patients with petroclival meningiomas can develop nonspecific symptoms due to raised intracranial pressure (ICP), either from the tumor mass or obstructive hydrocephalus, or specific symptoms due to cranial nerves compression, mass effect on the cerebellum and brainstem.[10,11] Headache is the most frequent complaint, and cerebellar signs are the most common clinical signs.[12,13,14,15] Cranial nerves V (approximately 65%)[3,16] and VIII (51.5%)[3] are most frequently involved, presenting with face numbness, trigeminal neuralgia, or hearing loss.[13,17] Facial nerve palsy occurs in 24.4 to 50% of patients.[2,11,14,16] The lower cranial nerves are involved less frequently (28.6%), as well as III, IV, and VI (18.3%), in less than half of the cases.[2,11,18] Spastic weakness can appear due to brainstem motor pathway compression in 15 to 57% of patients.

10.4 Preoperative Evaluation

CT is usually the first examination in diagnosing intracranial lesions. It shows hyperdense lesions, usually with strong contrast enhancement. The CT sequence known as a "bone window" is useful in evaluating the anatomy of the skull base, identifying hyperostosis, bone erosion as well as tumor calcifications (▶ Fig. 10.1). Contrast-enhanced brain-MRI is standard for assessing tumor characteristics and evaluating relationship with neurovascular structures and brain tissue. Petroclival meningiomas usually appear T1-isointense, T2 and fluid attenuated inversion recovery (FLAIR) hyperintense, showing strong, homogenous gadolinium uptake. T2-weighted MRI is important to determine whether there is a good arachnoid plane between the tumor and brainstem, also brainstem edema, suggesting vascular engulfment that might be considered as an adverse prognostic sign.[3] Venography is useful to evaluate the size of the transverse and sigmoid sinuses as well as their collateral flow, anatomy of major venous blood vessels, mostly vein of Labbe. MR angiography, CT angiography, and digital angiography can be used to assess displacement, stenosis, or occlusion of the basilar or internal carotid arteries and their branches as well as blood supply of the tumor.[14] It can also give excellent assessment of venous structures (▶ Fig. 10.2).

Meningiomas are known for their extensive vascularization that sometimes can lead to massive blood loss during surgery; though when dealing with skull base tumors such as petroclival meningiomas, devascularization cannot be achieved before tumor debulking. In these lesions, blood supply is usually provided by clival branches of the meningohypophyseal trunk and by external carotid branches. In case of high-vascularized tumors, preoperative embolization should be considered preferably 7 to 10 days before the operation. Feeders from meningohypophyseal trunk are difficult to access, and care should be taken in cases of partial embolization of only external carotid branches, because it might cause increased blood flow in residual blood vessels and extensive bleeding during the surgery.[19,20] Embolization can cause sudden intratumoral necrosis and hemorrhage that can lead to tumor volume enlargement and worsening of mass effect, so that whether brainstem edema is already present on preoperative MRI, embolization should be avoided[21] Cranial nerve palsy can also occur as complication of accidental embolization of their feeders.

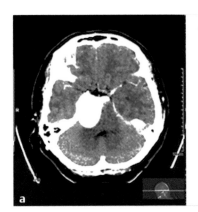
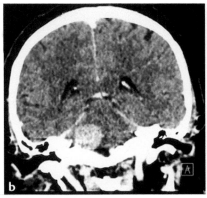

Fig. 10.1 (a, b) The CT scan shows a right spheno-petroclival hyperdense lesion with strong post-contrastographic enhancement, in absence of evident bone erosion or calcifications. It occupies the space between brainstem and right cerebellar hemisphere posteriorly, the pyramid of the temporal bone laterally and clivus anteriorly in the posterior cranial fossa. The tumor extends to the middle cranial fossa involving both cavernous sinus.

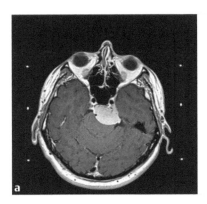
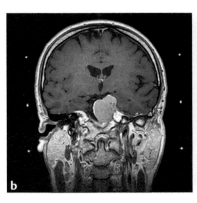

Fig. 10.2 Post-contrastographic brain-MRI study in a 62-year-old man: (a) axial spin-echo T1 weighted and (b) coronal spin-echo T1 weighted sequences showing a left petroclival lesion, with strong contrast enhancement. This lesion extends from the left lateral part of the clivus to the petroclival junction involving the posterior portion of the left cavernous sinus.

The authors attempted to reduce tumor vascularization of skull base meningiomas by mean of stereotaxic radiosurgery with targeted on tumor dural attachment. Operation was performed 2 to 3 months after irradiation, with significant reduction of blood supply, but with increased firmness of tumor.

Finally, it is mandatory for patients to undergo a baseline audiogram to evaluate preoperative hearing function as well as careful evaluation of other cranial nerve function since their assessment is crucial for the choice of operative approach.

10.5 Surgical Indications

Until 1970s petroclival meningiomas have been considered as unresectable lesions[1,22,23] and universally described as progressive, eventually lethal diseases. Nowadays, more data are available about natural history of these tumors. Volumetric analysis of untreated petroclival meningiomas showed annual growth rate from 0.81 to 2.38 cm/year, with 76% of patients diagnosed with progression, among which 63% presented with neurological worsening.[9,12]

This suggests that carefully designed treatment is necessary for this group of patients. Policy of "wait and see" might be justified only in elderly patients with very small tumors or with serious comorbidities that are suitable neither for operative treatment nor stereotaxic or conformal radiotherapy. In this group of patients, ventriculoperitoneal (VP) shunt might be considered if hydrocephalus is present.

A second important issue is the choice of therapeutic approach. In the era of expansion of stereotaxic radiosurgery, gamma knife treatment of small, deep-seated meningiomas might be reasonable. In several studies, good local control was achieved after stereotaxic radiosurgery, with tumor control rate of 80 to 91.2% after 5 years and 77.2 to 81% after 10 years.[24,25]

There is some concern about eventual anaplastic transformation but series with follow-up period of 10 to 15 years show a 2.2% rate of malignant transformation. As low rate of malignant transformation is also noticed in nonirradiated meningiomas only further investigation, that should consider detailed pathohistological analysis, can give accurate evaluation of late adverse effects of stereotaxic radiotherapy.

It can be concluded that stereotaxic radiosurgery, as sole treatment, can be ideal solution for small tumors in elderly, due to the good tumor control and low probability of malignant transformation in period of their life expectancy.

For young patients, radical surgery should be considered as the treatment of choice, because it gives a chance for cure without any further treatment. On the other hand, sacrifice of neurological function in order to maximize extent of resection (EOR) is not acceptable, and as mentioned before, stereotaxic radiosurgery is a comfortable single session treatment that provides good tumor control, especially in patients with very small tumor remnants. There have been a lot of suggestions for classification and therapeutic protocols for petroclival meningiomas, but none of them is univocally accepted.[15]

Presence of hydrocephalus at the time of diagnosis with signs of elevated ICP, in authors' experience, should be resolved with VP shunt placement. A period of 7 to 14 days is recommended between shunt procedure and tumor removal, which enables good brain relaxation and easier approach to these deep-seated tumors.

The choice of approach should be left to experienced surgical team. Optimal surgical approach for petroclival meningiomas is still controversial and depends on the location, size, and extension of the tumor as well as patient age, neurological status, particularly hearing and facial nerve function, and the neurosurgeon's preferences.[26,27,28,29]

Two main groups of approaches can be considered, the first including "standard" transcranial approaches as the retrosigmoid, for tumors localized in posterior fossa, and the pterional, subtemporal, and orbitozygomatic for tumors with middle cranial fossa extension. The second large group stands for skull base approaches that demand more extensive bone removal as the transpetrosal approach (anterior, posterior, and combined).

The best surgical route should give the widest exposure enabling maximal EOR with minimal approach-associated morbidity.

10.6 Surgical Techniques

10.6.1 Retrosigmoid Approach

In University of Naples "Federico II" and Clinic of Neurosurgery, Clinical Center of Serbia at Belgrade (authors' institutions), tumors without significant extension into middle cranial fossa are preferentially treated via a retrosigmoid approach, (▶ Fig. 10.3) while when a large middle fossa extension is noticed, a two-step approach with combination of the retrosigmoid and the frontotemporal is performed.[29,30] As brainstem decompression is a critical step in petroclival meningioma treatment, infratentorial part of tumor should be resected first (▶ Fig. 10.4). The major advantage of the retrosigmoid approach resides in its simplicity with avoidance of extensive petrous bone resection, reducing the risk of VII and VIII cranial nerves injury and eventually a postoperative cerebrospinal fluid (CSF) leak. Samii advocates the so called "retrosigmoid intradural suprameatal approach" that consists of intradural drilling of petrous bone above and anterior to internal acoustic meatus to extend the view of Meckel's cave and trigeminal nerve, with tentorial incision for tumors with supratentorial extension.[30]

In patients without hydrocephalus and VP shunt, preferred position is the semi-sitting, while the sitting position is choice for patient with small posterior fossa or

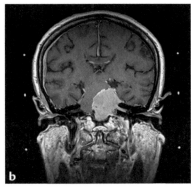

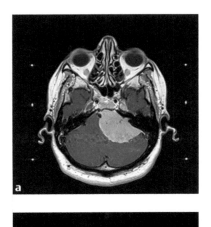

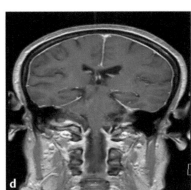

Fig. 10.3 Post-contrastographic brain-MRI in a 62-year-old woman: (**a**) axial spin-echo T1 weighted and (**b**) coronal spin-echo T1 weighted. The study shows a large left spheno-petroclival lesion with strong contrast enhancement. It originates from the left lateral part of the clivus and the petroclival junction extending to the middle cranial fossa. The tumor displaces posteriorly and contralaterally the brainstem and left cerebellar hemisphere encasing the origin of the left V cranial nerve as well as involving both cavernous sinus. (**c**) Postoperative axial spin-echo T1 weighted and (**d**) coronal spin-echo T1 weighted. These sequences show the subtotal removal of the lesion by retrosigmoid approach. The residual tumor remains in both cavernous sinus.

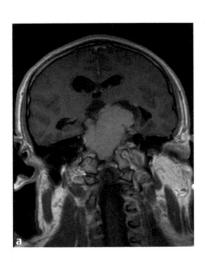

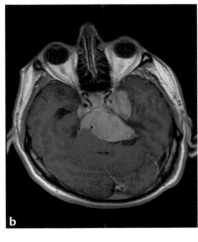

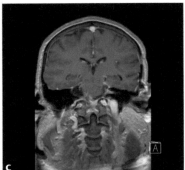

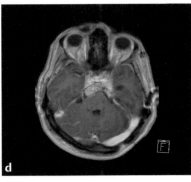

Fig. 10.4 Post-contrastographic brain-MRI study in a 32-year-old man: (**a**) axial spin-echo T1 weighted and (**b**) coronal spin-echo T1 weighted. It shows a large left spheno-petroclival lesion with strong contrast enhancement. The tumor extends from the left lateral part of the clivus and the petroclival junction to the contralateral side reaching the middle cranial fossa. It displaces posteriorly and contralaterally the brainstem and left cerebellar hemisphere involving the sella turcica and both cavernous sinus with compression on left temporal lobe. (**c**) Postoperative axial spin-echo T1 weighted and (**d**) coronal spin-echo T1 weighted sequences. These sequences underline the subtotal removal of the lesion by two surgical approaches. While the infratentorial portion of the tumor was removed by a retrosigmoid approach, the supratentorial component was then removed via a subtemporal route. The residual tumor remains in the upper part of the clivus, in the sella turcica and in both cavernous sinus.

with VP shunt. In these cases, the park bench position could demand the resection of lateral part (one-fourth) of the cerebellar hemisphere.

A suboccipital retrosigmoid craniotomy is performed in the standard manner, exposing the whole width of transverse and sigmoid sinuses, with removal of mastoid cells if necessary. For larger tumors with caudal extension, posterior rim of foramen magnum should also be removed, and posterior arch of atlas exposed, whether removal can be necessary. Somatosensory evoked potentials, facial electromyographic responses, and brainstem auditory evoked potentials are measured intraoperatively. After opening of the dura, the cerebello-medullary cistern is opened so that CSF can be evacuated and after that cerebellar hemisphere can easily be retracted to expose the tumor in the cerebellopontine angle. Then V and VII/VIII nerves should be identified, as they run across posterior side of tumor. Tumor resection should be performed from the upper pole, in the lateromedially direction, starting from the tentorium and bone, moving toward the brainstem (▶ Fig. 10.5).[31]

This approach permits earlier identification of the cranial nerves near their entrance or exit in bone or dura. If nerves cannot be visualized from the beginning, piecemeal dissection with frequent direct stimulation should be performed to avoid their injury. In smaller tumors, identification of lower group of cranial nerves should be easy, as well as tumor dissection in this part, but in the cases of larger tumor, caudal pole might be attached to, or encasing lower group, so meticulous care should be taken to preserve them. Tumor dissection is performed respecting the arachnoid planes. Preservation of arachnoid layer is mandatory while removing tumor from the cranial nerves and especially brainstem, because injury of brainstem and small perforating arteries can result in major morbidity.[26] After resection of their infratentorial portion, tumors with minor supratentorial extension and good arachnoid plane can be just peeled off upon the descent of the upper part of the lesion. Tentorial incision can be placed safely in order to extend the exposure, but care should be taken to avoid injury of trochlear nerve.[32]

Also tumors with extension into Meckel's cave can be resected with the retrosigmoid intradural suprameatal approach described by Samii.[31]

The same principles can be applied for the patients that are operated in park-bench, or lateral position, but retraction of cerebellar hemisphere might be a problem even after CSF evacuation from cisterna magna, so this approach is reserved for patients with comorbidities that might exclude sitting position and for the patients with previously implanted VP shunts. For better brain relaxation, preoperative external lumbar drainage should be performed in patients without VP shunt.

In the cases, with supratentorial extension a second surgery is performed via a frontotemporal approach. Patient is positioned supine, external lumbar drainage is placed in order to relax the brain and minimize the need for retraction, and standard frontotemporal craniotomy is performed. After dura opening and tumor exposure, an attempt is made to localize the carotid artery and optic nerve as they enter dura. Sometimes, it can be difficult because they are surrounded with tumor tissue, but with careful aid of low-power Cavitron Ultrasonic Surgical Aspirator (CUSA) in combination with sharp dissection, they can be preserved. It is important to preserve oculomotor and trochlear nerves that are running at the edge of tentorium. If it is necessary contralateral carotid artery and optic nerve can also be decompressed. We usually do not attempt the removal of tumor from cavernous sinus because it is associated with unacceptable cranial nerve morbidity.

10.6.2 Transpetrosal Approaches

This approach allows a wide skull base exposition with a better visualization of petroclival region, through a major bone removal and minor brain retraction, the vascularization of the tumor usually is better approached in this way. There are many variants of transpetrosal approaches and the choice depends on the amount of supratentorial extension of tumor, invasion of cavernous sinus, Meckel's cave, functional hearing before operation, and relationship

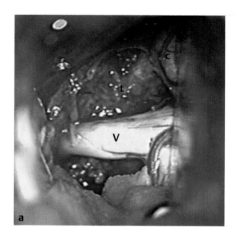
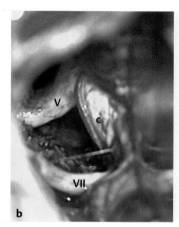

Fig. 10.5 Intraoperative photos showing the surgical field after opening the dura and cerebellomedullary cistern, during a retrosigmoid approach **(a)** before and **(b)** after removing the tumor. The cerebellar hemisphere (c) can easily be retracted to expose the tumor (t) in cerebellopontine angle. The V (V) and VII (VII) nerves should be identified as they run across posterior side of tumor.

of tumor with internal auditory canal. Although these approaches can be demanding with increased risk of cranial nerve injury, CSF leak fistula and infection, when performed by experienced skull base neurosurgeon, can be very effective permitting good EOR of supra/infratentorial meningiomas in a single stage procedure.[33]

10.6.3 Anterior Petrosal Approach

The anterior petrosal approach exposes the petroclival region from the above and can be used in the cases without major infratentorial extension and without lateral extension to internal auditory meatus.[28] It gives good view of the middle fossa, Meckel's cave, upper third of clivus, and ventral portion of the brainstem, providing direct approach to dural attachment and devascularization of the meningohypophyseal trunk feeders. It was originally defined by Kawase for the aneurysms of the basilar tip and it might be considered the best approach for the surgical management of lesions involving mostly the Meckel's cave.[34]

The patient is placed in the supine position and the head is rotated, so that the zygoma is the highest point of the surgical field. In this way, gravity facilitates the retraction of the temporal lobe. For additional brain relaxation, external lumbar drainage can be placed. Standard skin incision is made to expose zygomatic arch and temporal region. The zygomatic arch is cut and craniotomy is made along the floor of the middle fossa and crossing the sphenoid wing. The dura is detached from the floor of the middle fossa until the middle meningeal artery is encountered, coagulated, and cut. Further detaching of dura should allow visualization of important anatomical landmarks, third division of the trigeminal nerve at the foramen ovale, greater superficial petrosal nerve (GSPN), lateral wall of cavernous sinus, and the third and second divisions of the trigeminal nerve. Care should be taken to avoid extensive manipulation with GSPN because it can cause traction injury to the geniculate ganglion. At this point, Gasserian ganglion is visible (Meckel's cave) and the Glasscock's and Kawase's triangles can be identified. The bone of the petrous apex is drilled medially to the carotid artery, extending from the trigeminal impression to the internal auditory meatus and exposing the posterior fossa dura. The dura mater is opened along the base of the temporal lobe. The superior petrosal sinus is coagulated and cut, tentorium is resected, avoiding the injury of trochlear nerve. In this way, posterior fossa is entered and tumor is exposed. The resection should be performed in piecemeal fashion, respecting the arachnoid and without aggressive pulling tumor off thickened arachnoid layer covering the neurovascular structures and brainstem. Also, removal of the portion of tumor in the cavernous sinus is not advisable because of high morbidity as this part of tumor can be successfully treated at later stage with stereotaxic radiosurgery. The careful closure and reconstruction of all layers is necessary to avoid CSF leakage.

10.6.4 Posterior Petrosal Approach

Posterior petrosal approach gives extended view on posterior fossa, compared with anterior transpetrosal approach.[28] Although many variations of this approach have been described in the literature, all are modifications of the conventional mastoidectomy. It binds temporal craniotomy, presigmoid bone drilling, and a small lateral retrosigmoid craniotomy. The retraction of temporal lobe is minimal. The amount of petrous drilling is determined by hearing functions; in the patients with preserved hearing, retrolabyrinthine approach is preferred while the translabyrinthine is performed if hearing function is already lost. The transcochlear approach requires resection of cochlea and exposure of the facial nerve with occlusion of the auditory canal, so it can be performed in rare cases without functional hearing and with irreversible facial palsy because of high risk of facial nerve injury. The mobilization of sigmoid sinus is crucial so it should be widely exposed to the jugular bulb and anatomic variations, such as dominant or single sigmoid sinus on the side of operation, disconnection of transverse sinus with torcular, and abnormal vein of Labbe anatomy might complicate the approach.

The patient's position is similar to that in the anterior petrosal approach. Zygoma is cut, a temporal craniotomy and retrosigmoid craniectomy are performed with burr holes placed on both sides of transverse sinus. Mastoid bone is drilled and the air cells are removed to expose the presigmoid dura, with sigmoid sinus and bony labyrinth should be left intact. The dura is opened along the base of the temporal lobe and curves down in the presigmoid space. A gentle traction between temporal lobe and cerebellum allows the section of the superior petrosal sinus. Care should be taken to avoid injury to the vein of Labbe. Finally, the incision of the tentorium is performed into the incisura at a point posterior to entrance of the trochlear nerve. This approach connects middle and posterior cranial fossa and gives the opportunity to resect petroclival meningiomas with significant mass in both supra- and infratentorial compartments in single surgery. After tumor resection, the dura is closed with sutures, autologous or synthetic graft and fibrin glue. Open mastoid air cell and the middle ear cavity are closed by fat graft, muscle, and fibrin glue.

Combined transpetrosal approach is a synthesis of anterior and posterior petrosal approaches and gives opportunity to take advantages of each individual approach.

In the era of modern surgery, attempts have been made toward minimally invasive exposures so that these techniques for petroclival meningiomas removal are developing. Combined subtemporal and retrosigmoid keyhole approach[35] and endoscopic or endoscopically assisted approaches[36] have been satisfactorily introduced in the clinical practice.

10.7 Complications

After introduction of modern technology and improvement of neurosurgical technique and intraoperative monitoring during the last decades, the outcomes of surgically treated petroclival meningiomas have remarkably improved, along with reduction of mortality and morbidity rates.

In recent series, surgical mortality dropped below 5%[3] and it is mostly likely to occur after brainstem manipulation, with injury of perforating blood vessels, leading to edema and ischemia.[37] Severe swallowing and breathing disorders may also be caused by lesion of lower cranial nerve group. It is of great importance to avoid extensive "radical" tumor removal in this region, and surgeon has to respect the cleavage plane made of the thick arachnoid layer over brainstem and neurovascular structures which should be left in place. Temporal lobe and cerebellar hemisphere swelling are caused by prolonged and indelicate retraction. Transpetrous approaches minimize brain manipulation and the space is gained with bone drilling rather than brain retraction. In standard transcranial approaches, extra space can be gained with external lumbar drainage. Special care should be taken to preserve venous channels, in particular the vein of Labbe; on the other hand, veins in lateral and superior surface of cerebellum can be sacrificed without complications.

Fatal complications may be associated with ligation of the sigmoid sinus, when the patency of the opposite sigmoid sinus and normal flow through the torcular herophili is not assured.[2]

Cranial nerves from III to XII are at risk during petroclival meningioma resection.[10] Surgeon should keep in mind that nerves are displaced or encased by tumor, and careful preoperative MRI analyzing is necessary to assume their localization. Oculomotor nerve is rarely involved and injured. Tentorial splitting may cause trochlear nerve injury, because of its fragility.

Trigeminal nerve paralysis results in painful anesthesia, trigeminal neuralgia or corneal anesthesia, and subsequent keratitis.

From the retrosigmoid approach, facial nerve can be visualized at the beginning of the resection, so it should not be a problem to preserve it, and although some transitory palsy can occur due to surgical manipulation, but with very good recovery. The risk of facial injury is unacceptably high in transcochlear approach, so it is rarely used.

In patients with normal hearing, the VIII cranial nerve, the inner ear and their blood supply should be preserved, and pyramid drilling is limited to retrolabyrinthine approach.

CSF leakage is a well-known complication of skull base approaches and can be avoided with appropriate closure. The incidence of meningitis is about 20% in patients with CSF leak, so in our opinion, antibiotic therapy should be administered prophylactically. Head elevation, spinal taps, or continuous spinal drainage are useful to stop the leakage. In case of persistence of CSF leak, hydrocephalus should be evaluated as underlying factor and properly treated with shunting.

10.8 Early and Long-term Postoperative Management

Treatment of complex lesions, such as petroclival meningiomas, requires close collaboration between neurosurgeon and anesthesiologists, along with a well-equipped intensive care unit. Despite modern technology and experienced surgical team, early postoperative course of these patients might be troublesome. Authors advice for patient awakening immediately after operation, when possible. If external lumbar drainage has been placed, it can be left in place for few days to help CSF diversion. In case of patients who underwent tumor removal via an approach that required them to be in a sitting position, hyperoxic therapy against pneumochephalus is advised.

Prolonged orotracheal intubation and/or in cases with postoperative swallowing disturbances, tracheostomy and percutaneous endoscopic gastrostomy are mandatory in order to avoid complications as pneumonia, aspiration, and malnutrition.

Early mobilization can prevent pulmonary complications, deep venous thrombosis, and normalize CSF flow.

Long-term postoperative management is tailored individually, based on general neuro-oncological principles.[38] It is advisable to perform a baseline MRI within 48 hours or after 3 months from operation in order to assess the EOR. Thereafter, we propose annual MRI controls until 5 years post treatment, then every 2 years for patients without evidence of residual tumor.

In cases with small volume residual tumor, it can be observed or treated with stereotaxic radiosurgery with a 6-month MRI follow-up. A series of 35 retrospective studies showed a 5-year progression-free survival of 86 to 100% after primary stereotactic radiosurgery.[39]

For grade II meningiomas that are rarely found in this localization, 6-month follow-up is recommended after complete resection and fractioned or stereotaxic irradiation if there is evidence of residual tumor, with similar follow-up protocol.

After progression, reoperation should be considered, but with lower chances for radical resection because of adhesions and scars from previous operations.

10.9 Conclusion

Petroclival meningiomas are one of the most challenging pathology because of the peculiar localization; the most important aspect for successful treatment of these lesions does not only concern the choice of the approach, rather the fact that they should be treated by an experienced neurosurgeon, who knows how to foresee and avoid the complications. The treatment planning should be individualized according to tumor and patient characteristics; radical resection should be the goal, but never in spite of a neurological damage. Stereotaxic radiosurgery is an effective and safe tool that gives good control of small residual tumor. We advocate retrosigmoid approach, sole or in combination with frontotemporal craniotomy for tumors with extensive supratentorial extension, as this is the simplest and effective surgical strategy. Follow-up should be carried out according to neuro-oncological principles.[33]

References

[1] Castellano F, Ruggiero G. Meningiomas of the posterior fossa. Acta Radiol Suppl. 1953; 104:1–177

[2] Al-Mefty O. Operative atlas of meningiomas. Philadelphia, PA: Lippincott-Raven; 1998

[3] Almefty R, Dunn IF, Pravdenkova S, Abolfotoh M, Al-Mefty O. True petroclival meningiomas: results of surgical management. J Neurosurg. 2014; 120(1):40–51

[4] Mayberg MR, Symon L. Meningiomas of the clivus and apical petrous bone. Report of 35 cases. J Neurosurg. 1986; 65(2):160–167

[5] Kshettry VR, Lee JH, Ammirati M. The Dorello canal: historical development, controversies in microsurgical anatomy, and clinical implications. Neurosurg Focus. 2013; 34(3):E4

[6] Yoshino M, Abhinav K, Yeh FC, et al. Visualization of cranial nerves using high-definition fiber tractography. Neurosurgery. 2016; 79(1):146–165

[7] Yang K, Ikawa F, Onishi S, et al. Preoperative simulation of the running course of the abducens nerve in a large petroclival meningioma: a case report and literature review. Neurosurg Rev. 2017; 40(2):339–343

[8] Pirayesh A, Petrakakis I, Raab P, Polemikos M, Krauss JK, Nakamura M. Petroclival meningiomas: magnetic resonance imaging factors predict tumor resectability and clinical outcome. Clin Neurol Neurosurg. 2016; 147:90–97

[9] Van Havenbergh T, Carvalho G, Tatagiba M, Plets C, Samii M. Natural history of petroclival meningiomas. Neurosurgery. 2003; 52(1):55–62, discussion 62–64

[10] Landriel F, Black P. Meningiomas. In: Ellenbogen RG, Abdulrauf SI, Sekhar LN, ed. Principles of Neurological Surgery. Philadelphia, PA: Elsevier Saunders; 2012

[11] Ramina R, Fernandes YB, Neto CM, da Silva Jr LFM. Petroclival meningiomas: diagnosis, treatment, and results. In: Ramina R, de Aguiar PHP, Tatagiba M, ed. Samii's Essential in Neurosurgery. Berlin: Springer; 2008

[12] Hunter JB, Yawn RJ, Wang R, et al. The natural history of petroclival meningiomas: a volumetric study. Otol Neurotol. 2017; 38(1):123–128

[13] Kaku S, Miyahara K, Fujitsu K, et al. Drainage pathway of the superior petrosal vein evaluated by CT venography in petroclival meningioma surgery. J Neurol Surg B Skull Base. 2012; 73(5):316–320

[14] Zhao X, Yu RT, Li JS, Xu K, Li X. Clinical value of multi-slice 3-dimensional computed tomographic angiography in the preoperative assessment of meningioma. Exp Ther Med. 2013; 6(2):475–478

[15] Coppens J, Couldwell W. Clival and petroclival meningiomas. In: DeMonte F, McDermott MW, Al-Mefty O, eds. Al-Mefty's Meningiomas. New York, NY: Thieme; 2011:270–282

[16] Park CK, Jung HW, Kim JE, Paek SH, Kim DG. The selection of the optimal therapeutic strategy for petroclival meningiomas. Surg Neurol. 2006; 66(2):160–165, discussion 165–166

[17] Yasargil MG, Mortara RW, Curcic M. Meningiomas of basal posterior cranial fossa. Vienna, Austria: Springer; 1980

[18] Kim JW, Kim DG, Se YB, et al. Gamma Knife radiosurgery for petroclival meningioma: Long-term outcome and failure pattern. Stereotact Funct Neurosurg. 2017; 95(4):209–215

[19] Hirohata M, Abe T, Morimitsu H, Fujimura N, Shigemori M, Norbash AM. Preoperative selective internal carotid artery dural branch embolisation for petroclival meningiomas. Neuroradiology. 2003; 45(9):656–660

[20] Shah A, Choudhri O, Jung H, Li G. Preoperative endovascular embolization of meningiomas: update on therapeutic options. Neurosurg Focus. 2015; 38(3):E7

[21] Kusaka N, Tamiya T, Sugiu K, et al. Combined use of TruFill DCS detachable coil system and Guglielmi detachable coil for embolization of meningioma fed by branches of the cavernous internal carotid artery. Neurol Med Chir (Tokyo). 2007; 47(1):29–31

[22] Cushing H. Meningiomas: their classification, regional behaviour, life history, and surgical end results. New York, NY: Hafner Pub. Co.; 1962

[23] Krenkel, et al. Handbuch der Neurochirurgie. 1968

[24] Starke RM, Nguyen JH, Rainey J, et al. Gamma Knife surgery of meningiomas located in the posterior fossa: factors predictive of outcome and remission. J Neurosurg. 2011; 114(5):1399–1409

[25] Starke RM, Przybylowski CJ, Sugoto M, et al. Gamma Knife radiosurgery of large skull base meningiomas. J Neurosurg. 2015; 122(2):363–372

[26] Xu F, Karampelas I, Megerian CA, Selman WR, Bambakidis NC. Petroclival meningiomas: an update on surgical approaches, decision making, and treatment results. Neurosurg Focus. 2013; 35(6):E11

[27] Abdel Aziz KM, Sanan A, van Loveren HR, Tew JM, Jr, Keller JT, Pensak ML. Petroclival meningiomas: predictive parameters for transpetrosal approaches. Neurosurgery. 2000; 47(1):139–150, discussion 150–152

[28] Erkmen K, Pravdenkova S, Al-Mefty O. Surgical management of petroclival meningiomas: factors determining the choice of approach. Neurosurg Focus. 2005; 19(2):E7

[29] Terasaka S, Asaoka K, Kobayashi H, Yamaguchi S, Sawamura Y. [Natural history and surgical results of petroclival meningiomas]. No Shinkei Geka. 2010; 38(9):817–824

[30] Samii M, Gerganov V, Giordano M, Samii A. Two step approach for surgical removal of petroclival meningiomas with large supratentorial extension. Neurosurg Rev. 2010; 34(2):173–179

[31] Samii M, Tatagiba M, Carvalho GA. Retrosigmoid intradural suprameatal approach to Meckel's cave and the middle fossa: surgical technique and outcome. J Neurosurg. 2000; 92(2):235–241

[32] Watanabe T, Katayama Y, Fukushima T, Kawamata T. Lateral supracerebellar transtentorial approach for petroclival meningiomas: operative technique and outcome. J Neurosurg. 2011; 115(1):49–54

[33] Little KM, Friedman AH, Sampson JH, Wanibuchi M, Fukushima T. Surgical management of petroclival meningiomas: defining resection goals based on risk of neurological morbidity and tumor recurrence rates in 137 patients. Neurosurgery. 2005; 56(3):546–559, discussion 546–559

[34] Ichimura S, Kawase T, Onozuka S, Yoshida K, Ohira T. Four subtypes of petroclival meningiomas: differences in symptoms and operative findings using the anterior transpetrosal approach. Acta Neurochir (Wien). 2008; 150(7):637–645

[35] Zhu W, Mao Y, Zhou LF, Zhang R, Chen L. Combined subtemporal and retrosigmoid keyhole approach for extensive petroclival meningiomas surgery: report of experience with 7 cases. Minim Invasive Neurosurg. 2008; 51(2):95–99

[36] Beer-Furlan A, Abi-Hachem R, Jamshidi AO, Carrau RL, Prevedello DM. Endoscopic trans-sphenoidal surgery for petroclival and clival meningiomas. J Neurosurg Sci. 2016; 60(4):495–502

[37] Pintea B, Kandenwein JA, Lorenzen H, Blume C, Daher F, Kristof RA. Differences in clinical presentation, intraoperative findings and outcome between petroclival and lateral posterior pyramid meningioma. Clin Neurol Neurosurg. 2016; 141:122–128

[38] Goldbrunner R, Minniti G, Preusser M, et al. EANO guidelines for the diagnosis and treatment of meningiomas. Lancet Oncol. 2016; 17(9):e383–e391

[39] Rogers L, Barani I, Chamberlain M, et al. Meningiomas: knowledge base, treatment outcomes, and uncertainties. A RANO review. J Neurosurg. 2015; 122(1):4–23

11 Olfactory Groove Meningiomas

Daniel M. Prevedello, Alaa S. Montaser, Matias Gómez G., Bradley A. Otto, Ricardo L. Carrau

Abstract

Olfactory groove meningiomas (OGMs) are unique tumors with special characteristics differentiating them from other brain lesions, including clinical presentation, neurological findings, surgery planning, outcomes, and complications related to their treatment.

Generally, the definitive treatment of OGMs, like all other anterior skull base meningiomas, is surgical resection. Planning the surgical strategy to attack these tumors while achieving the optimum outcome with minimal complications is challenging, especially when attempting to preserve olfaction. Different approaches have been described for OGMs resection including: (i) subfrontal access, either through unilateral/bilateral frontal craniotomy or transbasal approach, (ii) anterolateral access through frontolateral approach (combination of pterional and subfrontal), (iii) lateral access through a pterional approach, and (iv) ventral access through endoscopic endonasal approach (EEA). Each of these approaches has potential advantages and drawbacks.

During preoperative planning of the surgical strategy, the surgical team must determine the main goals of surgery keeping in mind both the tumor and patient characteristics. Additionally, surgical experience, a multidisciplinary approach, adequate instruments and equipment, appropriate patient selection, and thorough preoperative planning are fundamental for achieving best results.

With the current microsurgical techniques, the overall rate of complications related to resection of OGMs is decreased. Long-term follow-up following surgical resection of OGMs is crucial to detect recurrence. The most significant factor influencing the rate of early and late recurrence is the extent of initial surgical resection of the tumor. Therefore, Simpson grade I resection should always remain the utmost goal of surgery for OGMs.

In practice, the authors favor the utilization of unilateral frontolateral approaches for resection of large OGMs with normal olfaction. EEAs are utilized primarily for resection of small and large OGM for patients who have lost sense of smell. Small eyebrow incisions with supraorbital subfrontal approaches are reserved for small OGM for patients with normal sense of smell. For giant OGM, a stage 1 endonasal approach should be utilized followed by a stage 2 frontolateral craniotomy for complete resection of the tumor.

Keywords: olfactory groove meningioma, anterior skull base meningioma, surgical approaches, endoscopic endonasal approach, endoscopic skull base surgery, outcomes, complications, recurrence

11.1 Introduction

Meningiomas are benign slow-growing tumors that account for approximately 20% of primary intracranial tumors, however, OGMs account for 8 to 13% of intracranial meningiomas. The first OGM was described in Cruveilhier's Traite d'Anatomie in 1835, while the first successful resection of an OGM was performed in 1885 by Francesco Durante.[1,2,3,4]

OGMs are unique tumors with special characteristics differentiating them from other brain lesions, including clinical presentation, neurological findings, surgery planning, outcomes, and complications.[1] OGMs are generally classified according to their size (maximum diameter) into small (< 2 cm), medium (2–4 cm), large (4–6 cm), and giant (> 6 cm). Giant OGMs are especially problematic and represent a surgical challenge owing to the possible postoperative morbidity and parenchymal damage.[5]

11.2 Preoperative Definition of the Lesion Features

11.2.1 Anatomical Consideration

The understanding of growth pattern and relationship with the surrounding critical neurovascular structures is very crucial for a successful surgical resection of OGMs. OGMs arise in the midline from the meningothelial cap cells at the region of the cribriform plate and the frontosphenoid suture and may extend from the crista galli to the planum sphenoidale, involving the whole anterior skull base. Although OGMs originate in the midline, they often have a tendency to extend unilaterally.[1,3,6,7]

The site of origin may be uncertain when they are large and extend back to the sella turcica, therefore, posteriorly extending OGMs and tuberculum sellae meningiomas pose some similarities. They can be differentiated mainly by the location of the optic apparatus in relationship to the tumor. As OGMs grow, they displace the chiasm and optic nerves downward and posteriorly. On the contrary, because tuberculum sellae meningiomas occupy a subchiasmal position, they tend to elevate the chiasm and pushes the optic nerve superolaterally.[1,7,8]

In large and giant OGMs, the olfactory tracts are likely invaded and/or destroyed on both sides, thus, preservation of olfaction may be impossible. However, in smaller lesions, the olfactory tracts are laterally displaced over the orbital roofs and there is often a good chance to preserve both or at least one of the olfactory tracts.[7,8] However, anatomical preservation of olfactory nerves doesn't imply functional preservation of olfaction. Loss of smell after anatomic preservation of the olfactory tracts could be related to direct manipulation or ischemia.

OGMs usually produce hyperostosis of the anterior skull base (28.3–62% of cases) that is thought to be due to microinvasion by the tumor rather than an inflammatory reaction to it, therefore, incomplete resection of unrecognized bony invasion is associated with high rates of tumor recurrence. However, these neoplasms may also erode the skull base bone and extend into the nasal cavity, paranasal sinuses, and orbits.[1,2,9,10]

OGMs, like all other anterior skull base meningiomas, are usually highly vascular and their resection may be complicated with significant bleeding. The vascularity of OGMs is derived from pial, dural, transosseous supply. Although the anterior and posterior ethmoidal arteries constitute the main arterial supply for OGMs, these tumors can also receive collaterals from several arteries such as anterior branches of the middle meningeal artery, meningeal branches of the ophthalmic artery and internal carotid artery (ICA), small branches of the anterior communicating artery (ACoA), and the distal maxillary artery. Encasement of critical vascular structures is not uncommon. The most common artery to be encased is the A2 segment of anterior cerebral artery (ACA) and its smaller branches such as the frontopolar or medial orbitofrontal artery, and ACoA.[1,8,11,12,13]

11.2.2 Clinical Presentation and Workup

Due to the slow growth nature of OGMs and their location, the clinical diagnosis is usually delayed. Thus, most of OGMs are diagnosed when they have attained larger size. In some series, 50 to 60% of the OGMs were larger than 6 cm in diameter at the time of surgery.[1,8]

It is important from clinical and surgical perspectives to differentiate OGMs from planum sphenoidale and tuberculum sellae meningiomas. Typically, the latter presents at an early stage (smaller size) with visual deficits, while OGMs are usually clinically silent in the early stage and visual deterioration is often a late presentation. Additionally, OGMs frequently extend into the paranasal sinuses and the nasal cavity, which is a rare feature of meningiomas arising at the planum sphenoidale or tuberculum sellae.[4]

The most frequently encountered symptoms are frontal lobe manifestations (such as personality changes, psychiatric symptoms, concentration difficulties, and apathy), headache, alteration of olfaction (hypo- or anosmia, often noted in retrospect by many patients), and finally visual disturbance (visual acuity and/or field changes). Typically, onset of these symptoms is very gradual that they are underestimated or may not be noted early in their course.[1,3,13,14] Vision loss is usually only noted when these tumors achieve a very large size (large and giants).

Other common presenting symptoms are seizures, mental status changes, and incontinence. Although originally described in OGMs, Foster-Kennedy syndrome (unilateral optic atrophy with contralateral papilledema) occurs only in small number of cases.[7,8,15]

In general, the diagnosis is mainly made based on radiographic imaging. MRI is the imaging modality of choice for all meningiomas, including OGMs. CT is particularly important for assessment of skull base bony anatomy, including areas of hyperostosis and erosions that helps in diagnosis and preoperative planning of surgical strategy as well.

The appearance of OGMs in MRI and CT is similar to meningiomas located elsewhere. On MRI, OGMs are typically iso- to hypointense on T1-weighted imaging (T1WI) and iso- to hyperintense on T2-weighted imaging (T2WI). They typically show avid homogeneous gadolinium enhancement. Most meningiomas show the characteristic "dural tail", a marginal dural thickening that tapers peripherally. MRI and magnetic resonance angiography (MRA) are helpful in defining the relationship of the tumor to the surrounding vascular structures such as ACA and ACoA. These are critical for surgical planning as vascular encasement may require a specific strategy.

On CT, OGMs appear as well-defined extra-axial lesions abutting the dura and displacing the normal brain. They are iso- to hyperdense on noncontrasted CT, with intense homogenous enhancement after contrast administration. OGMs are smooth in contour, however, multilobulated lesions are not uncommon. Calcification is another common finding. Cyst formation, atypical pattern of necrosis, or hemorrhage can be found in approximately 15% of cases.[1,8,14]

A thorough preoperative evaluation of the radiographic imaging is crucial for planning the surgical strategy, as it provides important information about the tumor such as its size and extent, presence of pial invasion, vascular encasement, hyperostosis, extent of frontal lobes edema, and hemodynamic and metabolic characteristics of the tumor.[16,17]

11.3 Surgical Indications

As a general rule, the definitive treatment of meningiomas, including OGMs, is surgical resection. However, observation may be an option in patients with small OGMs that are accidentally discovered, and in elderly patients with asymptomatic lesions or who cannot withstand the surgical intervention due to their comorbidities.[8] Radiation therapy is usually reserved for cases with recurrent and/or high grade (atypical or anaplastic) lesions.[2,18]

11.3.1 Planning the Surgical Strategy

Planning the surgical strategy to attack these tumors while achieving the optimum outcome with minimal complications is challenging, especially when attempting to preserve the olfaction.[19] Since the old report of first successful surgery of an OGM performed by Durante via a left frontal craniotomy in 1885, skull base surgeons have been trying to determine a surgical approach that allows safe and complete resection of OGM. However, this is still a matter of controversy.[1,4,13,15]

Goals of Surgery

Indeed, a total gross resection of the tumor, its dural attachment, and the involved bone (Simpson grade I resection) is the utmost goal of surgical intervention for meningiomas. This goal applies also to OGMs and can be achieved in most cases, despite the large size of the tumor, since OGMs often have an arachnoid membrane separating the tumor from practically all critical neurovascular structures, thus facilitating a complete resection.[1,8] Nevertheless, total gross resection may not be a possibility in many cases, especially if there is vascular encasement of the ACA, ACoA, and/or ICA. Nonetheless, the extent of resection varies widely depending on the patient and tumor characteristics.

Other fundamental goals of surgical intervention are the preservation of neurological function, avoidance of new neurological morbidities, avoidance of approach-related complications, and achieving good cosmetic outcome.

Having said that, the surgical team must determine the goal of surgery during preoperative planning, taking into consideration not only the tumor characteristics, such as the tumor size, extension in different planes, pial invasion, and vascular encasement, but also the patient characteristics such as the patient's age, comorbidities, clinical manifestations, and functional outcomes as such as olfaction presence and preservation.[20,21]

Selecting the Surgical Approach

While considering the most suitable approach for each patient, it is important to consider the approach that:
- Provides a more direct and early access to the nourishing vessels of the tumor. The main advantage of early attacking the blood supply of the tumor is reduction of intraoperative bleeding by transforming a highly-vascularized tumor into an avascular mass, thus, shortening the operative time and reducing the surgical morbidity.[22]
- Achieves a wide exposure enough to allow gross total resection of the tumor, affected bone, and dura, leading to better outcomes and less possibilities of recurrence. It should provide convenient exposure of the anterior skull base permitting better reconstruction as well.
- Minimizes brain retraction and manipulation of critical neurovascular structures, thus, decreasing the surgical morbidities.

It is crucial to consider whether there is pial invasion and/or vascular encasement. It is also important to keep in mind that the frontal lobes (especially when there is pial invasion, massive edema, and/or venous engorgement) and the optic apparatus (especially when there is chronic compression and secondary ischemia), are more vulnerable in certain situations that even minimal manipulations can cause a functional compromise.[23] Furthermore, the surgical team experienced and familiar with different approaches plays a key role in selecting the most suitable approach for each case.

11.3.2 Preoperative Embolization

Embolization techniques are performed in some centers prior to the surgery to promote devascularization, with or without bilateral ligation of anterior and posterior ethmoidal arteries.[11] However, the rule of preoperative embolization for OGMs is controversial.[12] In our opinion, preoperative embolization is not indicated in most cases as the blood supply is often directly encountered and disconnected earlier in the case.

While it is true that preoperative embolization of the ethmoidal arteries reduces intraoperative blood loss, surgery time, and the need for blood transfusion, it has some drawbacks. One of the major drawbacks is that it carries a very high risk of blindness due to the risk of retrograde migration of particles through the multiple anastomoses between the external and internal carotid arteries in this territory with high possibility of occlusion of the ophthalmic artery. Another disadvantage is the technical difficulty in gaining access to the ethmoidal arteries, which is sometimes not possible, because of the anatomical distortion caused by the tumor.[12]

11.4 Surgical Techniques

Different approaches have been described to achieve the best outcome with the least complications possible for OGM resection. These include a subfrontal access, either through unilateral/bilateral frontal craniotomy or transbasal approach, an anterolateral access through frontolateral approach, a lateral access through pterional approach, and a ventral access through EEA. A brief description of the potential advantages and disadvantages of each approach follows.

11.4.1 Subfrontal Approach with Unilateral or Bilateral Frontal Craniotomy

The subfrontal approach through unilateral or bilateral frontal craniotomy has been advocated for OGM by many authors and is one of the most commonly used approaches for OGMs. This approach is more suitable for large and giant OGMs as it provides a short surgical corridor with a broad exposure of the tumor and its basal dural attachment. It provides a good view for closure and reconstruction of the skull base with a pericranial flap. It allows also for drilling the hyperostotic anterior skull base bone and decompressing the optic nerves by deroofing of the optic canals if necessary.[14,19]

In many cases, especially in large and giant high-riding OGMs, orbital rim osteotomy can be added to unilateral or bilateral subfrontal approaches to gain extra basal access and minimize brain retraction. However, this is more time consuming and may increase the risk of complications, therefore, it should be only performed in selected cases.[7,13,24]

In small lesions, early devascularization of the tumor at the basal dural attachment can be achieved easily without significant brain retraction. However, in case of large and giant OGMs, which is more common, devascularization is very difficult unless a sizeable internal debulking of the tumor is achieved first, otherwise, the brain cannot be retracted or relaxed, especially when there is a considerable tumor-induced frontal lobe edema.[11]

Overexposure and significant retraction of the frontal lobes is one of the main drawbacks of this approach increasing the risk of frontal lobe contusions and edema with resultant cognitive and emotional impairment. Excessive brain retraction is mainly due to the increased intracranial pressure (ICP) and the difficulty of releasing cerebrospinal fluid (CSF) early in the procedure. Additionally, there is increased risk of injury to the critical surrounding neurovascular structures such as the optic apparatus, ICA, ACA, and ACoA, because they are only visualized late during tumor dissection. Other disadvantages include ligation of the superior sagittal sinus and the inevitable opening of frontal sinus with the risk of CSF leak and meningitis.[1,6,19,21,25]

Compared to bifrontal craniotomy, a unilateral frontal craniotomy provides the advantage of avoiding contralateral frontal lobe retraction and superior sagittal sinus violation. It is more suitable for tumors with predominant unilateral extension. In addition to difficulty of decreasing the ICP by releasing CSF prior to tumor dissection, and late visualization of critical neurovascular structures, unilateral frontal craniotomy has the disadvantage of smaller working window and narrower surgical corridor.[1,19]

11.4.2 Transbasal Approach

This approach is more suitable for tumors extending caudally into the paranasal sinuses and/or the orbits as it provides excellent access to the paranasal sinuses (frontal, ethmoidal, and sphenoidal) and the orbits as well.

Ligation of the anterior ethmoidal arteries can be achieved early during the procedure, which contributes to devascularization of the tumor to great extent. The

transbasal approach offers a lower basal access with less brain retraction, thus permitting early devascularization of the tumor at its basal dural attachment as well, and providing an excellent exposure of the anterior skull base for drilling the infiltrated bone and for skull base repair with pericranial flap.[2,6,11]

The disadvantages of this approach include prolonged surgical time, risk of long-term cosmetic defects due to removal of fronto-orbital bars, and higher CSF leak rates due to the wide exposure of the cranial base.[2,6,26] Furthermore, it also allows the visualization of the optic nerves only later in the case, and it could potentially put them in risk for damage.

11.4.3 Pterional Approach

The pterional approach have been advocated only for resection of small and medium size OGMs with pure intracranial extension and without skull base involvement, however, some authors suggest its use even for giant OGMs.[5] In cases of large and giant high-riding OGMs, orbital rim osteotomy can be added to gain extra basal access and minimize brain retraction.[24]

Compared to the subfrontal approach, the pterional approach provides several advantages including lower rates of postoperative CSF leak due to preservation of the frontal sinus, less brain retraction due to brain relaxation following CSF release by opening the basal cisterns prior to tumor manipulation, preservation of venous drainage of the frontal lobes leading to less congestion and edema, early identification and protection of the neurovascular structures, and potential sparing of the olfaction on the contralateral side.[5]

One of the major drawbacks of utilizing the pterional approach in large and giant OGMs is that there may be blind areas on the contralateral side especially when the tumor has a significant superior extension requiring more retraction of the brain and/or falx to achieve a good control and resection, or in cases in which the planes of the orbital roofs and the ethmoid are different along the vertical axis.[1,5,6]

11.4.4 Frontolateral Approach

This approach combines the advantage of subfrontal and pterional approaches. It provides a wide angle of exposure to the tumor with the possibility of attacking the basal dural blood supply of the tumor early in the procedure (as in subfrontal approach), and it allows for early identification of the optic nerve and the ICA, avoidance of ligation of the superior sagittal sinus, and early brain relaxation by opening the basal cisterns and releasing CSF (as in pterional approach).[24,27] Olfaction could be preserved by anatomic preservation of the contralateral olfactory nerve.

The disadvantages of this approach include longer operative time, and the higher possibility of CSF leak due to opening of the frontal sinus. Total gross resection may be limited through frontolateral approach in cases of large and giant OGMs encasing the ACA.[27] Another downside of this approach is related to brain herniation through the craniotomy in very large and giant OGM with substantial brain edema. Contralateral hyperostosis can be difficult to drill and contralateral reconstruction can be challenging.

11.4.5 Supraorbital Keyhole Approach

The supraorbital keyhole craniotomy is a minimally invasive approach that provides access to a wide range of disease processes along the anterior skull base, including OGMs. Typically, an eyebrow incision is often used and the bone flap required is 3 × 2 cm.

This approach allows direct visualization of the lesion and the surrounding critical neurovascular structures. Compared to the subfrontal and pterional approaches, the supraorbital key hole approach necessitates much less brain retraction and avoids the need of splitting the Sylvian fissure. It offers the advantages of a minimally invasive surgery such as less operative time and improved postoperative pain. It also provides an excellent cosmetic outcome.

Additionally, the application of endoscopy through this approach allows for enhanced illumination and improved visualization, especially of hidden areas around the anatomic corners of the surgical field that were not adequately visualized by the microscope.

The main drawbacks of the supraorbital keyhole approach are the limited maneuverability of instruments, the possibility of violating the frontal sinus during performing the craniotomy (especially if the frontal sinus is large and well-pneumatized), and the risk of damage to the frontotemporal branch of the facial nerve. It is very difficult to expose the basal dural attachment of the tumor at the midline if the ethmoid and the orbital roofs lies in different planes which should be kept in mind while preoperatively planning the surgical strategy.[26,28] The visualization of the olfactory groove can be compensated by the utilization of endoscopes, but it definitely increases the complexity of these cases.

11.4.6 Endoscopic Endonasal Approach

During the last two decades the extended EEAs to the ventral skull base have been advanced to great extent. Nowadays, EEA is considered one of the safe alternatives on the armamentarium of surgery to anterior skull base lesions, including OGMs.

EEA is an excellent option when the tumor is extending into the paranasal sinuses and/or the orbits. EEA is also more suitable in recurrent OGMs with paranasal sinuses extension especially when the first surgery was done through transcranial approach where the cribriform plate was not adequately drilled out and the pericranial flap has been used for previous skull base reconstruction.

It is to be emphasized that when approaching OGMs via EEA, the same microneurosurgical techniques and principles are applied during the procedure, such as internal debulking followed by capsule mobilization, extracapsular dissection of neurovascular structures, focal coagulation, and capsule removal.[21,23]

In case of OGM, the main advantage of EEA is that it provides a wide ventral corridor with the most direct access to the anterior skull base, specifically the cribriform plate and planum sphenoidale, allowing early vascular control of the anterior and posterior ethmoidal arteries. Once the ethmoidal arteries are coagulated and cut, the tumor is significantly devascularized.[23] Additionally, EEA allows for better drilling of the hyperostotic bone and complete resection of the dural attachment of the lesion, which are integral parts of the approach, leading to more complete (Simpson grade I) resection and lower rates of tumor recurrence. Furthermore, complete decompression of chronically compressed optic nerves without manipulating them and without damaging the perforating vessels to the chiasm are feasible through EEA leading to improved visual outcomes[1,11,28,29].

Other advantages of EEA include better visualization with near field magnification, avoidance of brain retraction, and minimal manipulation of the critical neurovascular structures, Therefore, EEA is associated with less morbidities and improved outcomes. Being minimally invasive surgery, EEA also carries the advantages of shorter hospital stay, less postoperative pain, and better cosmosis.[2]

The main drawback of EEA is the higher risk of postoperative CSF leak,[1,29] however, with the recent innovations in techniques used for skull base repair, including the vascularized nasoseptal flaps, the postoperative CSF leak rates have markedly decreased in experienced centers at rates between 5 and 10%.[28,30]

In our opinion, the major limitations of EEA for OGMs include the inevitable risk of anosmia, especially in patients with some preoperative preserved olfaction, the risk of cerebrovascular accidents and/or hemorrhage in case of vascular encasement, and limited resection in cases of lateral extension of the lesion and/or its basal dural attachment beyond the medial orbital walls bilaterally.

Nevertheless, surgical experience, a multidisciplinary approach, adequate instruments and equipment, appropriate patient selection, and thorough preoperative planning are mandatory for achieving best results with these approaches.

11.4.7 Algorithm for Surgical Management of Olfactory Groove Meningiomas (Endoscopic Endonasal Approaches vs. Craniotomy vs. Two-stages Strategy)

Since there is no consensus regarding the best approach to resect OGMs, the authors have developed an algorithm for surgical management of OGMs (▶ Fig. 11.1). This algorithm is based on thorough preoperative evaluation of the tumor and patient characteristics as mentioned before (see subsection *Planning the surgical strategy*).

In patients with small and medium size OGMs with caudal extension into the paranasal sinuses with no significant lateral extension of the tumor and/or its dural attachment beyond the orbital walls, no vascular encasement, no pial invasion, and if the patient is ano- or hyposmic, opt for EEA.

Craniotomy is chosen mainly for patients that have preserved olfaction and there seems to be a possibility for preservation. Eyebrow incision/supraorbital approach is recommended for small and medium sized lesions and frontolateral or pterional approaches with or without orbital rim removal for larger lesions. Ideally the authors come from the side that presents less edema and larger component of the tumor.

In patients with giant tumors and anosmia, a two-stage approach is planned. Since total resection is impossible

through EEA due to the lateral extension of the tumor, a second stage is planned through a craniotomy. The craniotomy is then performed after the tumor is devascularized and debulked with correspondent decrease on the amount of brain edema. The EEA is performed initially and all the ethmoidal arteries are coagulated and cut. The hyperostotic bone is completely drilled out and the tumor is debulked internally. It is important not to try to dissect the tumor from the brain, as it will generate scar in that plane, which will make the second stage more difficult or impossible. The second stage is then planned according to the patient's symptoms. If the patient was having vision loss and the initial debulking through the EEA was not enough to improve the patient's symptoms, then the second stage should be performed sooner than later (couple of weeks). If the patient improves from the vision loss, at least a 3-month wait has been observed for brain edema improvement in order to allow for less manipulation of the friable brain.

11.5 Illustrative Cases

11.5.1 Case 1

A 60-year-old male presented with headache, nausea, vomiting, weight loss, and difficulty with gait and balance. He also complained of altered taste and smell for the past 2 years. On examination, the patient was found to be anosmic. MRI brain (▶ Fig. 11.2a and b) revealed an OGM measuring 3.3 × 3.2 × 3 cm in the axial, sagittal, and

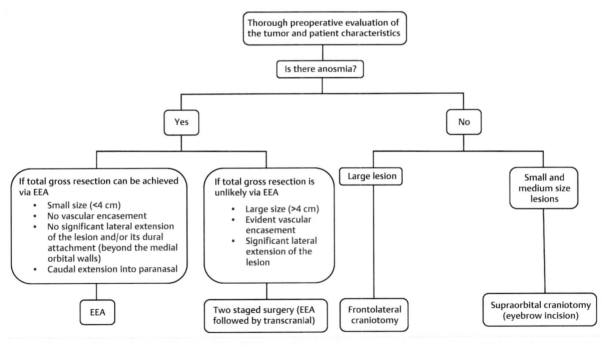

Fig. 11.1 Algorithm for surgical management of OGM

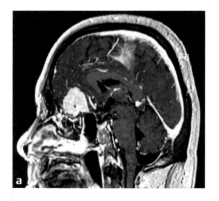

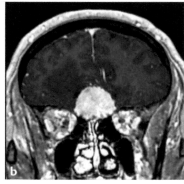

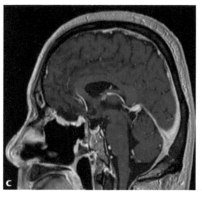

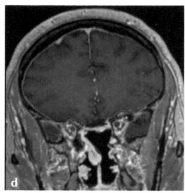

Fig. 11.2 Preoperative brain MRI.
(a) Sagittal and **(b)** coronal T1-weighted imaging (T1WI) with gadolinium contrast demonstrating medium-sized OGM. The tumor extends posteriorly over the planum sphenoidale. At 9 months follow-up, MRI brain **(c)** sagittal and **(d)** coronal T1WI with gadolinium contrast confirms the gross total resection of the tumor and shows no evidence of recurrence. Note the enhanced nasoseptal flap used for the skull base reconstruction.

coronal planes, centered in the midline. The mass was abutting the dura overlying the cribriform plate and fovea ethmoidalis. The tumor extended posteriorly over the planum sphenoidale and displaced branches of the ACA. There were associated mass effect and vasogenic edema within the adjacent frontal lobes.

Given both the clinical and radiographic findings, surgical intervention was indicated. After discussing different alternatives suitable for the surgical approach with the patient, a decision was made to proceed with EEA.

The patient underwent surgery via endoscopic endonasal transcribriform/transplanum approach. Once the whole anterior skull base was exposed from the frontal sinus to the sella, the hyperostotic bone was removed by drilling the cribriform plate and the planum sphoinadale. With the aid of neuronavigation, it was confirmed that the bony opening was enough to expose the entire tumor. The anterior and posterior ethmoidal arteries were coagulated and cut to devascularize the tumor and reduce the bleeding during intracranial dissection. After gross total resection of the tumor and its dural attachment, the anterior skull base was reconstructed using multilayered technique. Duragen was placed as an inlay layer followed by a pedicled nasoseptal flap, then the skull base reconstruction was buttressed with Gelfoam and Nasopore.

There were no intra- or postoperative complications. Histopathological analysis confirmed the diagnosis of meningioma WHO grade I with a Ki-67 labeling index (LI)

of 4%. Before discharging the patient, an MRI was obtained that confirmed gross total resection of the tumor. At 9-months follow-up, the patient was neurologically intact except for olfaction, and brain MRI showed no evidence of recurrence (▶ Fig. 11.2c and d).

11.5.2 Case 2

A 59-year-old male was evaluated in authors' skull base clinic with complaints of headache and visual disturbances more on the right side, in the form of visual field defect. Brain MRI was obtained revealing a large OGM arising from the left olfactory groove and measuring 5.5 × 3.3 × 4.4 cm in the axial, sagittal, and coronal planes. The lesion was predominantly extending to the left side and compressing the chiasm and optic nerves bilaterally (▶ Fig. 11.3a and b). His olfaction was evaluated preoperatively and it was normal (most likely due to no tumor present in the right olfactory groove area).

The patient underwent surgery via left fronto-orbital craniotomy with removal of the left orbital rim. The authors were able to preserve the olfactory nerve and tract contralaterally. There was encasement of the ACA on one side, however, the authors were able to separate the tumor from the vessel. A total gross resection of the tumor was achieved.

The patient tolerated the procedure well and the postoperative period was uneventful. The olfaction, which

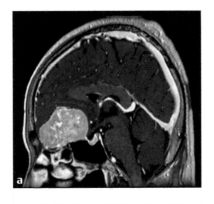
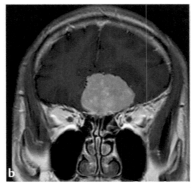
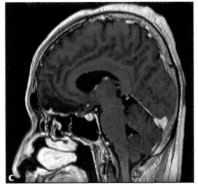
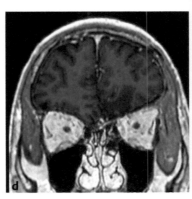

Fig. 11.3 Preoperative brain MRI.
(a) Sagittal and **(b)** coronal T1-weighted imaging (T1WI) with gadolinium contrast showing a large OGM extending from the posterior wall of the frontal sinus all the way to the tuberculum sellae. Note the tumor shows predominant extension to the left side. Follow-up MRI brain **(c)** sagittal and **(d)** coronal T1WI with gadolinium contrast after 30 months demonstrating gross total resection with no evidence of recurrence.

was intact preoperative, was preserved. Histopathological examination demonstrated atypical meningioma WHO grade II with a Ki-67 LI of 10%, and up to 20% focally in smaller fields, away from areas of necrosis. Prior to discharging the patient, brain MRI was obtained that confirmed total resection of the lesion. A decision was made not to perform any radiation and surveillance MRIs were planned. At 30-months follow-up, brain MRI showed no evidence of recurrence (▶ Fig. 11.3c and d).

11.5.3 Case 3

A 48-year-old female was presented to our emergency department complaining of severe headache that was not relieved with pain medication. She had history of chronic headaches and nonspecific nasal symptoms, initially attributed to seasonal allergies, for the past 2 years. In addition, she reported blurry vision and decrease in visual acuity for 1 year and decreased smell over the past 6 months prior to presentation. On examination, she had anosmia, subjective bilateral blurred vision with normal visual acuity and visual field.

MRI brain (▶ Fig. 11.4a and b) demonstrated a large OGM measuring 4.6 × 4.8 × 4.5 cm in the axial, sagittal, and coronal planes extending caudally into the ethmoidal sinus and anteroposteriorly all the way from the crista galli to the tuberculum sellae compressing the optic nerves and chiasm. There was significant associated right frontal lobe edema.

The risks and benefits of three different surgical approaches were discussed with the patient: EEA, unilateral fronto-orbital craniotomy, and two-stage combined approach. A two-stage combined procedure was chosen, with EEA as stage I with the main goal of tumor devascularization, drilling out of the affected skull base bone, and mass effect relief by tumor debulking. The rationale for fronto-orbital craniotomy as a second stage was to complete resection of the tumor that was devascularized and to perform the brain-tumor interface dissection on a less edematous frontal lobe, which ultimately would result in less morbidity and possibly better outcome.

An endoscopic endonasal transcribiform/transplanum approach was uneventful. The predefined goals of this first stage procedure were achieved. The patient tolerated the surgery well with no complications and stated improvement of the headache and the blurry vision bilaterally. Histopathological examination confirmed the diagnosis of meningioma WHO grade I with Ki-67 LI of 8%.

The second stage was then performed 4 months later when the patient came back complaining of worsening blurry vision bilaterally (more on the right side). A new MRI was performed that showed postoperative changes and a large central defect in the tumor corresponding to the previous surgery (▶ Fig. 11.4c). There was edema in the right frontal area. There was no hemorrhage, hydrocephalus, or acute brain infarct. Head CT demonstrated complete resection of the affected anterior skull base bone (▶ Fig. 11.4d).

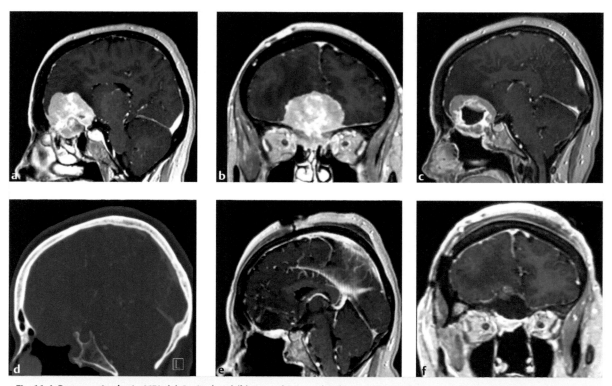

Fig. 11.4 Preoperative brain MRI. (a) Sagittal and **(b)** coronal T1-weighted imaging (T1WI) with gadolinium contrast showing a large OGM extending from the posterior wall of the frontal sinus all the way to the tuberculum sellae. **(c)** Sagittal T1WI with gadolinium contrast and **(d)** head CT sagittal view, following the first stage procedure (endoscopic endonasal approach). Note that all the infiltrated anterior skull base bone is drilled out. The skull base is reconstructed with a vascularized nasoseptal flap which is enhancing. Brain MRI **(e)** sagittal and **(f)** coronal T1WI with gadolinium contrast after the second stage procedure (fronto-orbito-temporal craniotomy) demonstrating complete resection of the tumor.

At this point, it was decided to proceed with stage II procedure via right fronto-orbito-temporal craniotomy. Gross total resection and adequate decompression of the optic nerves were achieved. The procedure was uneventful and the patient recovered with no complications.

The immediate postoperative MRI showed complete resection of tumor and no signs of complications. On late postoperative follow-up, MRI brain confirmed gross total resection of the lesion (► Fig. 11.4e and f) and the patient reported an improvement of the blurred vision of the left eye and a stationary condition of the right eye.

11.6 Complications

Postoperative complications vary according to the type of approach, however, with the current microsurgical techniques, the overall rate of complications related to resection of OGMs is decreased. The common reported complications related to surgery for OGMs in general include loss of olfaction, frontal lobe syndrome, postoperative CSF rhinorrhea, subdural hygroma, cerebrovascular accidents, postoperative seizure, infections, and systemic complications. In case of delayed recovery from anesthesia, immediate head CT should be obtained to rule out hematoma, pneumocephaly, significant cerebral edema, and ischemic stroke.[3,7,8]

Frontal lobe syndrome may result from edema or cerebral ischemia and is more common in larger lesions associated with significant parenchymal edema which is worsened by brain retraction especially when bilateral and even unilateral subfrontal approaches are utilized.[7]

Postoperative CSF rhinorrhea is more common in approaches where the frontal sinus is trespassed and in cases with tumor invading the paranasal sinuses, especially the ethmoid sinus. It usually results from inadequate skull base reconstruction.[14] Additionally, the probability of postoperative CSF rhinorrhea is higher with transbasal approach and EEA.

Visual impairment can result from manipulation of the optic nerves and chiasm, especially with large and giant OGMs. Because of the ischemic insult from the long-standing compression by the tumor, the optic apparatus becomes more vulnerable in these cases.[7]

The reported mortality rates related to surgery for OGMs in the old series ranged between 0 and 33%, however, with the advance in microsurgical techniques, these rates are markedly declined. The mortality rates related to surgery for OGMs reported in the literature in the last two decades ranged from 0 to 15%.[3,14]

11.7 Early and Long-term Follow-up

Postoperative follow-up of patients is very crucial for detecting complications and recurrence. In our practice, a head CT is obtained within the first 2 hours to exclude postoperative hematomas, brain edema, and/or pneumocephaly. Brain MRI with and without contrast administration is obtained before the patient is discharged in the first 24 hours postoperative to assess the extent of resection and to have a baseline for long-term follow-up.

The patient is followed up both clinically and radiographically. Our follow-up strategy is to obtain a brain MRI (with and without contrast) at 3 and 9 months postoperative, then annually for the first 5 years. Afterwards, MRI can be obtained every 2 years. It is to be emphasized that in case of recurrence or growth of any residual tumor is noted, a close clinical and radiographic follow-up is initiated according to the situation, followed by appropriate management.

11.7.1 Functional Outcomes

Olfactory Function

Olfactory function is very important for the quality of life and should be considered while planning and performing surgical intervention for OGMs. Although chances of preservation of olfaction is higher in small-sized lesions and in patients without preoperative olfactory dysfunction, unfortunately, preservation of olfaction in OGM patients has been generally disappointing regardless of the surgical approach performed.

Chances of preserving the olfaction in patients with intact preoperative olfactory function are better when approaching the tumor transcranially (subfrontal, frontolateral, and pterional) than endoscopic endonasally. However, even with anatomical preservation of at least one of the olfactory tracts, functional preservation is often hard to achieve.[4,30,31] Nevertheless, its emphasized that its always worthy to attempt preserving the olfaction in patients with preoperative normal or partial olfactory function.

Many theories for pathogenesis of anosmia related to OGMs have been proposed. Anosmia may be caused by degeneration of olfactory nerve cells by the long-standing compression by the lesion, direct infiltration of the olfactory nerves by the lesion, ischemic insult caused by deprivation of blood supply to the olfactory nerves during surgical intervention, or transection of olfactory fimbria during surgical manipulation.[4]

Frontal Lobe Manifestations

In majority of cases, frontal lobe manifestations show definitive improvement during the postoperative follow-up. Since these symptoms are generally caused by tumor mass effect exerted on the frontal lobes, tumor- or surgery-related parenchymal edema, and excessive traction of the frontal lobes, these symptoms improve much following resection of the tumor, subsidence of the parenchymal edema, and convalescence from surgery.

Visual Improvement

The duration of visual deterioration and the size of OGMs are the main determinants of visual outcome. The rate of postoperative visual acuity improvement is reported in the literature to be 26 to 83%, while the rate of postoperative visual field improvement is 29 to 100%.[13]

However, in our opinion, the surgical approach also has a significant influence on the visual outcome. Surgical approaches that allow for early visualization and adequate decompression of the optic nerves and chiasm, such as EEA, are associated with better visual outcomes. Additionally, a recent comparative meta-analysis has shown that the rates of postoperative visual improvement associated with EEA are significantly higher compared to conventional transcranial approaches.[28]

11.7.2 Recurrence

The recurrence-free survival after total gross resection of OGMs varies widely among surgical series published in the literature. Although some series with short-term follow-up of OGMs reported 0% recurrence rates, the recurrence rates reported by series with long-term follow-up (10–20 years) vary between 5 and 41%. The recurrence rate is believed to be strongly proportional to the duration of follow-up.[3,9,10] Therefore, long-term follow-up following surgical resection of OGMs is crucial to detect recurrence.

The incidence of recurrence of OGMs is highly affected by the extent of surgical resection and the histological grade of the tumor. However, the most significant factor influencing the rate of early and late recurrence is the extent of initial surgical resection of the tumor. Therefore, surgical trends have shifted in favor of more radical resection. It is thought by some authors that the main site of recurrence, other than the residual tumor if any, is the infiltrated skull base bone that has not been completely resected during the surgery.[2,3,9,14,18,32] Having said that, Simpson grade-I resection should always remain the utmost goal of surgery for OGMs. The authors believe that the two-stage approach for the large and giant OGM allows a more complete resection of the hyperostotic bone through the EEA while allowing a whole resection of the lateral and posterior component of the tumor on the second stage through the craniotomy.

References

[1] Adappa ND, Lee JYK, Chiu AG, Palmer JN. Olfactory groove meningioma. Otolaryngol Clin North Am. 2011; 44(4):965–980, ix

[2] Pepper J-P, Hecht SL, Gebarski SS, Lin EM, Sullivan SE, Marentette LJ. Olfactory groove meningioma: discussion of clinical presentation and surgical outcomes following excision via the subcranial approach. Laryngoscope. 2011; 121(11):2282–2289

[3] Nakamura M, Struck M, Roser F, Vorkapic P, Samii M. Olfactory groove meningiomas: clinical outcome and recurrence rates after tumor removal through the frontolateral and bifrontal approach. Neurosurgery. 2007; 60(5):844–852, discussion 844–852

[4] Bassiouni H, Asgari S, Stolke D. Olfactory groove meningiomas: functional outcome in a series treated microsurgically. Acta Neurochir (Wien). 2007; 149(2):109–121, discussion 121

[5] Tomasello F, Angileri FF, Grasso G, Granata F, De Ponte FS, Alafaci C. Giant olfactory groove meningiomas: extent of frontal lobes damage and long-term outcome after the pterional approach. World Neurosurg. 2011; 76(3–4):311–317, discussion 255–258

[6] Pallini R, Fernandez E, Lauretti L, et al. Olfactory groove meningioma: report of 99 cases surgically treated at the Catholic University School of Medicine, Rome. World Neurosurg. 2015; 83(2):219–31.e1, 3

[7] Aguiar PH, Almeida AN. Surgery of olfactory groove meningiomas. In: Samii's Essentials in Neurosurgery. Berlin: Springer; 2008:69–75

[8] Hentschel SJ, DeMonte F. Olfactory groove meningiomas. Neurosurg Focus. 2003; 14(6):e4

[9] Obeid F, Al-Mefty O. Recurrence of olfactory groove meningiomas. Neurosurgery. 2003; 53(3):534–542, discussion 542–543

[10] Romani R, Lehecka M, Gaal E, et al. Lateral supraorbital approach applied to olfactory groove meningiomas: experience with 66 consecutive patients. Neurosurgery. 2009; 65(1):39–52, discussion 52–53

[11] Manjila S, Cox EM, Smith GA, et al. Extracranial ligation of ethmoidal arteries before resection of giant olfactory groove or planum sphenoidale meningiomas: 3 illustrative cases with a review of the literature on surgical techniques. Neurosurg Focus. 2013; 35(6):E13

[12] Cecchini G. Anterior and posterior ethmoidal artery ligation in anterior skull base meningiomas: a review on microsurgical approaches. World Neurosurg. 2015; 84(4):1161–1165

[13] Nanda A, Maiti TK, Bir SC, Konar SK, Guthikonda B. Olfactory groove meningiomas: comparison of extent of frontal lobe changes after lateral and bifrontal approaches. World Neurosurg. 2016; 94:211–221

[14] Ciurea AV, Iencean SM, Rizea RE, Brehar FM. Olfactory groove meningiomas: a retrospective study on 59 surgical cases. Neurosurg Rev. 2012; 35(2):195–202, discussion 202

[15] Bitter AD, Stavrinou LC, Ntoulias G, et al. The role of the pterional approach in the surgical treatment of olfactory groove meningiomas: a 20-year experience. J Neurol Surg B Skull Base. 2013; 74(2):97–102

[16] Connor SEJ, Umaria N, Chavda SV. Imaging of giant tumours involving the anterior skull base. Br J Radiol. 2001; 74(883):662–667

[17] Nishiguchi T, Iwakiri T, Hayasaki K, et al. Post-embolisation susceptibility changes in giant meningiomas: multiparametric histogram analysis using non-contrast-enhanced susceptibility-weighted PRESTO, diffusion-weighted and perfusion-weighted imaging. Eur Radiol. 2013; 23(2):551–561

[18] Fischer BR, Brokinkel B. Surgical Management of Skull Base Meningiomas–An Overview. INTECH Open Access Publisher; 2012. Available at: http://cdn.intechweb.org/pdfs/30677.pdf. Accessed March 14, 2018

[19] Wang Y, Zhao J. Approach selection for the giant olfactory groove meningiomas. World Neurosurg. 2011; 76(3–4):257–258

[20] da Silva CE, de Freitas PE. Large and giant skull base meningiomas: The role of radical surgical removal. Surg Neurol Int. 2015; 6(1):113

[21] Raheja A, Couldwell WT. Microsurgical resection of skull base meningioma-expanding the operative corridor. J Neurooncol. 2016; 130(2):263–267

[22] Dhandapani S, Sharma K. Is "en-bloc" excision, an option for select large vascular meningiomas? Surg Neurol Int. 2013; 4(1):102

[23] Gardner PA, Kassam AB, Thomas A, et al. Endoscopic endonasal resection of anterior cranial base meningiomas. Neurosurgery. 2008; 63(1):36–52, discussion 52–54

[24] Spektor S, Valarezo J, Fliss DM, et al. Olfactory groove meningiomas from neurosurgical and ear, nose, and throat perspectives: approaches, techniques, and outcomes. Neurosurgery. 2005; 57(4) Suppl:268–280, discussion 268–280

[25] Gazzeri R, Galarza M, Gazzeri G. Giant olfactory groove meningioma: ophthalmological and cognitive outcome after bifrontal microsurgical approach. Acta Neurochir (Wien). 2008; 150(11):1117–1125, discussion 1126

[26] Rachinger W, Grau S, Tonn J-C. Different microsurgical approaches to meningiomas of the anterior cranial base. Acta Neurochir (Wien). 2010; 152(6):931–939

[27] El-Bahy K. Validity of the frontolateral approach as a minimally invasive corridor for olfactory groove meningiomas. Acta Neurochir (Wien). 2009; 151(10):1197–1205

[28] Lucas JW, Zada G. Endoscopic endonasal and keyhole surgery for the management of skull base meningiomas. Neurosurg Clin N Am. 2016; 27(2):207–214

[29] Fernandez-Miranda JC, Gardner PA, Prevedello DM, Kassam AB. Expanded endonasal approach for olfactory groove meningioma. Acta Neurochir (Wien). 2009; 151(3):287–288, author reply 289–290

[30] Liu JK, Hattar E, Eloy JA. Endoscopic endonasal approach for olfactory groove meningiomas: operative technique and nuances. Neurosurg Clin N Am. 2015; 26(3):377–388

[31] Jang W-Y, Jung S, Jung T-Y, Moon K-S, Kim I-Y. Preservation of olfaction in surgery of olfactory groove meningiomas. Clin Neurol Neurosurg. 2013; 115(8):1288–1292

[32] Liu JK, Christiano LD, Patel SK, Tubbs RS, Eloy JA. Surgical nuances for removal of olfactory groove meningiomas using the endoscopic endonasal transcribriform approach. Neurosurg Focus. 2011; 30(5):E3

12 Middle Fossa Floor Meningiomas

Roberto Delfini, Benedetta Fazzolari, Davide Colistra

Abstract

Little is known regarding meningiomas that primarily arise from the floor of the middle fossa as opposed to the other middle fossa meningiomas. In this chapter, we treat this relatively new entity, including primary Meckel's cave (MC) meningiomas because they respect similar anatomical landmarks.

Meningiomas of the middle cranial fossa can be approached by two distinct routes: an anterolateral approach or a lateral approach; in other words, via a pterional or a subtemporal approach. Both approaches can be further extended by means of additional osteotomies, such as the cranio-orbital zygomatic approach and the temporo-zygomatic approach. "Extended" approaches and adequate cerebrospinal fluid drainage, are helpful to achieve a "retractorless" surgical technique. It is also mandatory to achieve good surgical outcomes to preserve venous structures, as the vein of Labbè.

The aim of this chapter is to treat "middle fossa floor" meningiomas as a clinical entity that is distinct from meningiomas arising from the sphenoid wing and cavernous sinus, which have been already described in other chapters of this book, and to include in authors' classification primary MC meningiomas as well.

Keywords: middle fossa floor meningioma, Meckel's cave meningioma, pterional approach, subtemporal approach, fronto-temporo-orbito-zygomatic approach

12.1 Introduction

The middle cranial fossa is the site of several tumors. These tumors are primarily intracranial, arising from the meninges or cranial nerves, such as meningiomas or schwannomas, while other tumors, such as chordomas and chondrosarcomas, may arise from the bones and cartilages. Lastly, some tumors can originate from extracranial tissues and secondarily invade the middle cranial fossa structures, for example, nasopharyngeal carcinoma, esthesioneuroblastoma, lymphoma, and systemic metastasis. The majority of middle cranial fossa tumors are meningiomas; among these, sphenoid wing meningiomas are the most common.

The first successful removal of a lateral sphenoid wing meningioma was described in 1774 by Louis A. In 1918, Heuer GJ pioneered the pterional approach as a surgical technique to approach lesions of the middle cranial fossa, although Dandy W is frequently credited with inventing this operation. As regards trigeminal tumors, Cushing in 1938 stated: "It is possible of course that a method may some day be evolved whereby a Gasserian ganglion neuroma or meningioma may be safely approached and removed. Should this come to pass, it will be another conquest for neurosurgery."

More recently, many surgeons have modified the pterional approach to gain a more direct working distance and minimize brain retraction. The orbitozygomatic approach and its various other osteotomies have been proposed as extensions of the pterional approach to wider exposure of the middle cranial fossa and enable entry into the adjacent compartments (orbit, posterior fossa, pterygopalatine space).

Moreover, the subtemporal approach has been proposed as a safe surgical strategy for removing middle fossa tumors.

To sum up, many advanced methods have been introduced to treat tumors of the middle fossa, based on the standard pterional and subtemporal surgical routes, resulting in a better outcome.

Meningiomas arising primarily from the floor of the middle fossa are an uncommon occurrence, representing only 1.1% of all meningiomas in the series described by Sughrue et al.[1] However, many of these tumors in the past may have been grouped with other meningiomas of the convexity dura, sphenoid wing, lateral wall of the cavernous sinus, and tentorium.

In this chapter the authors emphasize that "middle fossa floor meningiomas" are a clinical entity distinct from meningiomas arising from the sphenoid wing and cavernous sinus (already described in other chapters of this book), and this denomination includes primarily MC meningiomas too.

12.2 Preoperative Definition of Lesion Features

12.2.1 Surgical Anatomy of the Middle Cranial Fossa

The middle cranial fossa is formed by the sphenoid and temporal bones. The anterior border of this fossa consists of the sphenoid wing and anterior clinoid process. Posteriorly, it is limited by the superior border of the petrous temporal bone with the sulcus for the superior petrous sinus, and the dorsum sella of the sphenoid bone. The floor is formed by the greater wing of the sphenoid anteriorly and the squamosal temporal bone posteriorly. The middle cranial fossa is divided into medial and lateral portions. The medial part is formed by the body of the sphenoid bone. The cavernous sinus occupies a significant portion of this region but its anatomy will be described elsewhere in this book. The lateral part is formed by the lesser and greater sphenoid wings, with the superior orbital fissure between them. The lesser wing is connected to the body of the sphenoid bone by an anterior root, which forms the roof of the optic canal, and by a posterior root, also called the optic strut, which forms the floor of the optic canal, and separates the optic canal from the superior orbital fissure. The greater wing forms the largest part of the middle fossa, with the squamosal and the petrosal parts of the temporal bone completing this surface. The superior orbital fissure transmits the oculomotor, trochlear, ophthalmic, and abducens nerves, a recurrent meningeal artery, and the superior and inferior ophthalmic veins. The maxillary nerve passes through the foramen rotundum of the greater sphenoid wing, which connects the middle cranial fossa to the pterygopalatine fossa. The mandibular nerve passes through the foramen ovale of the greater sphenoid wing, which connects the middle cranial fossa with the infratemporal fossa. The upper surface of the petrous bone is grooved along the course of the greater and lesser petrosal nerves.[2] The greater superficial petrosal nerve (GSPN) arises from the geniculate ganglion in the petrous bone, pierces the hiatus fallopii, then runs parallel to the lateral wall of the horizontal internal carotid artery in a groove called the sulcus of the GSPN, exiting the middle cranial fossa through the foramen lacerum and the pterygoid (vidian) canal.[3] The lesser petrosal nerve arises from the tympanic branch of the glossopharyngeal nerve (Jacobson's nerve), the nervus intermedius of the facial nerve and the auricular branch of the vagus nerve (Arnold's nerve), pierces the hiatus accessorius and then runs above the tensor tympani muscle anterior and parallel to the GSPN in a groove called the sulcus of the lesser petrosal nerve: it leaves the middle cranial fossa passing through the canaliculus innominatus (foramen of Vesalius), the foramen spinosum or the sphenopetrosal suture.[4] The carotid canal extends upward and medially and allows a passage to the internal carotid artery and carotid sympathetic nerves along their courses to the cavernous sinus. The roof of the carotid canal is formed by the petrous bone. However, this bony roof is frequently dehiscent for a variable degree. In many cases, the internal carotid artery in the carotid canal is covered only by the dura of the middle cranial fossa. The internal carotid artery reaches the middle cranial fossa passing through the inner opening of the carotid canal, located near the foramen lacerum at the petrous apex. The foramen lacerum may be covered by a cartilaginous sheet and is laterally delimited by the lingula, a protrusion of the sphenoid bone located at the junction of body and greater wing which provides an attachment to the petrolingual ligament, that divides the horizontal petrous carotid from vertical cavernous carotid segment.[5] The arcuate eminence indicates the position of the superior semicircular canal. A thin lamina of bone, the tegmen tympani, roofs the area above the middle ear and auditory ossicles on

the anterolateral side of the arcuate eminence. The internal auditory canal can be identified below the floor of the middle fossa by drilling along a line approximately 60° medial to the arcuate eminence, near the middle portion of the angle between the GSPN and arcuate eminence. The petrous apex, anteromedial to the internal acoustic meatus, is free of important structures. The middle cranial fossa is covered by dura and is fed by the middle meningeal and accessory meningeal arteries; it is innervated by the trigeminal nerve. The middle meningeal artery, branch of the maxillary artery of the external carotid artery circle, reaches the middle cranial fossa from the infratemporal fossa passing through the foramen spinosum, located in the greater wing of the sphenoid, posterior and lateral to the foramen ovale. The accessory meningeal artery rises from the middle meningeal artery or directly from the maxillary artery and reaches the middle cranial fossa passing through the foramen ovale.[2]

MC is a 10-mm-long, tunnel-shaped subdural cavity; it contains the plexiform segment of the roots of the trigeminal nerve and the Gasserian ganglion. The walls of the cave are composed of thin meningeal dura. The lateral wall is formed by the tentorium, the superior half of the medial wall is formed by the inner reticular layer of the cavernous sinus, the inferior half of the medial wall is formed by the petrolingual ligament and by the trigeminal impression on the petrous apex, which separate the MC from the internal carotid artery. The Gasserian ganglion lies in the anterior part of MC, while the posterior part of MC communicates with the prepontine cistern. Before the trigeminal nerve enters MC, it forms an angle of 60° as it crosses over the petrous apex. The nerve fibers are loose within the cave.[6]

12.2.2 Middle Cranial Fossa Floor Meningiomas

The middle cranial fossa is a common site of origin for meningiomas. This region can be represented as a rectangular open bowl rising to terminate in three distinct "ridges" and an open back.[1] The three ridges include the sphenoid wing anteriorly, the cavernous sinus medially, and the convexity dura laterally; the open back is the portion posterior to the petrous ridge that includes the tentorium. In this analogy, the concavity of the bowl consists of the floor of the middle fossa. The clinical behavior of meningiomas originating from each of these "ridges" and the tentorium is well-described, but very little is known regarding meningiomas that arise primarily from the floor of the middle fossa. Prior to the work of Sughrue et al, only 5 reports documenting the clinical outcome of a total of 19 cases of primarily middle fossa floor meningiomas could be identified in the literature.[7,8,9,10,11] In 2010, Sughrue et al defined a "middle fossa floor" meningioma as a meningioma with more than 75% of its radiographic attachment on the floor of the middle fossa and with less than 25% of attachment on either the sphenoid wing, cavernous sinus, petrous ridge, or lateral convexity dura, which form the four anatomic boundaries of the middle fossa concavity as determined by MRI (▶ Fig. 12.1 a, b and ▶ Fig. 12.2 a, b). As reported in this paper, between 1991 and 2006, 1,228 patients were treated at the University of

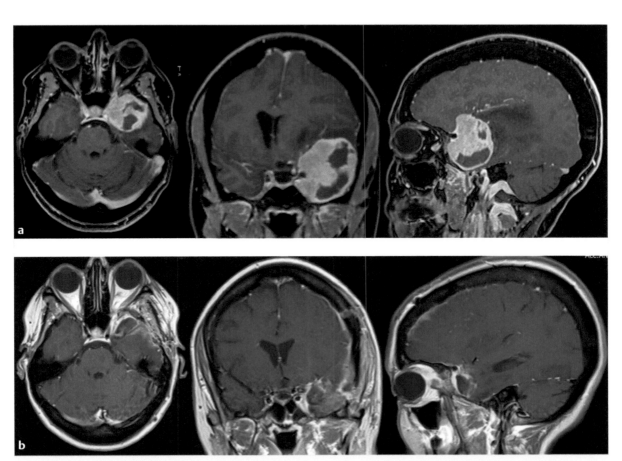

Fig. 12.1 (a) Middle fossa floor meningioma. An example of preoperative MRI showing a middle cranial fossa floor meningioma, defined as meningioma with more than 75% of its attachment on the floor of the middle fossa and with less than 25% of attachment on either the sphenoid wing, cavernous sinus, petrous ridge, or lateral convexity dura. **(b)** Postoperative MRI of a middle cranial fossa floor meningioma. Postoperative MRI showing total resection of a middle fossa floor meningioma.

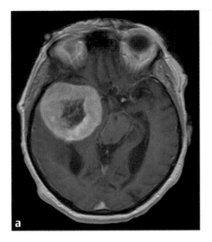
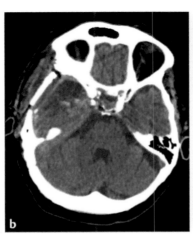

Fig. 12.2 (a) Middle fossa floor meningioma. Another example of preoperative MRI showing a huge middle cranial fossa floor meningioma. **(b)** Early postoperative CT scan of a middle cranial fossa floor meningioma.

California, San Francisco for meningiomas: of these, 17 (1.1%) patients met their criteria for a "middle fossa floor" meningioma. Two of these patients had had previous surgery and were excluded because it was unclear where the initial site of their tumor was located. Thus, only 15 patients were included in that series, bringing the total number of middle fossa floor meningiomas cases described in the literature to 34.

Primary meningiomas originating from the MC represent approximately 1% of all intracranial meningiomas. In 1992, Delfini et al divided primary MC meningiomas into two major groups: small meningiomas restricted to MC (group I) and large meningiomas arising from MC and extending beyond this area (group II).[12] In 1996, Samii et al reclassified primary MC meningiomas according to the tumor extension into four different types: type I, tumors mainly confined to MC; type II, MC meningiomas with extension into the middle fossa; type III, MC meningiomas with extension into the posterior fossa; type IV, MC meningiomas with extension into both the middle and posterior fossae.[13] In authors' opinion, middle fossa floor meningiomas should include "true" primary MC meningiomas, classified as group I according to supramentioned classifications.

12.3 Preoperative Management

MRI and CT are complementary procedures for evaluating middle cranial fossa meningiomas: on CT scans meningiomas are mostly hyperdense, and sometimes present calcification, marked and homogeneous enhancement, often associated with bony changes such as hyperostosis. CT with bone window exposure of the skull base detects any calcification and the effect of the meningioma on the bone (hyperostosis or erosion). MRI demonstrates the relationship of a skull base meningioma with the cranial nerves and vascular structures. On MRI, these tumors are isointense on both T1 and T2 weighted-images. Contrast enhancement is marked and homogenous, and a dural tail can be identified. Nowadays magnetic resonance angiography has supplanted cerebral angiography for establishing the relationship between the tumor and the major intracranial arteries and their branches and for preoperative evaluation of the vein of Labbé and venous sinus patency. However, for those few meningiomas that require endovascular embolization, cerebral angiography remains necessary to determine the feasibility and safety of the procedure. Preoperative angiography consistently identifies the internal maxillary artery, via the middle meningeal artery, as they supply blood to these tumors in most of cases. Balloon test occlusion of the ipsilateral internal carotid artery can be performed to evaluate the collateral circulation in the event that temporary or permanent occlusion become necessary during surgery.

12.4 Surgical Indications

The decision to refer patients with middle cranial fossa meningiomas to surgery is determined by two hinge points: mass development documented by neuroimaging and the presence of neurological symptoms. The most common presenting symptoms are headache, seizures, trigeminal nerve dysfunction, hearing loss, gait disturbance, and cognitive decline. In addition, the relative distance between the attachment point of these tumors and the cranial nerves, or owing to other pressure sensitive structures, these tumors present a different clinical behavior compared to other meningiomas, in that they can grow rather large before diagnosis, and frequently present with nonspecific symptoms.

12.5 Surgical Approaches

Tumors of the middle cranial fossa can be approached by two distinct routes: an anterolateral approach or a lateral approach; in other words, via a pterional or a subtemporal approach. Both approaches can be further extended by means of additional osteotomies, such as the cranio-orbital zygomatic approach and temporo-zygomatic approach. Generally speaking, zygomatic arch osteotomy is used in large tumors with a deep middle fossa and/or more posterior position. An adequate craniectomy of the squamous temporal bone makes it possible to obtain a flush approach angle with the middle fossa floor[1] without the need for inferior-middle temporal gyrus corticectomy, a procedure that, in authors' opinion, should be always avoided.

12.5.1 Pterional Approach

The pterional approach offers exposure of the Sylvian fissure and the superior orbital fissure, in addition to the temporal pole, with respect to a pure temporal approach. Via this route, the tumor can be approached from the transylvian, pretemporal, or subtemporal surgical trajectory.

The patient is placed supine and the ipsilateral shoulder can be elevated to reduce head rotation. The head is rotated 45° away from the side of the tumor, elevated by 15° to the trunk to favor venous drainage and hyperextended for brain relaxing. The head is fixed in a three point Mayfield headrest. The skin incision begins 1 cm anterior to the tragus at the level of the zygomatic arch and extends behind the hairline, as far as 1–2 cm before the midline (▶ Fig. 12.3).

The frontal branch of the facial nerve passes 1 cm from tragus, parallel and anterior to the superficial temporal artery which should be also preserved because it supplies the forehead. Moreover, to preserve the frontal branch of the facial nerve, the subgaleal flap is dissected no further than 3 cm from the eyebrow line. The superficial temporal fascia and temporal muscle are cut following the scalp

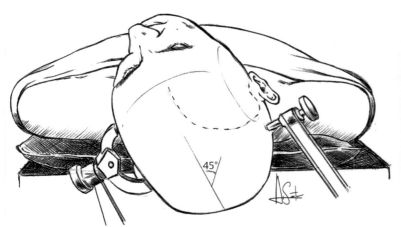

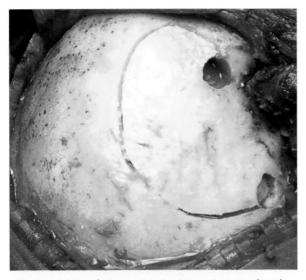

Fig. 12.4 Pterional craniotomy. Craniotomy is centered on the pterion. The first burr-hole is made on the "key-hole" and another burr-hole is made at the posterior limit of the zygomatic bone. The craniotomy is wider on the temporal side than on the frontal one.

remaining bone is drilled to expose the floor of the middle cranial fossa. During closure, the temporal muscle is returned to its original position and secured to the bone.

12.5.2 Fronto-temporo-(orbito)-zygomatic Approach

The orbitozygomatic approach is an extension of the pterional approach, which augments exposure via several routes, including the frontotemporal and transsylvian ones.[14] In authors' experience, additional exposure can never be gained by orbit removal, but only by zygomatic arch removal, as occurs when the middle cranial fossa is concave and its floor is below the zygoma level. The role of zygomatic arch osteotomy in these cases is primarily to achieve a flatter trajectory along the middle fossa floor (▶ Fig. 12.5 a, b).

The skin incision and craniotomy are localized more posteriorly than for sphenoid wing meningiomas, and the craniectomy of the squamous temporal bone is continued until flush with the middle fossa floor to approach this lesion subtemporally.

The subgaleal flap is dissected no further than 3 cm from the eyebrow line. The superficial temporal fascia, composed of a superficial and a deep layer, is cut following the scalp incision and dissected from the temporal muscle. The superficial temporal fascia remains attached to the frontal scalp, preserving the frontal branch of facial nerve. In fact, at this level, the frontal branch of facial nerve runs in the connective tissue of the *innominate fascia* between superficial temporal fascia and galea (90% of cases). We prefer this safer subfascial dissection because in 10% of the cases, the frontal branch of the facial nerve runs between the two layers of the superficial temporal fascia.

In correspondence of the zygomatic arch, the facial nerve runs superficially to its periostium, so a subperiosteal dissection is mandatory. Then, the temporal muscle is cut and the subperiosteal dissection is continued to

incision. The temporal muscle with its superficial fascia remain partially attached to the frontal scalp. Then, a subfascial subperiosteal dissection of the temporal muscle is performed and the frontotemporal bone is exposed to the pterion. A blunt subfascial dissection of the temporal muscle, carried out in a caudo-cranial manner, preserves the deep temporal fascia, which contains the vessels and nerves that supply the muscle. Craniotomy is centered on the pterion. The first burr-hole is made on the "key-hole" (McCarty point) and another burr-hole is made at the posterior limit of the zygomatic bone. The craniotomy is wider on the temporal side than on the frontal one (▶ Fig. 12.4). The lesser sphenoid wing makes it difficult to use the craniotome to connect the two burr-holes, therefore, a microdrill can be used. The bone flap is removed and the

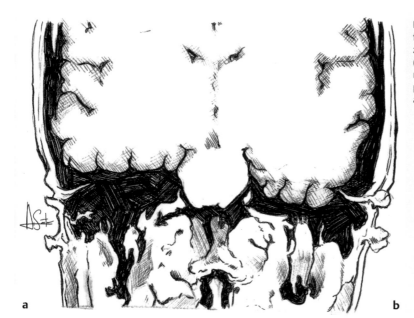

Fig. 12.5 **(a)** A flat middle cranial fossa floor. For the surgical exposure, the zygomatic arch osteotomy is not necessary. **(b)** A concave middle cranial fossa floor. The role of zygomatic arch osteotomy is primarily to achieve a flatter trajectory along the middle fossa floor.

a

b

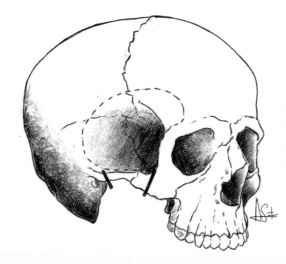

Fig. 12.6 Fronto-temporo-zygomatic approach. The zygomatic arch is sectioned with oblique cuts in its most posterior end and anteriorly where the zygomatic arch meets the lateral wall of the orbit. Then, a frontotemporal craniotomy is performed.

expose the zygomatic arch and zygomatic process of the frontal bone. Using an oscillating saw, the zygomatic arch is sectioned with oblique cuts in its most posterior end and anteriorly where the zygomatic arch meets the lateral wall of the orbit (▶ Fig. 12.6). Bone preplating is performed, then the zygoma is displaced inferiorly. The attachment of the masseter muscle on the inferior border of the zygomatic arch is preserved. It is strictly advised not to detach the masseter muscle from the inferior site of the zygomatic arch to avoid motility dysfunction of the temporomandibular articulation. The temporal muscle is reflected inferiorly. A frontotemporal craniotomy is performed.

12.5.3 Temporal Approach

The patient is positioned supine; Mayfield pins are inserted into the frontal and occipital bones and the head rotated by 90° (parallel to the floor). The vertex is tilted down 10–20° so that the zygoma becomes the highest point: this provides a natural retraction of temporal lobe. The question mark shaped incision starts 1 cm anteriorly to the tragus, curves posteriorly along the ear, and ends anteriorly on the mid-pupil line. Superficial temporal fascia and temporal muscle are cut and dissected together with the skin flap. The first hole is made just posteriorly and inferiorly from the McCarty point and the second posterior to the external acoustic meatus. A pure temporal craniotomy is then performed in order to obtain a flat working angle to the floor of middle cranial fossa, thus minimizing temporal lobe retraction. Removal of the zygomatic arch is indicated not only when the middle cranial fossa presents concave and its floor is below the zygoma level, but also for lesions that extend from the middle cranial fossa to the infratemporal fossa (▶ Fig. 12.7).

12.5.4 Operative Techniques

Approaching middle cranial fossa meningiomas usually requires brain retraction to expose the tumor. Although the best means of reducing brain retraction is to eliminate its need by using basal approaches, several methods can be used to minimize it. Spinal drainage is of paramount importance for ensuring brain relaxation.

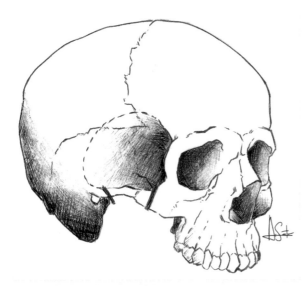

Fig. 12.7 Temporal approach. Craniotomy is performed in order to obtain a flat working angle to the floor of middle cranial fossa, thus minimizing temporal lobe retraction. Removal of the zygomatic arch is indicated not only when the middle cranial fossa presents concave and its floor is below the zygoma level, but also for lesions that extend from the middle cranial fossa to the infratemporal fossa.

Cerebrospinal fluid (CSF) drainage is performed using a lumbar subarachnoid drain inserted after induction and intubation of the patient. Gradual withdrawal of fluid (about 25 mL) is carried out during the operation as required. A flow-control clamp is applied to the drainage tube to prevent rapid loss of CSF. Other techniques include patient positioning to take advantage of the effects of gravity, hyperventilation, and osmotic diuretics that allow "*retractorless*" surgery.

It is imperative to preserve venous structures during surgery, and especially during temporal lobe mobilization, care must be taken to the course of the vein of Labbè. Although skull base approaches provide access to skull base tumors with the least possible manipulation of the brain and its vasculature, there are certain situations where injury to the venous drainage may be inevitable.[15] No pre- or intra-operative test or maneuver can decide for the surgeon whether a vein can be sacrificed or not: there are no reliable tests to assess the vitality of any venous structure because venous insufficiency leading to infarction is often delayed (24–48 h). Al-Mefty et al consider the dominant lateral sinus, draining the vein of Labbè or the Sylvian vein, to be "dangerous" veins: since the temporal lobe is liable to hemorrhagic venous infarction on their ligation, they advocate ligation of the vein as close as possible to the dura in order to preserve the anastomotic channels.[16]

Intraoperative electrophysiological monitoring during middle cranial fossa surgery is based mainly on trigeminal and facial nerve monitoring. These monitoring systems are able to detect several types of physiological activity in the muscle, which are indicative of mechanical stimulation of the nerves or nerve trauma.

Surgical removal requires firstly reaching and detaching the base of the tumor from middle fossa floor attachments, thus devascularizing the tumor in the process. Standard internal debulking is then performed followed by peripheral dissection. In authors' experience, preoperative embolization was never needed.

12.6 Complications

The overall surgical mortality rate for meningiomas of the middle cranial fossa is very low (1%); the incidence of neurological deficits depends on the tumor location, varying in published series from 9 to 11%[1] Preoperative cranial nerve deficits may worsen after surgical treatment, and varies from transient to permanent VI cranial nerve palsy, trigeminal deficit, hypo/hypesthesia in the V2 distribution, V1 deficit, or V3 numbness; patients may develop seizures and motor deficits. The most frequent complications related to the surgical approach are: temporal muscle atrophy, cranial nerve palsies, CSF leakage, epidural hematoma, brain edema, and laceration or thrombosis of the vein of Labbè.

12.6.1 How to Avoid Complications?

When performing the pterional approach (operative technique described above), care must be taken to avoid damaging the frontal branch of the facial nerve, which supplies the frontal muscle and mimic muscles of the orbit. The frontal muscle raises the ipsilateral eyebrow and denervation produces an obvious cosmetic deformity. Another complication that may occur during the pterional approach is atrophy of the temporal muscle, which impairs elevation of the mandible.

CSF leakage may occur if the frontal sinus or mastoid cells are entered during the pterional or subtemporal approach. In this case, any gap must be plugged with fat or muscle taken from the patient and biological glue. CSF leakage can be resolved by positioning a spinal lumbar drainage for 5 to 7 days.

During the subtemporal approach, the meningeal artery must be well-cauterized at the foramen spinosum, to avoid epidural hematomas. Epidural hematomas can also be prevented by anchoring the dura peripherally to the bone or to the periostium.

During the initial devascularization, care must be taken to avoid monopolar electrode cauterization or excessive bipolar forceps use on the middle fossa floor which could damage the cranial nerves passing through middle fossa floor foramina.

Brain edema during the pterional and subtemporal approach is the result of impaired venous drainage. This is particularly true during the subtemporal route as a result of obstruction of the venous flow in the vein of Labbè during temporal lobe retraction, already discussed in "Operative techniques" paragraph of this chapter. Moreover, brain edema can, in part, be prevented by reducing brain retraction through extensive osteotomy, adequate CSF drainage, and a correct patient positioning.

12.7 Long-term Outcome

Total excision of middle cranial base meningiomas can be achieved at most locations with a recurrence rate of 0 to 5%.[17] In cases of radical resection, there is no evidence of recurrence of MC meningiomas (type I according to Samii's classification) to date.[13]

The most advanced recurrent tumors were found in patients with inferior (caudal) transcranial regrowth through the foramina ovale or rotundum and infraorbital fissure. While many patients present clinical manifestations suggestive of tumor recurrence, almost one-third of patients are asymptomatic at the time of diagnosis.[18] Surgical removal of neoplastic hyperostosis or bone erosion is necessary to reduce the recurrence rate. Tumor regrowth may occur medially to involve the cavernous sinus, posteriorly along the petrous ridge, or inferiorly to invade the infratemporal fossa. Radiosurgery has proved to be an extremely important and valuable adjunct to the treatment of meningioma remnants or recurrences after surgery, with a very high rate of tumor control from 85 to 98% at 5 years.

12.8 Conclusion

As Cushing observed regarding meningiomas: "all said and done, it is the final result that counts, and having been brought up to believe that convalescence is shortened by attention to the technical details while the patient is on the operating table, I have no dread of a long session", the outcome of surgical treatment of middle cranial fossa meningiomas often depends on technical and time-consuming details. In the last three decades, a better understanding of microsurgical anatomy, refinements in imaging techniques and neuroanesthesia, as well as the development of innovative skull base approaches, have significantly improved the surgical management of middle cranial fossa tumors, resulting in a lower rate of mortality, morbidity, and recurrence. In addition, stereotactic radiosurgical techniques may offer more modalities for treatment and for preventing recurrences.

12.9 Acknowledgment

The authors would like to thank the illustrator, Di Santo L., for his contribution to this chapter.

References

[1] Sughrue ME, Cage T, Shangari G, Parsa AT, McDermott MW. Clinical characteristics and surgical outcomes of patients presenting with meningiomas arising predominantly from the floor of the middle fossa. Neurosurgery. 2010; 67(1):80–86, discussion 86

[2] Rhoton AL, Jr. The anterior and middle cranial base. Neurosurgery. 2002; 51(4) Suppl:S273–302

[3] Shao YX, Xie X, Liang HS, Zhou J, Jing M, Liu EZ. Microsurgical anatomy of the greater superficial petrosal nerve. World Neurosurg. 2012; 77(1):172–182

[4] Kakizawa Y, Abe H, Fukushima Y, Hongo K, El-Khouly H, Rhoton AL, Jr. The course of the lesser petrosal nerve on the middle cranial fossa. Neurosurgery. 2007; 61(3) Suppl:15–23, discussion 23

[5] Martins C, Campero A, Yasuda A, et al. Anatomical Basis of Skull Base Surgery: Skull Osteology. In: Kalangu KKN, Kato Y, Dechambenoit G, eds. Essential Practice of Neurosurgery. Nagoya: Access Publishing; 2009

[6] Muto J, Kawase T, Yoshida K. Meckel's cave tumors: relation to the meninges and minimally invasive approaches for surgery: anatomic and clinical studies. Neurosurgery. 2010; 67(3) Suppl Operative: ons291–8, discussion ons298–ons299

[7] Davies HT, Neil-Dwyer G, Evans BT, Lees PD. The zygomatico-temporal approach to the skull base: a critical review of 11 patients. Br J Neurosurg. 1992; 6(4):305–312

[8] Graziani N, Bouillot P, Dufour H, et al. Meningioma of the floor of the temporal fossa. Anatomo-clinical study of 11 cases [in French]. Neurochirurgie. 1994; 40(2):109–115

[9] Nakaguchi H, Suzuki I, Taniguchi M, et al. A case of middle cranial fossa meningioma extending into the infratemporal fossa: an approach to the pterygoid extension of the sphenoid sinus via the infratemporal fossa [in Japanese]. No Shinkei Geka. 1996; 24(7): 643–648

[10] García-Navarrete E, Sola RG. Clinical and surgical aspects of meningiomas at the base of the skull. II. Meningiomas of the middle fossa [in Spanish]. Rev Neurol. 2002; 34(7):627–637

[11] Honda M, Baba S, Kaminogo M, Tamaru N, Nagata I. Rapidly growing microcystic meningioma of the middle fossa floor. Case report. Neurol Med Chir (Tokyo). 2005; 45(6):311–314

[12] Delfini R, Innocenzi G, Ciappetta P, Domenicucci M, Cantore G. Meningiomas of Meckel's cave. Neurosurgery. 1992; 31(6):1000–1006, discussion 1006–1007

[13] Samii M, Carvalho GA, Tatagiba M, Matthies C. Surgical management of meningiomas originating in Meckel's cave. Neurosurgery. 1997; 41(4):767–774, discussion 774–775

[14] Schwartz MS, Anderson GJ, Horgan MA, Kellogg JX, McMenomey SO, Delashaw JB, Jr. Quantification of increased exposure resulting from orbital rim and orbitozygomatic osteotomy via the frontotemporal transsylvian approach. J Neurosurg. 1999; 91(6):1020–1026

[15] Savardekar AR, Goto T, Nagata T, et al. Staged 'intentional' bridging vein ligation: a safe strategy in gaining wide access to skull base tumors. Acta Neurochir (Wien). 2014; 156(4):671–679

[16] Al-Mefty O, Krisht A. The dangerous veins. In: Hakuba A, ed. Surgery of the Intracranial Venous System. New York, NY: Springer Verlag; 1996

[17] Delfini R. Management of tumors of middle fossa. In: Sindou M, ed. Practical Hanbook of Neurosurgery. New York, NY: Springer Verlag; 2009

[18] Leonetti JP, Reichman OH, Smith PG, Grubb RL, Kaiser P. Meningiomas of the lateral skull base: neurotologic manifestations and patterns of recurrence. Otolaryngol Head Neck Surg. 1990; 103(6): 972–980

13 Cerebellopontine Angle Meningiomas

Marcos Tatagiba, Toma Yuriev Spiriev, Florian H. Ebner

Abstract

The cerebellopontine angle (CPA) is the most common location of infratentorial meningiomas. Their origin in relation to the inner auditory canal (IAC) is an important landmark in their classification into five groups: (1) ventral to the IAC; (2) inside the IAC; (3) superior to the IAC; (4) inferior to the IAC; (5) posterior to the IAC. Different symptoms occur according to the location. However, frequently these meningiomas show a slow but progressive growing pattern and reach large volumes before causing signs of brainstem compression. On magnetic resonance imaging (MRI), CPA meningiomas are hypo-to isointense on T1-weighted images and show strong enhancement after contrast medium. T2-weighted images, and particularly high-resolution Constructive Interference in Steady State (CISS) sequences, depict arachnoid cleavage planes between the tumor and brainstem and detect possible areas of pial invasion.

Careful evaluation of several aspects is recommended in patient counseling. Options include follow-up with MRI, microsurgery, radiotherapy, or multimodality treatment.

Close follow-up in asymptomatic patients can be the initial treatment of choice. However, it seems that small or medium sized tumors grow more rapidly and treatment should be offered as soon as growth is documented or upon symptoms progression. The process of surgical decision making, selection of different skull base approaches as well as complication avoidance are described in detail in this chapter. The microsurgical goal is maximum safe resection with preservation of the patient's quality of life.

Keywords: cerebellopontine angle, meningioma, skull base, retrosigmoid approach, RISA, anterior petrosectomy

13.1 Introduction

Cerebellopontine angle (CPA) meningiomas comprise specific subset of tumors, which depending of their size, location, and growth pattern, can have various clinical presentations and prognosis, requiring individual approach to each patient in terms of treatment. Although infratentorial meningiomas are rare, comprising only about 10% of all intracranial meningiomas,[1] the CPA is the most common location of origin in the posterior cranial fossa, followed by the petroclival region.[2] Most of these lesions are benign, characterized by very slow growth, and only occasionally malignant histological types are found.[3,4] Meningiomas originate from arachnoid cap cells in this region and by growing, can compress and stretch cranial nerves, displace the brainstem, sometimes violating its pial plane, distort and encase vital brainstem vessels, even cause hydrocephalus. Their origin in relation to the internal acoustic canal is an important landmark in their classification in terms of surgical accessibility, choice of surgical approach, and possible risks for morbidity and mortality. According to the classification introduced by Nakamura et al, these lesions can be classified into five groups in relation to their location to the internal auditory canal[5]—anterior to the inner auditory canal (IAC) (group 1), involvement of the IAC (group 2), superior to the IAC (group 3), inferior to the IAC (group 4), posterior to the IAC, originating between the IAC and sigmoid sinus (group 5). This classification proved to be very accurate in predicting the outcome of facial and cochlear nerve function in CPA meningiomas, depending on the topographic classification of these tumors. There are other classifications of CPA meningiomas,[5,6,7,8] but we find the above mentioned the most convenient and useful in terms of surgical planning.

Historically, anterior CPA meningiomas and especially, the petroclival type had been related to higher morbidity and mortality when total removal was attempted.[7,9,10,11] In the recent years, with the advanced understanding of skull base anatomy, routine introduction of intraoperative neurophysiological monitoring techniques and advances of neuroimaging, a significant drop of mortality below 1% with notable reduced morbidity is reported.[12,13,14,15,16,17,18,19,20] On the other hand with the progress in radiosurgery,[21,22,23,24] and improvement in the understanding of the natural history of the tumors,[25,26,27,28,29] a multimodality treatment option with less aggressive surgery and a more conservative approach towards these lesions is aimed.[14,15,17]

Therefore, the decision for the treatment strategy for each particular case is very complex and numerous factors (from patient side, tumor characteristics, various treatment options including wait and see strategy, surgery, radiosurgery) have to be taken into consideration before a decision is made.

13.2 Clinical Presentation and Preoperative Evaluation

CPA meningiomas can have various presentations depending on their location, size, and aggressiveness (violation of brainstem arachnoid planes). Generally, the symptoms can be classified according to compression of cranial nerves, cerebellar signs (gait disturbance dyscoordination symptoms), brainstem symptoms (oculomotor symptoms and long tract signs), symptoms of increased intracranial pressure (ICP), and hydrocephalus. Headache is a common complain but is a nonspecific sign. Due to the indolent course of the disease symptoms and signs secondary to brain stem and cerebellar compression, are a late occurrence and often are not apparent even with very large tumors.

There is difference in the symptoms according to the location of the tumor in the CPA. If the meningioma originates posteriorly to the IAC, it manly presents with cerebellar compression, signs of cranial nerves VII and VIII deficit, and sometimes, symptoms of raised ICP. Tumors growing superior to the IAC can give symptoms of trigeminal neuralgia or numbness, due to compression of the trigeminal nerve. If the tumor is located in its main bulk inferior to the meatus, it may present with swallowing difficulties due to compression of the caudal group of cranial nerves.[12] However, in the case of petroclival meningiomas, located anteriorly to the IAC, it may have different clinical presentations. The symptoms often arise from brainstem compression, cranial nerve deficits—more often trigeminal nerve symptoms (45%) oculomotor disturbances (more often abducens nerve palsy—64%) and ataxia (37%).[30] According to Cho et al, hearing loss, facial weakness and trigeminal symptoms, gait disturbance, dysarthria, spasticity, and headache are among the predominant clinical findings in patients harboring petroclival meningiomas.[31]

More often due to very slow growth of tumor, it takes a lot of time before the diagnosis is established—between 2.5 and 4.5 years according to the literature.[7] Therefore, it is very important that proper radiological evaluation is done when a CPA tumor is suspected.

13.3 Neuroradiological Evaluation

A complete and thorough neuroradiological evaluation is essential for the correct decision-making when consulting a patient with CPA meningioma. This evaluation includes thin slice computed tomography (CT), gadolinium enhanced MRI including MRI angiography (▶ Fig. 13.1). Additional information can be obtained when using three-dimensional (3D) computed tomography angiography (CTA) and in selected cases, digital subtraction angiography (DSA).

CT is very useful for the initial diagnosis as it presents the meningioma as isodense before, and hyperdense after intravenous contrast administration. Calcification can be present, but are rare, and according to some authors, can be associated with slower growth pattern.[28,32,33] A bone erosion or hyperostosis may be present. It is generally accepted that bone hyperostosis represent tumor invasion and not reaction of the bone to the tumor. A bone window thin slice CT is useful for evaluation of the mastoid bone pneumatization and its extension over the sigmoid sinus. This is important for the planning of the extent of mastoid drilling in retrosigmoid craniotomy. The CT gives also information for the location and size of

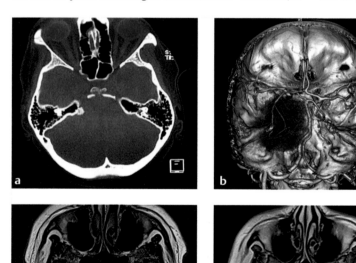

Fig. 13.1 Preoperative radiological workup. **(a)** Thin slice CT is required in order to carefully examine the petrous bone anatomy and pneumatization. This is important in retrosigmoid approaches (location and size of the sigmoid sinus as well as mastoid emissary veins) as well for transpetrosal approaches. Note the hyperostotic bone on the suprameatal tubercle caused by the meningioma. **(b)** CT angiography can give essential information about the displacement of the vessels by the tumor. Using software such as OsiriX software (Pixmeo, Bernex, Switzerland), a three-dimensional volumetric reconstruction can be created representing a large petroclival meningioma (this is an overlay of two images). Note the displacement of the superior cerebellar artery and basilar artery by the tumor; **(c and d)** T1 contrast enhanced and T2-weighted MRI are very useful in examination of the tumor/brainstem interface and to estimate the arachnoid plane allowing safe surgical dissection.

the mastoid emissary veins, size and anatomy of the sigmoid sinus, location and size of the jugular bulb. If transpetrous approaches are planned, the bone CT provide information for the pneumatization of the mastoid and petrous apex, proximity of the labyrinthine block to the IAC, location of the cochlea, course of the fallopian canal, size of the presigmoid space (▶ Fig. 13.1a).

In some cases, 3D CTA can give additional information for the displacement or encasement (such as anterior inferior cerebellar artery or superior cerebellar artery) of the major brainstem vessels from the meningioma.[34,35] Meningiomas can be very vascular tumors and will be very well-presented on a CTA. Some modern programs with 3D rendering capabilities, like Osirix (Pixmeo, Bern Switzerland) or Horos, could be used for preoperative planning in order to volumetrically present the tumor and bony structures as well the displaced vessels[36,37,38,39] (▶ Fig. 13.1b). Another important feature for the CTA is that it can very well present the associated venous anatomy including the dominance of the transverse and sigmoid sinuses, size of the jugular bulb, superior and inferior petrosal sinuses, and temporal lobe drainage pattern.

The diagnostic method of choice for the evaluation of CPA meningioma is the MRI with and without gadolinium contrast enhancement. The MRI examination most often reveals an isointense or hyperintense lesion on T1-weighted imaging, which is heterogeneous on T2-weighted imaging. The MRI T1-weighted modality (with and without contrast) is useful for evaluation of the size of the tumor, its location, and displacement of the neural structures. The MRI T2-weighted modality is very informative about arachnoid cleavage planes between the tumor/brainstem, possible areas of pial invasion (a high-intensity signal in the brainstem noted on T2-weighted imaging is typical of peritumoral edema due to brainstem pial transgression), relation to the cranial nerves, major vessels, and tentorium (▶ Fig. 13.1c). The flow voids on the MRI-T2 modality can indicate vessel displacement or encasement by the tumor, associated venous anatomy (venous sinuses size and variation). MRI venography can be very informative about the sigmoid sinus dominance and anatomy, vein of Labbé size and location, which is important information for the planning of a transpetrous approach.

Advanced techniques such 3 Tesla MRI CISS (high T2 sequences) sequence provide much more details regarding the arachnoid plane between the tumor/brain interface, as well as the cranial nerve displacement and involvement in the tumor. Diffusion tensor imaging (DTI) could be used to present some of the important brain circuitry (pyramidal tracts, pontocerebellar fibers within the brachium pontis), as well as cranial nerves (V, VII), displaced by the tumor.

DSA is less frequently used nowadays given the diagnostic efficacy of noninvasive magnetic resonance angiography and venography, as well as the 3D CTA. DSA is only planed if tumor embolization will be attempted.

The CPA meningiomas are supplied by the tentorial artery of Bernasconi-Cassinari clone of meningohypophyseal trunk), posterior branch of the middle meningeal artery, meningeal branch of the vertebral artery, petrosal branches of the meningeal arteries, and ascending pharyngeal branches of the external carotid artery.[12,40] These arteries can be used in selected patients for preoperative embolization in order to decrease the intraoperative blood loss that often obscures the intraoperative view and makes the surgery even more challenging. Most authors agree that in order to have a clinical benefit complete or near complete embolization of the tumor feeders have to be achieved,[41,42,43] which is not always possible. Another important point is the timing of surgery after the embolization. One of the arguments for early surgery after embolization is the tumor swelling secondary to its necrosis, which is not always the case. More recent series advocate for delayed surgery after 24 hours.[42,43] Nevertheless, the embolization is an invasive procedure and is not without risks. Major complications of embolization include stroke, blindness, retroperitoneal hemorrhage, and cranial nerve palsies with estimated incidence between 0 and 16% of cases.[43,44,45]

In our experience, we rarely use preoperative embolization in case CPA of meningiomas. Intraoperative blood loss can usually be compensated, and the problem with blood filling the operative field is avoided with the use of semi-sitting position.[46]

13.4 Patient Evaluation and Decision-making

For selection of the appropriate treatment modality in each case, it is mandatory to understand the natural history,[25,26,27] take into consideration patient age and comorbidities, preoperative predictive factors indicating the degree of safe resection and radiological finding pointing the risks for postoperative complications,[47,48] as well as the results of radiosurgery.[21,22,23,24] Historically speaking, the natural history of these tumors was once associated with progressive neurological worsening and was ultimately fatal prognosis.[49,50] At present with the modern diagnostic tools, there is much better possibility for close follow-up of the patients and better estimate the degree of growth rate. A cooperative retrospective study of 21 untreated patients diagnosed with petroclival meningiomas, with clinical and radiological (MRI) follow-up, ranged from 4 to 10 years (mean, 82 months; median, 85 months) has shown radiological tumor growth in 76% of the cases.[26] With 63% of the growing tumors, there was functional deterioration. According to the authors of the study the mean growth rates were 1.16 mm/year in diameter and 1.10 cm³/year in volume. Rapid growth spurts were documented in small and medium-sized tumors. Moreover, a change in growth pattern preceded functional deterioration.

Another study by Tatasaka et al[27] followed 15 patients (median follow-up period was 40 months) diagnosed with petroclival meningiomas. Sixty percent of the cases showed radiological tumor growth during the follow-up period. There was functional deterioration in 47% of the cases.

A recent study by Hunter et al[29] volumetrically studied 34 untreated patients with petroclival meningiomas using consecutive MRI. The mean follow-up was 44.5 months. According to the results, 88.2% showed progressive growth, with estimated mean annual volumetric growth rate of 2.38 cm/year (−0.63 to 25.9 cm/year). Tumor volume, T2 hyperintensity within the tumor, peritumoral edema, and ataxia and/or cerebellar symptoms at presentation were all significantly associated with greater rates of tumor growth.

Therefore, these results suggest that untreated tumors show progressive growth over time and close follow-up in asymptomatic patients have to be the initial treatment of choice. However, it seems that small or medium sized tumors grow more rapidly and treatment should be offered when there is documented growth or upon symptoms progression.

In case of symptomatic patient, treatment modality vary from surgery alone, radiosurgery or combination from surgery and radiosurgery for the tumor remnant. Taking in mind the data from natural history of the disease, a possible treatment strategy would be surgical resection for younger and healthy patients and focused beam radiation therapy (stereotactic radiosurgery or radiotherapy) for elderly patients or unhealthy patients who cannot undergo surgery. Radiotherapy could be used as single treatment option for small tumors (< 3 cm). However, there are known complications from radiosurgery[51,52,53,54] and with the advances of modern microsurgical techniques and intraoperative monitoring, some authors advocate excision even for small CPA and petroclival meniniomas.[18,19]

If surgical treatment is the choice of approach, there are numerous factors that have to be taken into consideration in order to predict surgical resectability and possible complications including peritumoral edema, presence of nourishing pial vessels, age of the patient, location of the tumor, duration of symptoms, preoperative neurological status, vessel encasement, tumor size, presence and severity of the associated hydrocephalus, and comorbid conditions, such as hypertension and diabetes mellitus.[47,48,55,56] There are several proposed grading scales used in the evaluation of for the surgical risks in skull base meningiomas.

Sekhar et al[48] studied multiple preoperative variables such as preoperative Karnofsky scale score, previous radiosurgery, preoperative radiological findings, intraoperative findings and correlated them to postoperative outcome at early and late follow-up. Statistical analysis revealed significant correlations between early functional deterioration and preoperative Karnofsky scale scores,

absence of an arachnoid cleavage plane, between tumor and brainstem, edema of the brainstem, and direct blood supply from the basilar artery. Permanent functional deterioration was statistically associated with feeding from the basilar artery, tumor size, incomplete tumor resection, and early postoperative dysfunction. The authors proposed three stages of tumor relationship to the brainstem arachnoid and pial membranes: Stage 1 tumors show preservation of the arachnoid plane, presented as a high-intensity band between the meningioma and the brainstem on T2-weighted MRI. In stage 2 tumors, the arachnoid plane is lost, presented by absence of the high-intensity band between tumor and the brainstem on T2-weighted MRI. In stage 3 tumors, the pial membrane is violated and the arachnoid cleavage plane is absent, with presence of brainstem edema depicted on the MRI as hyperintensity signal on the T2-weighted images. In this stage, the dissection of the tumor from the brainstem can cause damage of the latter and injury of the basilar artery perforators which supply the pial brainstem surface.[47,48]

Based on the results of their study, the authors recommend that patients with small or medium size tumors should be offered treatment, due to the higher chance for postoperative worsening in large and giant tumors. Another important recommendation is that in case of brainstem pial invasion of the tumor, a subtotal or near total resection is warranted, because of higher chance of postoperative deterioration.

Other authors have also examined the risk factors associated with resection of skull base and particularly CPA meningiomas and devised a useful scale (the "ABC surgical risk scale") to predict the postoperative outcome and the possible degree of resection.[47] The authors identified five major variables in order to properly predicts the extent of tumor removal and postoperative neurological changes: (1) tumor attachment size; (2) arterial involvement; (3) brainstem contact; (4) central cavity location; and (5) cranial nerve group involvement.

These scoring scales as well the data from the natural history would help choosing the correct treatment approach for the patent.

In our experience, an important factor is tumor consistency. Firm and calcified tumors can be more difficult to dissect, with greater risk for postoperative cranial nerve deficit, compared to soft and aspirable tumors.

13.5 Preoperative Surgical Planning and Complication Avoidance

If the patient is selected for surgery, there are several factors that have to be considered in order to decrease the risk for morbidity and mortality. The detail preoperative clinical and radiological workup would reveal important factors for planning of the surgical strategy: location, extension, and size of the tumor, presence or absence of hydrocephalus, brainstem edema, tumor associated hyperostosis, venous anatomy, as well as patient age comorbidities, patent foramen ovale, preoperative hearing and facial nerve function, and surgeon's preference.[11,12,14,15,16,17,18,20,46,57,58,59,60,61,62,63]

Preoperative brain edema and hydrocephalus are factors that could potentially increase the complications rate and have to be managed before surgery. In case of severe brain edema, the patient has to be loaded preoperatively with dexamethasone (8 mg intravenously initially followed by 4 mg every 8 hours). It takes approximately 13 to 18 hours before the dexamethasone takes effect; therefore, this regiment has to be started several days before the operation.[64]

Obstructive hydrocephalus may present in case of very large tumors. Management options include preoperative ventriculoperitoneal (VP) shunt placement, endoscopic third ventriculostomy (ETV), temporary external ventricular drainage. We do not recommend preoperative insertion of ventriculoperitoneal shunt, due to potential infection, as well as potential postoperative hemorrhagic complications after surgery of the tumor itself. According to our experience, successful removal of the tumor usually manages the hydrocephalus and placement of permanent VP shunt can be avoided in most cases. ETV is a minimally invasive option for the management of obstructive hydrocephalus caused by the tumor.[65,66,67,68] An alternative is the external ventricular drain with possibility of monitoring intracranial pressure. Lumbar puncture has to be avoided due to the risk of tonsillar herniation.

If sitting or semi-sitting position is planned, preoperative echocardiography excludes a patent foramen ovale, is the main part of the diagnostic workup.[46]

Careful review of the radiological data in order to examine petrous bone pneumatization, associated venous anatomy, 3D volumetric reconstructions of the from the CTA data, tumor vascularity origin, presence or absence of hyperostosis have to be done in order to properly plan the surgical approach. (*See neuroradiological examination for more details.*)

13.6 Surgical Approaches

There are various surgical approaches designed for the treatment of CPA meningiomas.[7,10,11,12,13,14,16,17,18,20,48,57,60,63,69,70,71,72,73,74,75] General principles are adequate bony exposure, early eradication of vascular supply, tumor debulking, maintenance of the arachnoid plane between the neurovascular structures and avoidance of dissection where the tumor has violated the pial brainstem surface. Depending on the location and size of the tumor, there are several approaches that can be used. The transpetrosal

approaches can be subdivided into anterior (Kawase) approach, posterior–presigmoid retrolabyrinthine, translabyrinthine, transcochlear approaches, and combined petrosal approach. A variation of the retrosigmoid approach, the trans- and suprameatal type can also be included in the transpetrous approaches.

In order to better illustrate the area of the skull base that can be reached with the different petrosal approaches the clivus is divided into following zones (▶ Fig. 13.2)[12]:

- Zone I extend from the upper border of the dorsum sellae to the internal acoustic canal and is the area that can be reached using the anterior petrosectomy approach.
- Zone II extend from the IAC to jugular tubercle and is the area reachable by posterior petrosal approaches. Tumors involving both zone I and zone II require a combined petrosal approach.
- Zone III extends from the jugular tubercle to the lower edge of the clivus and is an area that can be reached by the lateral suboccipital-transcondylar approaches.

There are advantages and disadvantages of one or the other approach. The advantages of the transpetrous approaches are that they offer a more lateral and oblique angle of view toward the clivus and decrease brain retraction.

On the other hand, one of the main disadvantages of the transpetrous approaches is that they have higher morbidity due to the approach itself [cerebrospinal fluid (CSF) leaks, cranial nerve injuries, vascular complications] and they are time-consuming.

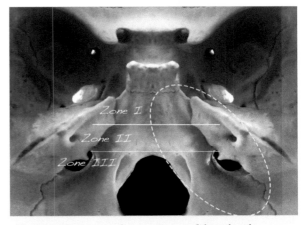

Fig. 13.2 Clivus zones demarcation, useful to plan the approach.[6] Zone I: Accessible through anterior petrosectomy; Zone II: Accessible through posterior petrosectomy; Zone III: Accessible through far lateral transcondylar approach. The combined petrosal approach allows exposure of zones I and II. The dashed area marks the area that is reachable with the retrosigmoid approach as well as its supratentorial extension (retrosigmoid intradural suprameatal approach).

According to our experience, most of the CPA meningiomas can be resected via the classic retrosigmoid approach or in combination with the suprameatal drilling [retrosigmoid intradural suprameatal approach (RISA)] gaining access to the petrous apex[5,11,20,60,61,62,63,74,76] (▶ Fig. 13.2, dashed area). The retrosigmoid approach offers a straight view to the whole CPA (from IIIrd to XIIth cranial nerve)[77] and in most cases, the medial clivus area can be reached owing to the displacement of the brainstem by the tumor. Moreover the RISA, with drilling of the petrous apex and splitting of the tentorium, provides additional exposure to the posterior part of the middle fossa.[60,61,72,73,74,78,79]

13.6.1 Anterior Petroesectomy Approach

The anterior petrosectomy approach is used for the treatment of petroclival meningomas arising at the petrous apex, but not extending below the VII/VIII nerve group (below the IAC) (▶ Fig. 13.2—Zone I). This is basically a subtemporal extradural middle fossa approach, where one exposes the Meckel's cave, lifts the trigeminal nerve and drills the petrous apex to the inferior petrosal sinus, up to the posterior fossa dura. This is followed by opening of the posterior and middle fossa dura, splitting of the tentorium and combining the two fossae.[70,80,81,82,83] One of the advantages of this approach is that it allows for early devascularization of the meningiomas because most of their blood supply originates from vessels traversing the petrous bone and the tentorium.

For each case, we use advanced electrophysiological monitoring including somatosensory evoked potentials (SEPs), motor evoked potentials (MEPs), facial nerve motor evoked potentials (FMEPs), direct intraoperative cranial nerve stimulation, auditory evoked potentials (AEPs), and electromyography (EMG)/MEP of the cranial nerve VII and the lower cranial nerves.

For antibiotic preoperative administration, we use second or third generation cephalosporin. Additionally, mannitol 1 g/kg and dexamethasone 20 mg is given before the skin incision to achieve maximum brain relaxation. Preoperative lumbar drain is placed in order to decrease temporal lobe retraction.

The patient is positioned supine on the operative table with the head fixed on a Mayfield pin-holder and rotated 45° towards the opposite shoulder, so as the zygomatic arch is the highest point of the operative field and the sagittal suture is parallel to the floor. Alternatively, in elderly patients with stiff and spondylotic cervical spine, the lateral position can be chosen.

We use a straight skin incision with minimal hair shave (▶ Fig. 13.3a). The incision starts from the root of the

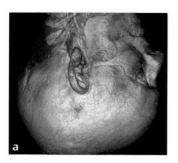
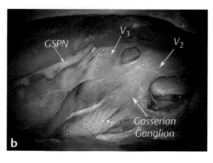
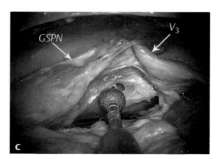
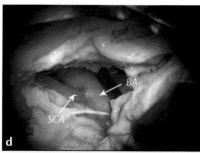
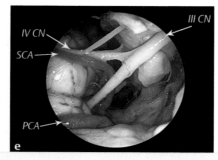

Fig. 13.3 Anterior petrosectomy approach. (a) 3D reconstruction using OsiriX software (Pixmeo, Bernex, Switzerland). This is an overlay of two images. A straight skin incision is used starting from the root of the zygoma to the linea temporalis superior. (b) Image representing middle fossa anatomy after the dura is elevated. (c) The V3 and Gasserian ganglion are displaced in order to expose the true petrous ridge. (d) The petrous apex is removed, the posterior fossa dura as well as the temporal dura are opened and the tentorium is divided. The basilar artery as well as the superior cerebellar artery are visible. (e) Endoscopic view of the approach demonstrating the third, fourth cranial nerves and the associated vessels. Note that the tentorium is sectioned before the dural entrance of the fourth cranial nerves (anatomical dissections made by Dr. Luigi Rigante). BA, basilar artery; GSPN, greater superficial petrosal nerve; PCA, posterior cerebellar artery; SCA, superior cerebellar artery.

zygomatic arch reaching 2 cm above the superior temporal line The dissection is made in anatomical layers. Care should be taken to preserve the superficial temporal artery (STA), which runs in the temporoparietal fascia, just below the skin.[84] Therefore, only the frontal or parietal branch of the artery have to be divided and the trunk is usually preserved.

The temporalis muscle fascia is incised using scalpel or scissors, not electrocautery, in order to be able to adequately close the fascia at the end of the surgery. The temporalis muscle is incised along the same line as the skin incision and retrograde muscle dissection is used, preserving the deep temporalis muscle fascia along with muscle blood supply and innervation.[85] The latter maneuver would potentially decrease the postoperative temporalis muscle atrophy.

A craniotomy centered over the root of the zygoma approximately 5/5 cm in size (below the superior temporal line) is done. After elevation of the bone flap, the remaining bone at the inferior end of the craniotomy is drilled until is flushed with the middle fossa floor. Some authors recommend dropping the zygomatic arch (left attached to the masseter muscle) in order to increase the exposure.[83] In our opinion, this is seldom necessary and adds additional morbidity to the approach. One of the main factors in this stage is preservation of the integrity of the dura.

The next step is extradural dissection and exposure of the middle fossa floor (▶ Fig. 13.3b). Dural elevation from back to front is recommended, which is aimed to preserve the greater superficial petrosal nerve (GSPN). This nerve emerges from its respective foramen just in front of the arcuate eminence and is a direct branch of the facial nerve (geniculate ganglion) between its labyrinthine and tympanic segments. It provides innervation to the lacrimal gland and its lesion results in dry eye.

After elevation of the dura from back to front, first the arcuate eminence and then GSPN are identified. The GSPN is followed anteriorly towards foramen spinosum (middle meningeal artery) and foramen ovale (V3 branch of the trigeminal nerve). Neuromonitoring plays essential role in this step of the operation—using monopolar stimulation probe at low intensity (0.1–0.3 mA), the geniculate ganglion can be identified on the petrous bone surface. Sometimes, it is difficult to differentiate the V3 entrance to the foramen ovale. With the help of the monopolar probe, the nerve can be directly stimulated and the contractions of the temporalis muscle are visible. Alternatively, for orientation over the middle fossa floor, the neuronavigation can be used. At some cases, dehiscence over the petrous bone are present and the petrous (C2) segment of the carotid artery can be seen laying just below the GSPN.

The transition zone between the periosteal and endosteal dural layers is the place to start the elevation of temporal dura from the dura propria of the lateral wall of the cavernous sinus and exposure of the Meckel's cave.[31,86]

The dissection and elevation of the dura is continued medially towards the superior petrosal sinus and the petrous ridge anteriorly. In order to expose the true petrous ridge, the Gasserian ganglion and V3 have to be gently lifted from the petrous bone.[87,88] At this stage, occasional bradycardia can be expected due to the occurrence of the trigeminocardiac reflex.[89,90] In such cases, temporary halt of the surgical activity usually resolves the symptoms.

The boundaries of the bone resection of the anterior petrosectomy (Kawase's triangle or more precisely quadrilateral) are the GSPN lateral, V3 anterior, superior petrosal sinus medial, and the arcuate eminence (harboring the superior semicircular canal) posterior (▶ Fig. 13.3c).[70,80] The location of the IAC can be found using the neuronavigation or can be estimated as a line bisecting a 120° angle between the GSPN and the arcuate eminence.[70,82] Drilling is started over the estimated position of the IAC. Care is taken not to damage the superior semicircular canal or the cochlea at the cochlear angle.[91,92,93,94] Drilling of the IAC continues to the Bill's bar, a small bone crest separating the facial from the superior vestibular nerve. After that the drilling is continued in anteromedial direction to the superior petrosal sinus until the posterior fossa dura is exposed.[12] The inferior limit of the drilling is the inferior petrosal sinus. The lateral limit of the drilling is the GSPN and petrous carotid artery.

After the drilling is completed, the temporal lobe dura is incised parallel to the superior petrosal sinus. The temporal lobe is gently lifted and the brain spatula is advanced to the ambient cistern, which is opened in order to evacuate CSF and achieve further brain relaxation. The trochlear nerve is identified at its point where it pierces the tentorium.

The next step is the tentorium splitting, which have to be done behind the dural entrance of the trochlear nerve. The superior petrosal sinus has to be ligated. The bleeding encountered during this maneuver can be controlled with bipolar coagulation, hemostatic sponge, or by injecting a small amount of fibrin glue onto the sinus bleeding edges.[95] The posterior fossa dura is also opened and the trigeminal nerve is visualized at its exit point from the brainstem. After completion of the dural and tentorial opening, one can have a wide view of the space between the IIIrd cranial nerve to the VIIth/VIIIth nerve complex, with the trigeminal nerve in the center of the surgical exposure (from the brainstem to the Meckel's cave) ▶ Fig. 13.3d, e.

As a general rule, safe removal of CPA meningioma requires extensive surgical debulking using microsurgical technique and ultrasonic aspirator first, which will decrease the volume of the tumor and allow for safer arachnoid dissection. Care has to be taken to identify and preserve the cranial nerves and respect the arachnoid layers which guide the dissection. Constant cooperation with the neurophysiological team is crucial for the safety of the surgery.

After completion of the surgical resection, measures have to be taken to assure adequate dural closure. For the purpose, we use temporalis fascia or pericranium as an onlay graft for closure of the posterior fossa. We place a fat graft in the petrous bone defect and a layer of fibrin glue. The dura is lifted to the bone with tack up sutures. A central tenting suture to the bone flap is placed.

The bone flap is repositioned. The soft tissues are closed in layers. No subgaleal drainage is used as to avoid CSF leaks. A compressive head wrap is applied. The spinal drain is removed at the end of the surgery.

13.7 Posterior and Combined Petrosal Approaches

Posterior petrosal approaches can be divided into retrolabyrinthine or translabyrinthine exposure depending on the preoperative hearing status of the patient and if the labyrinth is to be preserved during surgery. It is a combination with small posterior temporal craniotomy and mastoidectomy, which exposes the sigmoid sinus, superior petrosal sinus, presigmoid space. The combined petrosal approach incorporates the temporal craniotomy with possibility of adding anterior petrosectomy, with any of the posterior petrosal approaches, as well as transcochlear approach (▶ Fig. 13.4).

13.7.1 Retrolabyrinthine Approach

The patient is placed supine. Neuromonitoring settings including SEP, MEP, FMEP, direct intraoperative cranial nerve stimulation, AEP and EMG/MEP of the cranial nerve VII and the lower cranial nerves are used. A slightly curvilinear skin incision is made from level of the pinna of the ear, curving towards the projection of the asterion and reaching the mastoid tip (▶ Fig. 13.4a) The skin/galeal flap is elevated as a separate layer. Then the muscles are incised to the bone, at the same line as the skin incision, creating a muscle-fascial flap, which is very important for watertight fascial closure at the end of the surgery. The flap is elevated until the Henle's spine is seen (landmark for the mastoid antrum). The visible bony landmarks that make the boundaries of the mastoidectomy approach are the root of the zygoma, asterion, and mastoid tip.

The first step is the cortical mastoidectomy, with the boundaries described above. In order to create more space for sigmoid sinus mobilization, the bone behind the sinus is also removed. The bone opening is gradually widened. For the initial part of the approach, a large cutting drill bit is used. Advancing towards the sinus, the drill bit is changed to large diamond drill. Using larger drill is safer, because it has a wider working area and decreases the risk of inadvertent sinus injury.

The mastoid emissary veins can be important landmark for the location of the sinus. The bleeding from the

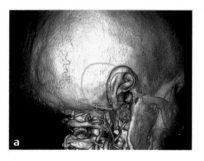
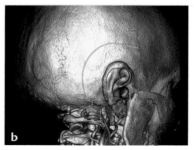
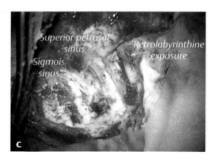
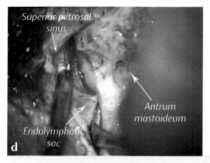
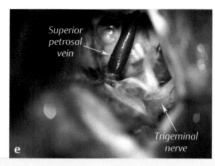

Fig. 13.4 Posterior and combined petrosal approaches. (a) The skin incision used for retrolabyrinthine and translabyrinthine approach. **(b)** The skin incision utilized for the combined petrosal approach. **(c)** Right combined petrosal approach in semi-sitting position. The temporal as well as posterior fossa dura are visible. The sigmoid as well as the superior petrosal sinuses are identified. Retrolabyrinthine exposure is done and the bone is removed until the endolymphatic sac is reached. **(d)** Retrolabyrinthine exposure is done and the bone is removed until the endolymphatic sac is reached. **(e)** Intradural exposure after sectioning of the tentorium. The petrosal vein as well as the trigeminal nerve are visible.

mastoid emissary veins is controlled by bone wax. Another option is to skeletonize the vein and coagulate it close to the sinus. Drilling over the sigmoid sinus has to be done very carefully. The sinus wall is thinner than the other sinuses and can be injured during bone removal, if care is not taken. We thin out the bone by diamond drill and leave only a small amount of bone over the sinus that can be removed with dissector.[96]

Dura of the presigmoid space and middle fossa is dissected and gradually revealed by drilling. The sigmoid, transverse, and superior petrosal sinuses intersection, named the Citelli's angle is identified. It is an important landmark during the dissection as it points to where the sigmoid sinus intersects the middle fossa dura.[97] The jugular bulb is positioned medial to the cortical bone overlying the mastoid digastric groove. The position of the jugular bulb and its variation (high jugular bulb) can be estimated on the preoperative CT scans.

There are two very important landmarks during drilling—the lateral semicircular canal (which is positioned above the tympanic segment of the facial nerve) and the spine of Henle which marks the position for the mastoid antrum. The floor of the antrum is the cortical bone of the lateral semicircular canal.

After removal of the superficial mastoid air cells, the antrum mastoideum and the compact bone of the labyrinth are reached. The space revealed posteriorly by the wall of the sigmoid sinus, superiorly by the tegmen tympani, and anteriorly by the prominence of the posterior and lateral semicircular canal is called the Trautmann's triangle.[97] This is the presigmoid dural space that is the surgical access to the CPA and anterior surface of the cerebellum. Above the prominence of the lateral semicircular canal, the antrum mastoideum communicates with the tympanic cavity. Reaching the antrum, mastoideum exposes the incus bone (▶ Fig. 13.1a).

It is very important during the dissection to identify the fallopian canal, where the mastoid segment of the facial nerve runs. Anatomically the genu of the facial nerve (tympanic segment) is just inferior to the lateral semicircular canal. Another landmark is the position of the incus, which short process points to the tympanic segment of the facial nerve.[97] A guide for the depth of drilling and distance to the nerve can be the monopolar stimulation probe of the neurophysiological monitoring. The depth towards the nerve decreases with the decrease of the level of the mA used to initiate nerve stimulus.

If a retrolabyrinthine approach is selected, the semicircular canals are not opened. After exposure of the Trautmann's triangle, the dura of the presigmoid space is incised parallel to the sigmoid sinus and along the superior petrosal sinus. Care is taken not to injure the vein of Labbé, which enters the superior petrosal sinus close to its junction with the sigmoid sinus. Preoperative evaluation of the venous anatomy is essential in order to preserve the Labbé vein and avoid postoperative venous

infarctions. The tentorium is incised perpendicular to the superior petrosal sinus in length of 3 cm, then medially parallel to the transverse sinus for additional 3 cm. This maneuver allows a wide exposure of the cerebellum separating it from the posterior aspect of the temporal lobe like "opening a book."[18] The tentorium incision is continued anterior to the entrance point of the IV nerve. This approach allows for exposure of the petroclival area from the III to VII/VIII cranial nerve complex. The trigeminal nerve is usually displaced posteriorly and superior.

13.7.2 Translabyrinthine Approach

This approach is indicated in patients with loss of hearing function. The exposure is similar to the one described for the retrolabyrinthine approach, however, it includes total labyrinthectomy.

The labyrinth is composed of the lateral, posterior, and superior semicircular canals. The anterior end of the superior canal projects upward below the arcuate eminence. The posterior canal faces the posterior fossa dura. The lateral canal is positioned above the tympanic segment of the facial nerve.[97] The posterior and superior semicircular canals join together to form the common crus. The latter with the lateral semicircular canal opening form the vestibule. The vestibule is the bone cavity that harbors the soft tissue part of the labyrinth utricle and saccule. Through the aperture of the vestibular aqueduct runs the endolymphatic duct that connects the utricle to the endolymphatic sac. The endolymphatic sac sits beneath the dura on the posterior surface of the temporal bone above and medial to the lower part of the sigmoid sinus.

In the translabyrinthine approach, first the lateral semicircular canal is drilled away followed by the posterior and superior canals to their entrance in the vestibule. A thin shell of bone is preserved over the facial nerve and the fallopian canal is not opened. After removing all three semicircular canals, the vestibule reached. Upon its removal, the area in the saccule marks the most lateral extent of the internal auditory meatus.[96] Adding labyrinthectomy to the approach will increase the exposure with about 1.5 cm, allowing for better visualization of the midline structures. Some authors recommend a partial labyrinthectomy, with removal of only the superior and a posterior semicircular canals with the so called "transcrucial approach."[97] This approach is made in an attempt of hearing preservation.

13.7.3 Combined Petrosal Approach

This approach includes a combination of temporal craniotomy with addition of retrolabyrinthine or translabyrinthine approach.[98,99] We use the semi-sitting position with the head tilted 30° to the side of the lesion is used. The extensive electrophysiological monitoring, as described for the previous approaches, is also utilized. A skin incision starting 2 cm above and anterior to the ear then curving down in a linear fashion posterior to the mastoid tip is made (▶ Fig. 13.4b). A vascularized fascia/temporalis muscle flap, used later for watertight closure, is reflected anteriorly and inferiorly. The bony landmarks—root of zygoma, asterion, Henle's spine, and mastoid tip are identified. We prefer to do the craniotomy first, then the mastoidectomy. A burr-hole is made over the asterion and a trough is created using the drill, over the mastoid bone, exposing the transverse-sigmoid junctions and medial edge of the sigmoid sinus. Then, a combined suboccipital and temporal craniotomy flap is tailored. The next step is to add a retrolabyrinthine or translabyrinthine exposure, depending on the case (▶ Fig. 13.4c). If a retrolabyrinthine approach is chosen and hearing is to be preserved, care should be taken not to enter the endolymphatic duct, or the labyrinth (▶ Fig. 13.4d, e).[100] The dura incision is carried in a T-fashion, along the superior petrosal sinus and sigmoid sinus. The temporal lobe is retracted superiorly with care to preserve the vein of Labbé. The superior petrosal sinus is ligated and transected to the free margin of the tentorium, behind the entrance of the trochlear nerve. The tumor is removed as previously described.

13.7.4 Closure of Posterior and Combined Petrosal Approaches

Meticulous closure at the end of the surgery is very important in order to avoid postoperative CSF leak complications. The T-shaped dural incision, described here for most of the cases allows for closure of the dura. Otherwise temporalis fascia or pericranium can be used. We do not recommend the use of artificial dural subsites, due to higher risk of infections.[101,102] The antrum mastoideum is plugged with a piece of muscle and sealed with fibrin glue. The mastoidectomy cavity is filled with abdominal fat graft and secured with additional fibrin glue and the vascularized muscle/fascia flap is placed over the opened air cells. Cranioplasty using bone cement is done to avoid cosmetic deformity. The skin is closed in layers.

The disadvantages of these approaches are that they are time-consuming and carry an increased risk of facial nerve palsy, hearing loss (in case of translabyrinthine approach), CSF fistula, and vein of Labbé injury. We rarely use the translabyrinthine or retrolabyrinthine approach as a single surgical exposure. In selected cases, we use the combined subtemporal presigmoid approach.

13.8 Retrosigmoid Approach for the Treatment of Cerebellopontine Angle Meningiomas

The retrosigmoid approach offers a fast and direct surgical corridor to lesions located in the CPA and petroclival

area, with low approach-related morbidity.[20,60,61,62,63,73,74,76,78] With gradual training, this approach can be safely performed by senior residents.[76] This approach can be extended inferiorly to foramen magnum through C1 hemilaminectomy or superiorly through the RISA.[103] Intradural extensions include transmeatal to IAC and inframeatal to the jugular foramen.

For small CPA meningiomas, we use the supine position with the head turned to the contralateral shoulder. For most CPA meningiomas, including the petroclival type, we prefer the semi-sitting position, which offers the advantages of spontaneous drainage of CSF and blood, bimanual dissection with fine forceps, minimal use of bipolar coagulation (which diminishes the risks of the associated morbidity), while the assistant constantly irrigates the operative field (the so-called "three-hands technique").[20,61,62,78,79,103]

Extensive neurophysiological monitoring is used in every case, which include bilateral AEP SEPs, MEPs, FMEPs, direct intraoperative facial nerve stimulation, AEPs, and EMG/MEP of the cranial nerve VII and the lower cranial nerves. A transesophageal echocardiography for immediate detection of air embolism is inserted. After the neurophysiological monitoring is set, the patient is placed in the semi-sitting position. Electrophysiological monitoring of SEP can decrease complications related to positioning (extensive head rotation or flexion with compression of the spinal cord, due to degenerative spinal changes). Any changes in the latency and amplitude can indicate that the head position has to be corrected.[103]

The head is secured on the three-point skull clamp. A single pin is placed on the lesion side at the level of the linea temporalis superior and the paired pins over the linea temporalis superior on the contralateral side. The operative table is bent forwards and the legs are raised above the level of the heart, which further reduces the risks of inadvertent air embolism and facilitates better venous return (▶ Fig. 13.5a). The head is fixed on the Mayfield skull clamp with the following order: extension, ante-position, rotation (30°), flexion.[75,79,103] Thus, the mastoid is the most prominent point of the surgical field. The anesthesiologist checks whether the lateral neck is accessible on both sides for jugular vein compression during the operation. A properly secured patient positioning is a team effort and when done in a routine manner, it offers very low complication rates in terms of venous air embolism, vascular complications, or position related neurologic compromise.[46,79]

The skin incision is centered over the anatomical projection of the asterion, two fingers behind the pinna of the ear and extending 1 cm below the mastoid tip (▶ Fig. 13.5a). The dissection is made in anatomical layers with respect of the lesser and greater occipital nerve. Neck muscles are divided in line with the skin incision and spread with a cerebellar retractor. Bleeding from the

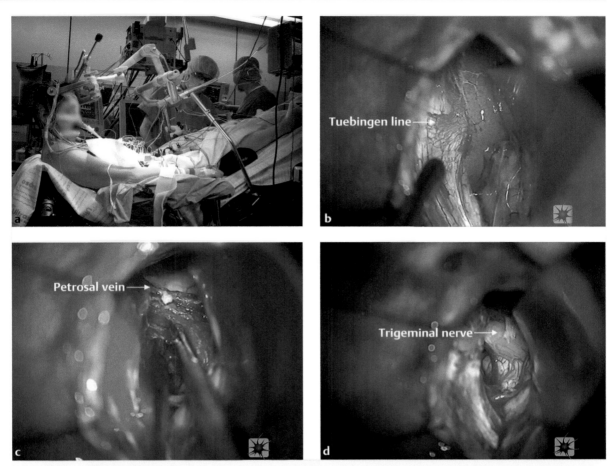

Fig. 13.5 Retrosigmoid approach. (a) Semi-sitting position and skin incision. **(b, c, d)** Removal of a cerebellopontine angle meningioma located superior to the IAC. The Tuebingen line is a landmark for the location of the IAC. The tumor is removed in a piecemeal fashion with aim to preserve the petrosal veins. (Reproduced from Campero, A, Martins C, Rhoton A Jr, Tatagiba M. Dural landmark to locate the internal auditory canal in large and giant vestibular schwannomas: the Tubingen line. Neurosurgery 2011; 69(1 Suppl Operative): p. ons99–102; discussion ons102.)

occipital artery and emissary veins is controlled by bipolar coagulation. Subperiosteal muscle elevation is done until the relevant bony landmarks are exposed—the asterion, mastoid tip, and digastric groove. During this step, the surgeon has to be aware of air embolism due to patent emissary veins. A jugular vein compression is carried out by the anesthesiologist and any opened bony canal that becomes visible is closed with bone wax.[79] Care should be taken also at the inferior pole of dissection at the passage from the vertical to the horizontal part of the occipital bone around the arch of C1, where the V3 segment of the vertebral artery is located. The vertebral artery can be with variable anatomy in this location (passing through a bone channel, surrounded by a bone ring, or located higher over the occipital bone), so care have to be taken during the dissection in order to avoid its injury.[104] A burr hole is placed just below the asterion which usually exposes the lower edge of sigmoid transverse junction and constitutes the superolateral limit of

the craniectomy.[105] Then, a second burr hole is placed just below the first one and a craniectomy is performed The bone over the sigmoid sinus is removed using rongeurs and a larger diamond drill until the medial edge of the sinus is reached. The extent of bone removal to the sigmoid sinus is estimated on the preoperative CT scan. Any opened mastoid air cells are closed with bone wax. The bleeding from emissary veins is controlled by bone wax. Intermittent jugular vein compression at this stage is important to avoid air embolism. In case of large emissary vein, a safer approach would be to skeletonize it with the diamond drill and coagulate it under direct visualization.

A bone opening of 3 cm in diameter is usually enough, exposing the sigmoid transverse junction, inferior border of the transverse sinus, medial border of the sigmoid sinus, and horizontal part of the occipital squama.[79,103]

After the bone work is completed, the operative field is prepared for the microsurgical work. The wound edges are covered with wet gauzes; cerebellar Apfelbaum retractor is mounted and supporting armrests are attached to the operating table, providing more comfort and accuracy for the surgeon.

The dura is opened under the microscope in a straight fashion, along and parallel to the sigmoid sinus. Tack-up sutures along the sinus dural edge are additionally placed in order to increase the view.

The next step is to evacuate CSF from the lateral cerebellomedullary cistern. After cerebellar relaxation, the cerebellum is gently displaced medially with the brain spatula mounted on cerebellar retractor. Depending on the localization of the tumor, different surgical strategies are applied (▶ Fig. 13.5b, c, d). If the tumor is posterior to the IAC and pushes the cranial nerves anteriorly, the lesion could be safely debulked and carefully dissected from the surrounding structures due to the arachnoid layer present between the tumor and cranial nerves. In this case, the general principles for meningioma surgery are applied—first the tumor is devascularized from its dural attachment, followed by intratumor debulking using the ultrasonic aspirator, and then bimanual dissection and resection respecting the arachnoid membranes. These operations are very well-tolerated by the patients, with low rates of postoperative complications.

On the other hand, if the tumor is anterior to the IAC (as in petroclival meningiomas), the microsurgical dissection is more difficult due to the depth of the approach, location of the tumor anterior to the cranial nerves (which may be involved by the tumor and displaced in unpredictable location). In such cases, the lower cranial nerves, cranial nerves VII and VIII, usually lie posterior to the tumor capsule or are sometimes embedded within the tumor. The trigeminal nerve is usually displaced at the superior pole of the tumor and the cranial nerve VI is located at the deepest anterior portion of the tumor. The trochlear nerve runs at the free edge of the tentorium.

Very careful meticulous microsurgical dissection under constant communication with the IOM team and frequent direct cranial nerve stimulation with the monopolar probe is recommended. There are several working corridors for resection of petroclival meningiomas:

Tentorium—cranial nerve V; Trigeminal nerve—cranial nerves VII/VIII; cranial nerves VII/VIII—cranial nerve IX-X-XI; Caudal cranial nerves and foramen magnum. Using these surgical corridors, piecemeal tumor resection and internal debulking is possible.[18,106] Care has to be taken to identify on the preoperative MRI images any involvement by the tumor of major brainstem vessels, which have to be protected during surgery. The tumor debulking is done using the ultrasonic aspirator only after identification of the major vascular structures. After sufficient internal debulking is achieved, the tumor capsule is dissected from the cranial nerves from the lateral to medial direction: from the bone toward the brainstem.[106] The dissection of the tumor from the brainstem is done last with constant communication with the IOM team and attention to the monitoring changes. The extracapsular tumor dissection has to be done in an arachnoidal plane. The goal of the surgery is to decompress the brainstem and affected cranial nerves. However, if the arachnoidal plane is violated and the brainstem pia matter is infiltrated by the tumor or the tumor is firmly adherent to the major vessels, no attempt is made to perform a complete resection.

For large petroclival meningiomas with extension to the Meckel's cave and supratentorial compartment, the RISA approach and endoscope-assisted techniques provide excellent exposure for removal of these tumors through a single retrosigmoid exposure (▶ Fig. 13.6).[60,61,72,73,74,75,78,103,106] Once the tumor in the CPA is removed, the petrous apex can be resected by intradural drilling of the bone located superior and anterior to the IAC and dorsolateral to the trigeminal nerve, which is named the suprameatal tubercle. Drilling of this piece of bone allows for mobilization of the trigeminal nerve and opening of the Meckel's cave. Great care has to be exerted not to cause inadvertent damage to the internal carotid artery anterolaterally, the petrosal sinus superiorly, and the superior and posterior semicircular canals laterally.[106] The presence of a tumor mass enlarges the working space within the CPA and creates an approach provided by the tumor itself, avoiding the risks of additional morbidity of complex cranial base approaches.[106]

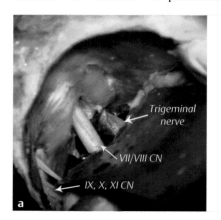
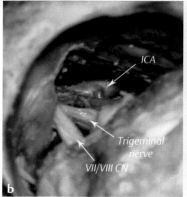

Fig. 13.6 Retrosigmoid intradural suprameatal approach. Left semi-sitting position. (a) A retractor is placed over the lateral cerebellar surface nerves of the cerebellopontine angle are isolated. The dura over the suprameatal tubercle is removed. **(b)** The suprameatal tubercle and the petrous apex are removed and the tentorium is split, thus allowing access to the middle cranial fossa. The internal carotid artery is exposed in the most anterior portion of the operative field.
CN, cranial nerve; ICA, internal carotid artery. Dissection is done by prof. Marcos Tatagiba.

If the tumor extends to the middle fossa, splitting of the tentorium, 2 cm distal and parallel to the superior petrosal sinus provide additional exposure to the posterior part of the middle fossa. The trochlear nerve, which runs at the free edge of the tentorium, has to be identified and protected.

After the tumor resection is completed, the surgical field is thoroughly irrigated with saline and a final jugular compression is applied in order to examine any point of discrete venous bleeding that may lead to a postoperative hemorrhage.

The dura is closed under the microscope with running continuous 4.0 silk suture. The linear dural incision usually allows for good reapproximation of the dura, without the need for dural graft repair. Any opened mastoid air cells are closed with muscle and fibrin glue. A methylmethacrylate or titanium cranioplasty is preferred not only for cosmetic purposes, but also to prevent the postoperative headaches associated with scarring of the suboccipital muscles to the dura.[106,107] The wound is closed in layers. No drain is used.

The patients spend usually the first night at the intensive care unit (ICU).

Our observations are that different than vestibular schwannoma hyperacusis can improve following surgery of CPA meningiomas. That is the reason that we do not recommend hearing destructive approaches, such as the translabyrinthine approach. In cases of cochlear nerve preservation, patients may benefit from cochlear implant, which can improve hearing capacity.

13.9 Postoperative Complications Avoidance

The most common postoperative complications are CSF leaks, infections, postoperative hematoma, hydrocephalus, brain edema, venous infarction, pulmonary complications (aspirator associate pneumonia), and thromboembolic events.

CSF leaks are one of the most common complications following skull base surgery with estimated incidence of 5 to 15%.[96] The leakage may occur either through the skin at the wound site or through the nose, when the mastoid air cells are not adequately closed.

Careful and meticulous suturing of the dura, tight fascia closure with locked running suture, as well as obliteration of the opened mastoid air cells with fat or muscle with fibrin glue are important measures to prevent the occurrence of CSF leaks. In case of wound CSF leakage, placement of additional suture and a lumbar drain for 3 to 5 days usually resolves the leak. If the CSF leak continues, wound re-exploration may be needed in order to close the leakage point. In some cases, persistent CSF leak can be indicator for hydrocephalus and the need for permanent CSF shunt have to be evaluated.

Infections prevention starts from the preoperative preparation. Some studies indicate that preoperative whole body disinfection with chlorhexidine containing shampoo may decrease the surgical site infections, but this data is not conclusive.[108,109,110] Some authors recommend the use of chlorhexidine-alcohol solution for intraoperative cleaning of the wound, which has shown superior results in randomized control trials compared to other solutions for disinfection and prevention of surgical site infections.[109] Preoperative shaving also have to be avoided because it increases the risk of surgical site infections.[110]

A large prospective study comprising 6,243 consecutive craniotomies as well as other studies of the same authors, indicated that independent risk factors for meningitis and surgical site infections were CSF leakage, concomitant incision infection, male sex, surgery duration, and repeated surgery.[108,111,112] Therefore, early management of the CSF leak before a fistula is formed is mandatory in order to avoid postoperative meningitis. Avoidance of the use of synthetic dural substitutes in dural closure can decrease the risk of postoperative infections.[101,102] Our practice is to use patient's own tissues (pericranium, fascia lata, abdominal fat) for reconstruction.

Meningiomas are correlated with higher risk for postoperative bleeding.[113,114,115] Postoperative hematomas can be within the operative field or present as distant supratentorial hemorrhages.[113,114,115,116,117] Postoperative hemorrhages at the site of the craniotomy can be caused by inadequate hemostasis at the end of surgery, compromise of major CPA veins, inadequate control of the blood pressure after the surgical procedure, preoperative administration of antiaggregation or anticoagulation medications, and coagulation disorders.[59,113,114,115]

Care should be taken to secure adequate hemostasis at the end of the surgery and preserve, if possible, major draining veins in the posterior fossa. Keeping the blood pressure at normal levels and a final jugular compression by the anesthesiologist before dural closure can reveal discrete bleeding sites.

Preservation of petrosal veins cannot always be possible in CPA meningioma surgery. However, an attempt has to be made because of the risk of postoperative venous infarctions, which can complicate the surgery.[59]

Risk factors for the development of postoperative hematoma formation are low platelet count, prolonged prothrombin time or partial thromboplastin time, recently administered anticoagulants, and aspirin therapy prior to surgery.[114] In one study, administration of antiplatelet agents was the most frequent risk factor; it was used by 43% of patients reoperated for hematoma.[114] Therefore, it is advisable to stop the aspirin at least 10 days before surgery, and when on anticoagulation, the international normalized ratio should be below 1.5. Low-molecular-weight heparin (LMWH) for prophylactic of deep venous thrombosis (DVT) is be avoided preoperatively and is administered after first postoperative day.[115,118,119,120,121]

According to some authors, most postoperative hematoma occurs in the first 6 hours after surgery.[122] Other authors indicated equal distribution of postoperative hematoma cases in the first 48 hours postsurgery.[115] We recommend close monitoring of the patient after surgery in the ICU in order to decrease the chance of complications.

In case of symptomatic postoperative hematoma in the CPA, the patient can deteriorate very rapidly due to compression of the IV ventricle, secondary hydrocephalus, and brainstem compression. In such cases, initial placement of ventriculostomy catheter is recommended followed by evacuation of the hematoma and close monitoring of the patient in the ICU postoperatively.

There are complications that can be attributed to the sitting position, such supratentorial hemorrhages, tension pneumocephalus, and venous air embolism.[46,123] However, if the sitting position is done on a regular basis, which adequate preoperative workup for patent foramen ovale, intraoperative precautions (transesophageal echocardiography and monitoring), correct intraoperative positioning from experienced team of neuroanesthesiologists, neurophysiologists, and neurosurgeons, the risks are estimated to be low (approximately 1,5%).[46,123]

The surgeries for CPA meningiomas can sometimes take very long hours, which increase the risks of postoperative thromboembolic incidents (DVT and pulmonary embolisms). Therefore, during surgery, every patient has compression stockings on the legs. We position the lower extremities in semi-sitting position above the level of the heart in order to have sufficient venous return.[46,78,79] With administration of LMWH, the risks of postoperative hematoma have to be balanced against risks of DVT. It is generally agreed that administration of LMWH the day after surgery is safe.[118,120,121] However, preoperative administration of LMWH is associated with increased risk of postoperative bleeding.[119]

In some large CPA meningiomas, after uneventful operation (gross total resection, no apparent venous injury), brain edema in the early postoperative period can sometimes be seen. The reason for this observation is not entirely clear, but aggressive management of elevated intracranial pressure with corticosteroids and mannitol has to be done.[2] In some cases, even reintubation and mechanical ventilation is indicated.

In large tumors, especially petroclival type, with involvement of the lower cranial nerves with brainstem pial invasion sometimes long postoperative stay in the ICU can be expected. In such cases, we recommend early tracheostomy and gastrostomy in order to decrease the risk for pulmonary complications and provide adequate nutrition to the patient.

Swallowing training program may become mandatory. The majority of the patients will need logopedic support at the immediate postoperative care to help the balance and facial nerve training.

13.10 Radiosurgery for Cerebellopontine Angle Meningiomas

The goal of meningioma surgery is total removal of the tumor, including dural attachment and involved bone. However, this is not always possible in patients with CPA lesion and especially in petroclival meningiomas due to the wide attachment of the tumor stretching the cranial nerves, involving vital arterial and brainstem structures. In such cases, gross total resection is associated with high risk of postoperative morbidity, despite the advances in microsurgery and routine introduction of the intraoperative monitoring. A literature review reveals that the gross total excision rates has dropped in the recent series to 20 to 40%,[12,13,14,15,16,17,25] compared to early reports pointing 70 to 80% gross total excision rates.[7,10,11,20,63,69,70,71] This paradigm shift is governed by the better understanding of natural history of the disease following surgery, the advances in radiosurgery in the recent years and the aim for better quality of life for the patients.

From the data of several published series for the natural history and long-term follow-up of CPA and petroclival meningiomas, the recurrence rate after subtotal and near total resection seem to be low.[13,16,25]

In the study of Natarajan et al of 150 patients operated for petroclival meningiomas with follow-up of 102 months, the reported recurrence-free survival rate was 85% at 12 years with Karnofsky Performance Scale 84 +/− 9 at the time of the latest follow-up evaluation.[16]

In the series of Little et al describing the surgical management of 137 petroclival meningioma patients only 17.6% of patients presented with radiological recurrence at a mean follow-up of time of 29.8 months.[13] The rate of gross total resection was achieved in 40% of patients, and near total resection was achieved in 40% of patients.

Other authors report long-term follow-up of subtotal resected CPA meningiomas with estimated growth rate of 0.37 cm/year with median progression free survival time of 66 months.[25]

This data indicates that multimodality treatment including radiosurgery, as adjunct to surgery, is accepted management option for these tumors.

The goals of radiotherapy are to prevent tumor progression, prolong the interval to recurrence, and improve survival whether administered as adjuvant or primary therapy. Conventional radiotherapy and stereotactic radiosurgery can be used as a single treatment option for small CPA tumors (up to 3 cm in diameter) or in combination with the surgical treatment.

Long-term follow-up in radiosurgery series data indicate tumor control rated of more than 90%.[21,22,23,24,124,125,126] Zachenhofer et al present a series of 36 patients with cranial base meningiomas treated with radiosurgery as a single treatment option or after surgery, with follow up of 103 months and 94% tumor control rate.[126]

Subach et al[124] present a series of 62 patients with petroclival meningiomas treated with radiosurgery with follow-up of 37 months. The authors report decrease in tumor volumes in 14 (23%) patients. Other 42 patients (68%), had no change is size of the tumor; increased in tumor size was noted in 5 (8%). Another paper by Roche et al[21] present patient series of 32 petroclival meningiomas treated with gamma-knife surgery (GKS) with follow-up from 24 to 118 months (mean 52.6 months) The authors report no change in tumor volume in 28 cases and a slight decreased in 4 cases. Other authors have presented series of 168 meningioma patients with mean follow-up of 72 months.[22] The authors report improvement in 44 patients (26%); in 98 (58%) patients, no change in pretreatment condition was noted, and 26 patients (15%) showed neurologic deterioration. Tumor volume decreased in 78 patients (46%). However, in 74 patients (44%), tumor remained stable but in 16 patients (10%) increased in size.

In another large series of 108 patients treated with low-dose gamma knife radiosurgery and follow-up of 86.1 months (range 20–144 months) a tumor volume decrease was seen in 50 patients (46%), 51 patients (47%) remained stable, and in 7 patients (6%), local recurrence was observed.[127]

These results show good tumor control rate and stable long-term results. However, it has to be noted that there are known complications with the administration of radiotherapy, such as malignant neoplasms,[51,52,53] as well as tumor progression after stereotactic radiosurgery.[54]

Therefore, according to our experience, the administration of radiotherapy as a single treatment modality or adjunct to microsurgery has to be weighted for the risks and natural history (operated and nonoperated patients) and reserved until documented tumor growth or clinical progression.

13.11 Conclusion

CPA meningiomas are lesions that require careful evaluation of numerous factors before a treatment can be recommended. Options include follow-up with MRI, surgery, radiotherapy, or multimodality treatment. If surgery is chosen as treatment option, detailed clinical and radiological examination is essential before the appropriate approach for each patient is selected. Such operations are team effort and require dedicated neuroanesthesiologists, specialized neuro-ICU, neuromonitoring specialists as well as active postoperative care in order to secure safe tumor resection and smooth follow-up period. The goal of surgery is maximum safe resection with preservation of the quality of life.

References

[1] Central Brain Tumor Registry of the United States (CBTRUS); 2006. Page 18 http://www.cbtrus.org/2010-NPCR-SEER/CBTRUS-WEBREPORT-Final-3-2-10.pdf

[2] Yamin B, Ryu S, Rock JP. Surgical management of posterior fossa meningiomas. Alfredo Quiñones-Hinojosa, ed. Schmidek & Sweet Operative Neurosurgical Techniques: Indications, Methods, and Results. 6th ed. Philadelphia, PA: Elsevier Saunders; 2012: 501–516

[3] Riemenschneider MJ, Perry A, Reifenberger G. Histological classification and molecular genetics of meningiomas. Lancet Neurol. 2006; 5 (12):1045–1054

[4] Sade B, Chahlavi A, Krishnaney A, Nagel S, Choi E, Lee JH. World Health Organization Grades II and III meningiomas are rare in the cranial base and spine. Neurosurgery. 2007; 61(6):1194–1198, discussion 1198

[5] Nakamura M, Roser F, Dormiani M, Matthies C, Vorkapic P, Samii M. Facial and cochlear nerve function after surgery of cerebellopontine angle meningiomas. Neurosurgery. 2005; 57(1):77–90, discussion 77-90

[6] Yasargil GM, Mortara R, Curcic M. Meningiomas of the basal posterior cranial fossa. Adv Tech Stand Neurosurg. 1980; 7:3–115

[7] Bricolo AP, Turazzi S, Talacchi A, Cristofori L. Microsurgical removal of petroclival meningiomas: a report of 33 patients. Neurosurgery. 1992; 31(5):813–828, discussion 828

[8] Schaller B, Merlo A, Gratzl O, Probst R. Premeatal and retromeatal cerebellopontine angle meningioma. Two distinct clinical entities. Acta Neurochir (Wien). 1999; 141(5):465–471

[9] Mayberg MR, Symon L. Meningiomas of the clivus and apical petrous bone. Report of 35 cases. J Neurosurg. 1986; 65(2):160–167

[10] Hakuba A, Nishimura S, Jang BJ. A combined retroauricular and preauricular transpetrosal-transtentorial approach to clivus meningiomas. Surg Neurol. 1988; 30(2):108–116

[11] Samii M, Tatagiba M. Experience with 36 surgical cases of petroclival meningiomas. Acta Neurochir (Wien). 1992; 118(1–2): 27–32

[12] Abdel Aziz KM, Sanan A, van Loveren HR, Tew JM, Jr, Keller JT, Pensak ML. Petroclival meningiomas: predictive parameters for transpetrosal approaches. Neurosurgery. 2000; 47(1):139–150, discussion 150–152

[13] Little KM, Friedman AH, Sampson JH, Wanibuchi M, Fukushima T. Surgical management of petroclival meningiomas: defining resection goals based on risk of neurological morbidity and tumor recurrence rates in 137 patients. Neurosurgery. 2005; 56(3):546–559, discussion 546–559

[14] Bambakidis NC, Kakarla UK, Kim LJ, et al. Evolution of surgical approaches in the treatment of petroclival meningiomas: a retrospective review. Neurosurgery. 2007; 61(5) Suppl 2:202–209, discussion 209–211

[15] Xu F, Karampelas I, Megerian CA, Selman WR, Bambakidis NC. Petroclival meningiomas: an update on surgical approaches, decision making, and treatment results. Neurosurg Focus. 2013; 35 (6):E11

[16] Natarajan SK, Sekhar LN, Schessel D, Morita A. Petroclival meningiomas: multimodality treatment and outcomes at long-term follow-up. Neurosurgery. 2007; 60(6):965–979, discussion 979–981

[17] Seifert V. Clinical management of petroclival meningiomas and the eternal quest for preservation of quality of life: personal experiences over a period of 20 years. Acta Neurochir (Wien). 2010; 152(7):1099–1116

[18] Ramina R, Fernandes Y, Neto M. a Sliva F, Petroclival meningiomas. diagnosis, treatment and results. Samii's Essentials in Neurosurgery. 2nd ed. Berlin: Springer Verlag; 2014:199–216

[19] Ramina R, Neto MC, Fernandes YB, Silva EB, Mattei TA, Aguiar PH. Surgical removal of small petroclival meningiomas. Acta Neurochir (Wien). 2008; 150(5):431–438, discussion 438–439

[20] Samii M, Tatagiba M, Carvalho GA. Resection of large petroclival meningiomas by the simple retrosigmoid route. J Clin Neurosci. 1999; 6(1):27–30

[21] Roche PH, Pellet W, Fuentes S, Thomassin JM, Régis J. Gamma Knife radiosurgical management of petroclival meningiomas results and indications. Acta Neurochir (Wien). 2003; 145(10):883–888, discussion 888

[22] Flannery TJ, Kano H, Lunsford LD, et al. Long-term control of petroclival meningiomas through radiosurgery. J Neurosurg. 2010; 112(5):957–964

[23] Starke RM, Nguyen JH, Rainey J, et al. Gamma Knife surgery of meningiomas located in the posterior fossa: factors predictive of outcome and remission. J Neurosurg. 2011; 114(5):1399–1409

[24] Starke RM, Williams BJ, Hiles C, Nguyen JH, Elsharkawy MY, Sheehan JP. Gamma knife surgery for skull base meningiomas. J Neurosurg. 2012; 116(3):588–597

[25] Jung HW, Yoo H, Paek SH, Choi KS. Long-term outcome and growth rate of subtotally resected petroclival meningiomas: experience with 38 cases. Neurosurgery. 2000; 46(3):567–574, discussion 574–575

[26] Van Havenbergh T, Carvalho G, Tatagiba M, Plets C, Samii M. Natural history of petroclival meningiomas. Neurosurgery. 2003; 52(1):55–62, discussion 62–64

[27] Terasaka S, Asaoka K, Kobayashi H, Yamaguchi S, Sawamura Y. [Natural history and surgical results of petroclival meningiomas]. No Shinkei Geka. 2010; 38(9):817–824

[28] Jadid KD, Feychting M, Höijer J, Hylin S, Kihlström L, Mathiesen T. Long-term follow-up of incidentally discovered meningiomas. Acta Neurochir (Wien). 2015; 157(2):225–230, discussion 230

[29] Hunter JB, Yawn RJ, Wang R, et al. The Natural History of Petroclival Meningiomas: A Volumetric Study. Otol Neurotol. 2017; 38(1):123–128

[30] Ichimura S, Kawase T, Onozuka S, Yoshida K, Ohira T. Four subtypes of petroclival meningiomas: differences in symptoms and operative findings using the anterior transpetrosal approach. Acta Neurochir (Wien). 2008; 150(7):637–645

[31] Cho CW, Al-Mefty O. Combined petrosal approach to petroclival meningiomas. Neurosurgery. 2002; 51(3):708–716, discussion 716–718

[32] Nakasu S, Fukami T, Nakajima M, Watanabe K, Ichikawa M, Matsuda M. Growth pattern changes of meningiomas: long-term analysis. Neurosurgery. 2005; 56(5):946–955, discussion 946–955

[33] Nakamura M, Roser F, Michel J, Jacobs C, Samii M. The natural history of incidental meningiomas. Neurosurgery. 2003; 53(1):62–70, discussion 70–71

[34] Li Y, Zhao G, Wang H, et al. Use of 3D-computed tomography angiography for planning the surgical removal of pineal region meningiomas using Poppen's approach: a report of ten cases and a literature review. World J Surg Oncol. 2011; 9:64

[35] Chen JQ, Guan Y, Li G, et al. Application of 3D-computed tomography angiography technology in large meningioma resection. Asian Pac J Trop Med. 2012; 5(7):577–581

[36] Rosset A, Spadola L, Ratib O. OsiriX: an open-source software for navigating in multidimensional DICOM images. J Digit Imaging. 2004; 17(3):205–216

[37] Vides CS, Azpíroz LJ, Jiménez AJ. Plugin for OsiriX: mean shift segmentation. Conf Proc IEEE Eng Med Biol Soc. 2007; 2007:3060–3063

[38] Jalbert F, Paoli JR. [Osirix: free and open-source software for medical imagery]. Rev Stomatol Chir Maxillofac. 2008; 109(1):53–55

[39] Horos software offical web page; Available from: https://www.horosproject.org/

[40] Marcos Tatagiba FE. Kleinhirnbrückenwinkelprozesse. In: Moskopp D, Wassmann H, eds. Neurochirurgie. Handbuch für die Weiterbildung und interdisziplinäres Nachschlagewerk, 2015:37

[41] Bendszus M, Rao G, Burger R, et al. Is there a benefit of preoperative meningioma embolization? Neurosurgery. 2000; 47(6):1306–1311, discussion 1311–1312

[42] Chun JY, McDermott MW, Lamborn KR, Wilson CB, Higashida R, Berger MS. Delayed surgical resection reduces intraoperative blood loss for embolized meningiomas. Neurosurgery. 2002; 50(6):1231–1235, discussion 1235–1237

[43] Nania A, Granata F, Vinci S, et al. Necrosis score, surgical time, and transfused blood volume in patients treated with preoperative embolization of intracranial meningiomas. Analysis of a single-centre experience and a review of literature. Clin Neuroradiol. 2014; 24(1):29–36

[44] Bendszus M, Monoranu CM, Schütz A, Nölte I, Vince GH, Solymosi L. Neurologic complications after particle embolization of intracranial meningiomas. AJNR Am J Neuroradiol. 2005; 26(6):1413–1419

[45] Carli DF, Sluzewski M, Beute GN, van Rooij WJ. Complications of particle embolization of meningiomas: frequency, risk factors, and outcome. AJNR Am J Neuroradiol. 2010; 31(1):152–154

[46] Feigl GC, Decker K, Wurms M, et al. Neurosurgical procedures in the semisitting position: evaluation of the risk of paradoxical venous air embolism in patients with a patent foramen ovale. World Neurosurg. 2014; 81(1):159–164

[47] Adachi K, Kawase T, Yoshida K, Yazaki T, Onozuka S. ABC surgical risk scale for skull base meningioma: a new scoring system for predicting the extent of tumor removal and neurological outcome. Clinical article. J Neurosurg. 2009; 111(5):1053–1061

[48] Sekhar LN, Swamy NK, Jaiswal V, Rubinstein E, Hirsch WE, Jr, Wright DC. Surgical excision of meningiomas involving the clivus: preoperative and intraoperative features as predictors of post-operative functional deterioration. J Neurosurg. 1994; 81(6):860–868

[49] Cushing HW, Eisenhardt L. Meningiomas: Their Classification, Regional Behaviour, Life History and Surgical End Results. Springfield, Charles C Thomas, 1938

[50] Castellano F, Ruggiero G. Meningiomas of the posterior fossa. Acta Radiol Suppl. 1953; 104 Suppl:1–177

[51] Yu JS, Yong WH, Wilson D, Black KL. Glioblastoma induction after radiosurgery for meningioma. Lancet. 2000; 356(9241):1576–1577

[52] Shamisa A, Bance M, Nag S, et al. Glioblastoma multiforme occurring in a patient treated with gamma knife surgery. Case report and review of the literature. J Neurosurg. 2001; 94(5):816–821

[53] Shin M, Ueki K, Kurita H, Kirino T. Malignant transformation of a vestibular schwannoma after gamma knife radiosurgery. Lancet. 2002; 360(9329):309–310

[54] Couldwell WT, Cole CD, Al-Mefty O. Patterns of skull base meningioma progression after failed radiosurgery. J Neurosurg. 2007; 106(1):30–35

[55] Levine ZT, Buchanan RI, Sekhar LN, Rosen CL, Wright DC. Proposed grading system to predict the extent of resection and outcomes for cranial base meningiomas. Neurosurgery. 1999; 45(2):221–230

[56] Saberi H, Meybodi AT, Rezai AS. Levine-Sekhar grading system for prediction of the extent of resection of cranial base meningiomas revisited: study of 124 cases. Neurosurg Rev. 2006; 29(2):138–144

[57] Campero A, Martins C, Rhoton A, Jr, Tatagiba M. Dural landmark to locate the internal auditory canal in large and giant vestibular schwannomas: the Tübingen line. Neurosurgery. 2011; 69(1) Suppl Operative:ons99–ons102, discussion ons102

[58] Gharabaghi A, Koerbel A, Löwenheim H, Kaminsky J, Samii M, Tatagiba M. The impact of petrosal vein preservation on post-operative auditory function in surgery of petrous apex meningiomas. Neurosurgery. 2006; 59(1) Suppl 1:ONS68–ONS74, discussion ONS68–ONS74

[59] Koerbel A, Gharabaghi A, Safavi-Abbasi S, et al. Venous complications following petrosal vein sectioning in surgery of petrous apex meningiomas. Eur J Surg Oncol. 2009; 35(7):773–779

[60] Koerbel A, Kirschniak A, Ebner FH, Tatagiba M, Gharabaghi A. The retrosigmoid intradural suprameatal approach to posterior cavernous sinus: microsurgical anatomy. Eur J Surg Oncol. 2009; 35(4):368–372

[61] Samii M, Tatagiba M, Carvalho GA. Retrosigmoid intradural suprameatal approach to Meckel's cave and the middle fossa: surgical technique and outcome. J Neurosurg. 2000; 92(2):235–241

[62] Tatagiba M, Acioly MA, Roser F. Petroclival tumors. J Neurosurg. 2013; 119(2):526–528

[63] Tatagiba M, Samii M, Matthies C, Vorkapic P. Management of petroclival meningiomas: a critical analysis of surgical treatment. Acta Neurochir Suppl (Wien). 1996; 65:92–94

[64] Stummer W. Mechanisms of tumor-related brain edema. Neurosurg Focus. 2007; 22(5):E8

[65] Feng H, Huang G, Liao X, et al. Endoscopic third ventriculostomy in the management of obstructive hydrocephalus: an outcome analysis. J Neurosurg. 2004; 100(4):626–633

[66] Gangemi M, Mascari C, Maiuri F, Godano U, Donati P, Longatti PL. Long-term outcome of endoscopic third ventriculostomy in obstructive hydrocephalus. Minim Invasive Neurosurg. 2007; 50(5): 265–269

[67] van Beijnum J, Hanlo PW, Fischer K, et al. Laser-assisted endoscopic third ventriculostomy: long-term results in a series of 202 patients. Neurosurgery. 2008; 62(2):437–443, discussion 443–444

[68] Oertel J, et al. Long-term follow-up of repeat endoscopic third ventriculostomy in obstructive hydrocephalus. World Neurosurg. 2016

[69] Al-Mefty O, Fox JL, Smith RR. Petrosal approach for petroclival meningiomas. Neurosurgery. 1988; 22(3):510–517

[70] Kawase T, Shiobara R, Toya S. Middle fossa transpetrosal-transtentorial approaches for petroclival meningiomas. Selective pyramid resection and radicality. Acta Neurochir (Wien). 1994; 129 (3–4):113–120

[71] Couldwell WT, Fukushima T, Giannotta SL, Weiss MH. Petroclival meningiomas: surgical experience in 109 cases. J Neurosurg. 1996; 84(1):20–28

[72] Seoane E, Rhoton AL, Jr. Suprameatal extension of the retrosigmoid approach: microsurgical anatomy. Neurosurgery. 1999; 44(3): 553–560

[73] Ebner FH, Koerbel A, Kirschniak A, Roser F, Kaminsky J, Tatagiba M. Endoscope-assisted retrosigmoid intradural suprameatal approach to the middle fossa: anatomical and surgical considerations. Eur J Surg Oncol. 2007; 33(1):109–113

[74] Ebner FH, Koerbel A, Roser F, Hirt B, Tatagiba M. Microsurgical and endoscopic anatomy of the retrosigmoid intradural suprameatal approach to lesions extending from the posterior fossa to the central skull base. Skull Base. 2009; 19(5):319–323

[75] S, H., Interne Fortbildung 2014: retrosigmoidaler Zugang. Department of Neurosurgery Tübingen, 2014

[76] Ebner FH, Dimostheni A, Tatagiba MS, Roser F. Step-by-step education of the retrosigmoid approach leads to low approach-related morbidity through young residents. Acta Neurochir (Wien). 2010; 152(6):985–988, discussion 988

[77] Rhoton AL, Jr. The cerebellopontine angle and posterior fossa cranial nerves by the retrosigmoid approach. Neurosurgery. 2000; 47(3) Suppl:S93–S129

[78] Tatagiba MS, Roser F, Hirt B, Ebner FH. The retrosigmoid endoscopic approach for cerebellopontine-angle tumors and microvascular decompression. World Neurosurg. 2014; 82(6) Suppl:S171–S176

[79] Tatagiba M, Roser F, Schuhmann MU, Ebner FH. Vestibular schwannoma surgery via the retrosigmoid transmeatal approach. Acta Neurochir (Wien). 2014; 156(2):421–425, discussion 425

[80] Kawase T, Shiobara R, Toya S. Anterior transpetrosal-transtentorial approach for sphenopetroclival meningiomas: surgical method and results in 10 patients. Neurosurgery. 1991; 28(6):869–875, discussion 875–876

[81] Kawase T, Toya S, Shiobara R, Mine T. Transpetrosal approach for aneurysms of the lower basilar artery. J Neurosurg. 1985; 63(6): 857–861

[82] Tummala RP, Coscarella E, Morcos JJ. Transpetrosal approaches to the posterior fossa. Neurosurg Focus. 2005; 19(2):E6

[83] Miller CG, van Loveren HR, Keller JT, Pensak M, el-Kalliny M, Tew JM, Jr. Transpetrosal approach: surgical anatomy and technique. Neurosurgery. 1993; 33(3):461–469, discussion 469

[84] Davidge KM, van Furth WR, Agur A, Cusimano M. Naming the soft tissue layers of the temporoparietal region: unifying anatomic terminology across surgical disciplines. Neurosurgery. 2010; 67(3) Suppl Operative:ons120–ons129, discussion ons129–ons130

[85] Oikawa S, Mizuno M, Muraoka S, Kobayashi S. Retrograde dissection of the temporalis muscle preventing muscle atrophy for pterional craniotomy. Technical note. J Neurosurg. 1996; 84(2):297–299

[86] Janjua RM, Al-Mefty O, Densler DW, Shields CB. Dural relationships of Meckel cave and lateral wall of the cavernous sinus. Neurosurg Focus. 2008; 25(6):E2

[87] Day JD, Fukushima T, Giannotta SL. Microanatomical study of the extradural middle fossa approach to the petroclival and posterior cavernous sinus region: description of the rhomboid construct. Neurosurgery. 1994; 34(6):1009–1016, discussion 1016

[88] Fukushima T, Day JD, Hirahara K. Extradural total petrous apex resection with trigeminal translocation for improved exposure of the posterior cavernous sinus and petroclival region. Skull Base Surg. 1996; 6(2):95–103

[89] Schaller B, Probst R, Strebel S, Gratzl O. Trigeminocardiac reflex during surgery in the cerebellopontine angle. J Neurosurg. 1999; 90 (2):215–220

[90] Koerbel A, Gharabaghi A, Samii A, et al. Trigeminocardiac reflex during skull base surgery: mechanism and management. Acta Neurochir (Wien). 2005; 147(7):727–732, discussion 732–733

[91] Wang J, Yoshioka F, Joo W, Komune N, Quilis-Quesada V, Rhoton AL, Jr. The cochlea in skull base surgery: an anatomy study. J Neurosurg. 2016; 125(5):1094–1104

[92] Tanriover N, Sanus GZ, Ulu MO, et al. Middle fossa approach: microsurgical anatomy and surgical technique from the neurosurgical perspective. Surg Neurol. 2009; 71(5):586–596, discussion 596

[93] Middle fossa. Anatomic view. Neurosurgery. 2007; 61(4): S4–S85

[94] Viale G, Middle fossa. The surgical approach to the posterior cranial fossa according to Galen. Neurosurgery. 2007; 61(5) Suppl 2:399–402, discussion 402–403

[95] Sekhar LN, Natarajan SK, Manning T, Bhagawati D. The use of fibrin glue to stop venous bleeding in the epidural space, vertebral venous plexus, and anterior cavernous sinus: technical note. Neurosurgery. 2007; 61(3) Suppl:E51–, discu–ssion E51

[96] Poulsgaard L. Translabyrinthine Approach to Vestibular Schwannomas. Alfredo Quiñones-Hinojosa, ed. Schmidek & Sweet Operative Neurosurgical Techniques: Indications, Methods, and Results. 6th ed. Philadelphia, PA: Elsevier Saunders; 2012

[97] Retrolabyrinthine. Translabyrinthine, and transcochlear approaches. Neurosurgery. 2007; 61(4):S4–S153

[98] Samii M, Ammirati M. The combined supra-infratentorial pre-sigmoid sinus avenue to the petro-clival region. Surgical technique and clinical applications. Acta Neurochir (Wien). 1988; 95(1–2): 6–12

[99] Ammirati M, Samii M. Presigmoid sinus approach to petroclival meningiomas. Skull Base Surg. 1992; 2(3):124–128

[100] Marcos Tatagiba MA. Chordomas and chordosarcomas. Samii's Essentials in Neurosurgery. 2nd ed. Berlin: Springer Verlag; 2014:192–196

[101] Malliti M, Page P, Gury C, Chomette E, Nataf F, Roux FX. Comparison of deep wound infection rates using a synthetic dural substitute (neuro-patch) or pericranium graft for dural closure: a clinical review of 1 year. Neurosurgery. 2004; 54(3):599–603, discussion 603–604

[102] Gaberel T, Borgey F, Thibon P, Lesteven C, Lecoutour X, Emery E. Surgical site infection associated with the use of bovine serum albumine-glutaraldehyde surgical adhesive (BioGlue) in cranial surgery: a case-control study. Acta Neurochir (Wien). 2011; 153(1): 156–162, discussion 162–163

[103] Marcos Tatagiba MA. Retrosigmoid approach to the posterior and middle fossa. In: Samii's Essentials in Neurosurgery, 2014:217–235

[104] Rhoton AL, Jr. The foramen magnum. Neurosurgery. 2000; 47(3) Suppl:S155–S193

[105] Ribas GC, Rhoton AL, Jr, Cruz OR, Peace D. Suboccipital burr holes and craniectomies. Neurosurg Focus. 2005; 19(2):E1

[106] Samii M, Gerganov VM. Surgery of extra-axial tumors of the cerebral base. Neurosurgery. 2008; 62(6) Suppl 3:1153–1166, discussion 1166–1168

[107] Teo MK, Eljamel MS. Role of craniotomy repair in reducing postoperative headaches after a retrosigmoid approach. Neurosurgery. 2010; 67(5):1286–1291, discussion 1291–1292

[108] Korinek AM, Baugnon T, Golmard JL, van Effenterre R, Coriat P, Puybasset L. Risk factors for adult nosocomial meningitis after craniotomy: role of antibiotic prophylaxis. Neurosurgery. 2008; 62 Suppl 2:532–539

[109] Darouiche RO, Wall MJ, Jr, Itani KM, et al. Chlorhexidine-alcohol versus povidone-iodine for surgical-site antisepsis. N Engl J Med. 2010; 362(1):18–26

[110] Broekman ML, van Beijnum J, Peul WC, Regli L. Neurosurgery and shaving: what's the evidence? J Neurosurg. 2011; 115(4): 670–678

[111] Korinek AM, Service Epidémiologie Hygiène et Prévention. Risk factors for neurosurgical site infections after craniotomy: a prospective multicenter study of 2944 patients. The French Study Group of Neurosurgical Infections, the SEHP, and the C-CLIN Paris-Nord. Neurosurgery. 1997; 41(5):1073–1079, discussion 1079–1081

[112] Korinek AM, et al. Risk factors for adult nosocomial meningitis after craniotomy: role of antibiotic prophylaxis. Neurosurgery. 2006; 59 (1):126–133, discussion 126–133

[113] Kalfas IH, Little JR. Postoperative hemorrhage: a survey of 4992 intracranial procedures. Neurosurgery. 1988; 23(3):343–347

[114] Palmer JD, Sparrow OC, Iannotti F. Postoperative hematoma: a 5-year survey and identification of avoidable risk factors. Neurosurgery. 1994; 35(6):1061–1064, discussion 1064–1065

[115] Lassen B, Helseth E, Rønning P, et al. Surgical mortality at 30 days and complications leading to recraniotomy in 2630 consecutive craniotomies for intracranial tumors. Neurosurgery. 2011; 68(5): 1259–1268, discussion 1268–1269

[116] Waga S, Shimosaka S, Sakakura M. Intracerebral hemorrhage remote from the site of the initial neurosurgical procedure. Neurosurgery. 1983; 13(6):662–665

[117] Brisman MH, Bederson JB, Sen CN, Germano IM, Moore F, Post KD. Intracerebral hemorrhage occurring remote from the craniotomy site. Neurosurgery. 1996; 39(6):1114–1121, discussion 1121–1122

[118] Agnelli G, Piovella F, Buoncristiani P, et al. Enoxaparin plus compression stockings compared with compression stockings alone in the prevention of venous thromboembolism after elective neurosurgery. N Engl J Med. 1998; 339(2):80–85

[119] Dickinson LD, Miller LD, Patel CP, Gupta SK. Enoxaparin increases the incidence of postoperative intracranial hemorrhage when initiated preoperatively for deep venous thrombosis prophylaxis in patients with brain tumors. Neurosurgery. 1998; 43(5):1074–1081

[120] Raabe A, Gerlach R, Zimmermann M, Seifert V. The risk of haemorrhage associated with early postoperative heparin administration after intracranial surgery. Acta Neurochir (Wien). 2001; 143(1):1–7

[121] Gerlach R, Scheuer T, Beck J, Woszczyk A, Seifert V, Raabe A. Risk of postoperative hemorrhage after intracranial surgery after early nadroparin administration: results of a prospective study. Neurosurgery. 2003; 53(5):1028–1034, discussion 1034–1035

[122] Taylor WA, Thomas NW, Wellings JA, Bell BA. Timing of post-operative intracranial hematoma development and implications for the best use of neurosurgical intensive care. J Neurosurg. 1995; 82 (1):48–50

[123] Himes BT, et al. Contemporary analysis of the intraoperative and perioperative complications of neurosurgical procedures performed in the sitting position. J Neurosurg. 2016:1–7

[124] Subach BR, Lunsford LD, Kondziolka D, Maitz AH, Flickinger JC. Management of petroclival meningiomas by stereotactic radiosurgery. Neurosurgery. 1998; 42(3):437–443, discussion 443–445

[125] Sheehan JP, Starke RM, Kano H, et al. Gamma Knife radiosurgery for posterior fossa meningiomas: a multicenter study. J Neurosurg. 2015; 122(6):1479–1489

[126] Zachenhofer I, Wolfsberger S, Aichholzer M, et al. Gamma-knife radiosurgery for cranial base meningiomas: experience of tumor control, clinical course, and morbidity in a follow-up of more than 8 years. Neurosurgery. 2006; 58(1):28–36, discussion 28–36

[127] Iwai Y, Yamanaka K, Ikeda H. Gamma Knife radiosurgery for skull base meningioma: long-term results of low-dose treatment. J Neurosurg. 2008; 109(5):804–810

14 Foramen Magnum Meningioma

Devi Prasad Patra, Anil Nanda

Abstract

Foramen magnum (FM) meningiomas are rare overall, yet relatively common specific to that region. These are slow growing tumors and therefore present late in the course due to involvement of adjacent brainstem and lower cranial nerves. Surgical resection provides the best chance for cure but is challenging due to its critical location. A detailed anatomical knowledge of bony anatomy around the FM, lower eight cranial nerves, and vertebral artery (VA) is essential for a safe surgical approach. The tumor location in relation to the brainstem dictates the surgical approach and is the main determinant for surgical difficulty and morbidity. Tumors located posterior and posterolateral to the brainstem are easily approached through a suboccipital approach. However, tumors ventral to the brainstem require complex surgical approaches including far-lateral approach or extreme lateral approach. The critical steps involved in these approaches are the occipital condylar resection and mobilization of the VA. However, majority of the FM meningiomas can be safely removed without the condylar resection, due to the significant brainstem shifting associated with these lesions. With the use of neuronavigation and neuromonitoring, the rate of complete resection has been reported to be more than 85%, with an acceptable recurrence rate of 0 to 12%. Gamma knife radiosurgery has emerged as a useful adjunct to surgery and has a promising role in complex and large tumors especially after subtotal resections.

Keywords: foramen magnum meningiomas, far lateral approach, extreme lateral approach, occipital condyle, vertebral artery, surgical resection, operative approach

14.1 Introduction

The foramen magnum (FM) region is a highly complex territory of the skull base and contains many important and vital structures. Meningiomas in this region though rare as compared to other intracranial locations, comprise more than three-fourth of the tumors.[1,2] Close proximity to the highly sensitive structures like medulla and lower cranial nerves poses formidable challenge in their surgical resection. The difficulty increases multifold especially in anteriorly located lesions which are anatomically hidden from the surgeon's view. Many new surgical approaches and modifications have been developed and compared to provide adequate access to deal with these lesions. With recent improvements in surgical techniques and image guidance, almost all lesions are now surgically resectable with acceptable complications.

14.2 History

The earliest description of a meningioma at the FM region was in 1872 by Hallopeau, he described his autopsy finding of a patient who died within 5 months of developing motor symptoms.[3] Surgery around this region was considered intimidating and less rewarding. Later, in 1922, Fraizier published his series of 14 patients of spinal cord tumors which included one FM meningioma.[4] He described his difficulty in achieving a total resection in a patient with a craniospinal tumor in which two-third of the tumor was intracranial. He described *"…had it not been for the fact that the respiratory act was sustained alone by the half of the diaphragm, its removal could have been accomplished."* Unfortunately, the patient developed respiratory arrest during the operation and died. Three years later, in 1925, Elsberg and Strauss could achieve the successful removal of a FM tumor in which the patient had a complete symptomatic improvement.[5] Literature on FM meningioma was sparse in the mid twentieth century and most of the cases have been described along with other spinal cord or intracranial tumors. Management of FM meningioma as a separate entity was discerned and described by Yasargil, who documented his series of 114 cases in 1980.[6] Subsequently, Bernard George and colleagues presented their series of 230 FM region tumors at 44th Annual Congress at Brussels in 1993, which contained 106 cases of meningioma.[7] Most of the patients in the early literature were operated by the classic posterolateral approach with variable degree of resection rate. The resection rates were less appealing for the anterior FM meningiomas. Subsequently, Heros described the feasibility of far lateral approach which revolutionized the surgical approaches to the FM region.[8] Since then, various modifications and nuances have been described and compared to increase the resectability of the tumors while reducing the complication rates.

14.3 Surgical Anatomy

On account of the invaluable contribution by Albert Rhoton, the microsurgical anatomy of the FM region has become more lucid for neurosurgeons.[9] The intricate anatomy at this location has been of great interest to neuroanatomist and multiple reports have been published on cadaveric dissections. Similarly, in quest of defining the optimal approach, various quantitative anatomical studies have been described, focusing on different skull base approaches and their modifications.[10,11,12,13,14,15,16,17] With respect to approaches for the FM meningiomas, it is important to understand the microsurgical anatomy of three basic yet most important structures in this region which include the occipital condyles, vertebral artery (VA), and the cranial nerves of the posterior fossa.

14.3.1 Occipital Condyle

The FM is ovoid in shape in its anterior posterior direction and occipital condyles occupy its anterior half. The occipital condyles face downward, anteriorly, and laterally, and slightly bulge into the foramen. It is attached to the superior facets of the atlas and forms the occipitoatlantal joint. The condylar fossa is a depression on the occipital bone that lies just above and posterior to the posterior lip of condyles. The condylar fossa contains the condylar vein which connects the vertebral venous plexus to the sigmoid sinus. The condylar fossa is the main bony structure that is removed during a far lateral approach that provides a great degree of intradural exposure. The occipital condyles are bean-shaped and for anatomical description have been divided into three thirds. The most important structure important in relation to the condyles is the hypoglossal nerve that runs in the hypoglossal canal which lies above the mid-third of the condyle. The hypoglossal nerve traverses anterolaterally at an angle of 45° to the sagittal plane after arising from the brainstem and is relatively fixed. During condylar resection, the safe limit (considered as the resection of medial one-third of condyle) is defined by the exposure of cortical bone over the hypoglossal canal. Other bony structures that are relevant to this area are the jugular process and jugular tubercle but are less commonly removed in meningioma resection.

14.3.2 Vertebral Artery

Detailed knowledge of the VA anatomy especially on its extradural course is of paramount importance during surgical approaches of the FM. The artery is less obvious in this region and due to its variable and complex course, it is more prone for injury during soft tissue dissection. During a routine far lateral approach, the VA is usually exposed from the transverse foramen of C2 to its intradural course (▶ Fig. 14.1a). The artery traverses vertically and slightly laterally from the transverse foramen of C2 to transverse foramen of C1. After exiting from C1 foramina, the artery curves medially and posteriorly around the atlanto-occipital joint. During this course, it rests on the superior surface of posterior arch of atlas called as the vertebral groove, which often gets ossified to form a canal. After exiting medially from the groove, the artery turns anteriorly and medially to pierce the dura. During its dural entry, a cuff of dura around the artery may form a sleeve which is an important anatomical point to realize during the dural incision. The artery gives rise to many meningeal branches during its extradural course. The posterior spinal artery and possibly the posterior inferior cerebellar arteries are important branches during its

dural entry and should always be searched for during dissection around this region. The VA may need to be mobilized during the course of surgery to expose the atlanto-occipital joint. The V2 segment is usually freed up by drilling the posterior ramus of transverse foramina of C1 which along with dissection from the vertebral groove allows the artery to be mobilized inferomedially. The extradural course of the VA, especially in its third segment, is surrounded by a vertebral venous plexus which can be a source of brisk bleeding while dissecting the VA. Therefore, a subperiosteal dissection is always advisable that avoids entry into the periarterial soft tissue containing the plexus. The intradural course of the VA is variable with formation of loops and curves while resting on anterior clival dura. After coursing anteromedially, it joins the opposite VA to form the basilar artery (BA) which usually lies at the pontomedullary junction. The posteroinferior cerebellar artery is an important branch from this segment of VA.

Cranial Nerves

After the dural opening, the dentate ligaments serve as the midline structure that divides the spinal canal into anterior and posterior compartments. The rootlets of C2, C1, and the spinal part of accessory nerve are the main neural structures found in the upper spinal canal. The first cervical nerve runs just below and posterior to the dural entry point of VA. Above this level are the important lower cranial nerves which run anterolaterally after origin from the brainstem (▶ Fig. 14.1b). The glossopharyngeal nerve arises as one or two rootlets, the vagus as series of seven or more rootlets and the cranial accessory as four to five rootlets and all of them form a fan-like structure running across the jugular tubercle into the jugular foramen. In most of the cases, the lower cranial nerves are displaced either anteroinferiorly or posterosuperiorly depending upon the origin of the tumor (described later). The hypoglossal nerve runs behind the VA into the hypoglossal canal after its origin from the medulla.

14.4 Epidemiology, Clinical Presentation, and Imaging

FM meningiomas are rare and only comprise about 0.3 to 3.2% of all meningiomas.[18] However, when compared to all posterior fossa pathologies, it accounts for a sizable proportion of all tumors. More specifically, in the FM region, this is the most common pathology encountered and comprises about 70% of the lesions.[19] Similarly, among spinal meningiomas, around 8.6% of the lesions are located in the FM region extending to the upper cervical spine. Most of the patients present in their fourth to sixth decade. However, pediatric patients have also been reported harboring FM meningiomas. Athanasiou et al in

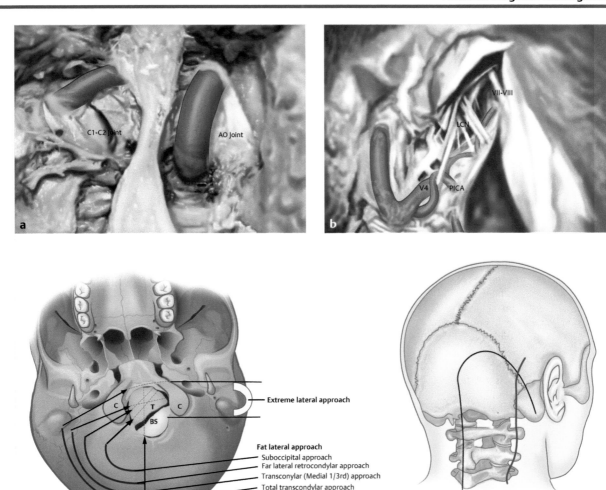

Fig. 14.1 (a) Illustration showing the course and bony relations of the V2 and V3 segment of vertebral artery. (b) Illustrations showing intracranial exposure after dural opening in far lateral approach. Note the course of the lower cranial nerves and the intracranial VA. (c) Schematic diagram showing various skull base approaches to foramen magnum region. Note that with subsequent lateral extension of the bony resection, the exposure to the contralateral side of anterior foramen magnum is getting increased. (d) Illustration showing the hockey stick skin incision in far lateral approach.

their literature review of 34 pediatric patients with FM meningiomas found that, the mean age of presentation is less (9.95 years) as compared to meningiomas at other locations (14–15 years) and attributed this to early development of increased intracranial pressure, brainstem compression and hydrocephalus inherent to its location.[20] Most of the FM meningiomas in the pediatric age group or at multiple locations are associated with neurofibromatosis type 2 (NF-2).[21] Similar to meningiomas at other locations, FM meningiomas are more common in female with male to female ratio of 2–4:1.

Meningiomas in the FM region are particularly slow growing and therefore present very late in the course of the disease.[22] Most of the symptoms are due to chronic compression brainstem and spinal cord and occasionally

the cranial or spinal nerves. The symptoms are initially vague and nonspecific that leads to initial misdiagnosis to cervical spondylotic myelopathy, cervical disk herniation, multiple sclerosis or other noncompressive myelopathy.[19] The diagnostic delay from the onset of symptoms was higher in older literatures that was as high as 6.5 years,[23,24] however, recent studies report an average delay of almost 30 months.[18] In a significant subset of patients, the lesion is totally asymptomatic and is detected during routine imaging for head trauma or other nonrelated causes. In symptomatic patients, the most common presentation is cervical pain and headache. The headache is related to the stretching of the cervical and posterior fossa dura. In few patients, the headache is progressive and is due to increased intracranial pressure secondary to hydrocephalus. The hydrocephalus is due to the obstruction of the CSF pathway from brainstem compression and usually does not need permanent CSF diversion. However, it is important to clinically differentiate the headaches due to raised intracranial pressure from other causes, which needs urgent intervention. The most common neurological manifestation due to brainstem compression is the gait ataxia followed by spastic quadriparesis. Typical patterns though not seen in all cases are the cruciate paresis and rotating palsy. In the former pattern, ipsilateral arm is involved followed by contralateral leg, contralateral arm, and ipsilateral leg, respectively. Rotating palsy involves extremities in a rotating sequential pattern from ipsilateral arm to ipsilateral leg, contralateral leg and then to contralateral arm. In tumors with significant caudal extension to the cervical spine, lower motor involvement is seen leading to atrophy of muscles of arm, forearm, or even of the intrinsic muscles of hands. Sensory involvement is not very common but is possible in larger tumors with significant compressions where features of dissociated sensory loss or a Brown-Sequard syndrome are seen. In tumors with more cranial extension, cranial nerves and cerebellar peduncles or hemispheres are likely to get compressed. The most common involvement is of the spinal accessory nerve which gives rise to atrophy of the trapezius and sternocleidomastoid muscles. Other infrequently involved nerves are the hypoglossal nerve leading to tongue atrophy and lower cranial nerves that gives rise to dysphagia or dysphonia. More proximal cranial nerves like vestibulocochlear, facial, or trigeminal nerves are very rarely involved. Cerebellar symptoms are mostly bilateral due to peduncular involvement or compression of crossing fibers in the brainstem. Unilateral appendicular ataxia is possible in laterally located tumors due to compression of cerebellar hemispheres.

The formal imaging studies required for these tumors are the nonenhanced computed tomogram including the bone windows and MRI with gadolinium. Imaging is very crucial in surgical planning and intraoperative navigation. Similar to meningiomas at other locations, these tumors are iso- to hypointense on T1, iso- to hyperintense on T2, and enhance brightly with gadolinium. The T2 hyperintensity is related to the tumor water content and softer and friable tumors appear brighter in this sequence. There is little confusion in getting a diagnosis of meningioma with presence of these typical imaging features. However, in few patients with atypical imaging findings other differential diagnoses of intradural and extradural tumors at FM meningiomas should be excluded. The sagittal and coronal images are important to define the tumor extension and surgical planning. Other important features to be looked in the imaging are the course of the VA, degree of compression, and shifting of the brainstem. CT scans are invaluable mostly to delineate the cranial anatomy especially the occipital condyle, jugular tubercle,

hypoglossal foramen, etc. In some cases, tumors are associated with calcifications which is easily detected by the CT scan. Angiograms like CT or MR are rarely necessary unless a detailed vascular anatomy needs to be studied. Such situations arise in patients with suspected VA encasement or invasion. Secondly, when a more lateral approach is planned a CT angiography is helpful to show the extracranial course of VA and to rule out any anomalous course or branch on the side of approach.

14.5 Classification of Foramen Magnum Meningioma

There have been several classification schemes for FM meningiomas all of which are centered on the description of tumor with respect to the tumor position in relation to the brainstem. The earliest classification put forward by Cushing and Eisenhard describe tumors based on their vertical extensions.[25] The "craniospinal meningiomas" comprised tumors arising from the dura over the clivus ventral to the brainstem with possible extension to upper spinal canal. The other variant "spinocranial meningiomas" comprised tumors arising from the spinal dura posterior to the spinal cord with possible intracranial extension dorsal and lateral to medulla. George and Lot[18] described tumors based on their position in a horizontal relation to the brainstem. They classified tumors into posterior, lateral, or ventral variants. Bruneau and George[26] included the relation of tumor to VA into their classification system and described four tumor types: type-A tumors arise below the VA and grow upwards, type-B tumors arise above the VA and grow downwards, and type-C tumors are described by the VA coursing across the lesion with or without encasement. The C1 type is intradural whereas C2 type has dural penetration with an extradural component. The origin of the tumor in relation the VA is important in two possible ways. Firstly, tumors originating from below the VA pushes the lower cranial nerves upward and posteriorly putting the surgeon in an advantageous position. However, tumors arising from above the VA pushes the nerves anteriorly and inferiorly and thereby are encountered early in the course and requires careful dissection. Secondly, it is important to estimate the involvement of the VA by the tumor. In most patients, encasement of the artery by intradural tumors are less problematic because of the presence of a well-preserved arachnoid plane between the tumor and artery. However, extradural tumors arising from the spinal dura can involve the extradural part of the VA. In such cases, tumors may involve the adventitia of the artery, thereby making surgical excision difficult.

Despite many proposed classifications, most of the surgeons group their cases into two types, i.e., the ventral type and posterolateral type.[22] This simplest categorization does have clinical utility while considering appropriate surgical approach. The vertical extension of the tumor has got a lesser contribution in choosing the right approach.

14.6 Operative Approaches

An important hindrance to all skull base approaches dedicated to this area is the significant high rate of intraoperative complications and postoperative morbidity. However, with better understanding of the anatomy, use of intraoperative monitoring, and intraoperative navigation tools there has been significant decrease in intraoperative adverse events with a resulting improved postoperative outcome. In addition, with advent of stereotactic radiosurgery, there has been a trend towards more conservative surgical resection. However still, many skull base surgeons are proponents of gross total resection in the index surgery itself as it gives the best chance of cure. With experienced hands, even complex tumors could be resected completely, with acceptable morbidity.

The primary determinant for a particular surgical approach over others is the location of the tumor in the horizontal axis with respect to midline. Generally, tumors located posterior and posterolateral to brainstem are easy to access from a posterior route. Tumors ventral to the brainstem are difficult to approach from a posterior perspective because of the brainstem and therefore requires more lateral approach. Overall, the surgical approaches to the FM meningiomas are divided into three types with various possible modifications. These approaches with progressively increased complexity and morbidity includes the posterior suboccipital approach, far lateral approach, and extreme lateral approach (▶ Fig. 14.1c). Ventral approaches like open transoral or endoscopic approaches have been described historically but rarely used nowadays.

14.6.1 Posterior Suboccipital Approach

This is the simplest and frequently used approach for posterior and posterolateral tumors in which the main bulk of the tumor displaces the brainstem anteriorly. The cranial nerves and the spinal nerves are displaced anteriorly and superiorly and therefore pose little risk while dissection. This approach is feasible even in more anteriorly located tumors because of the brainstem shift associated with most of the tumors.[27,28]

The patient is positioned in prone with the head slightly flexed to expand the suboccipital space. A skin incision is placed in the midline starting from just below the inion upto the spine of the third cervical vertebra. The skin incision is deepened and the posterior rim of the FM and posterior arch of atlas and axis are identified. The muscles are dissected laterally up to the condylar fossa. A

sub-occipital craniotomy is done including removal of posterior arch of atlas. In pure sub-occipital approach, identification of the vertebral artery is usually not required, however, its location should be confirmed to avoid its inadvertent injury. The tumor is usually identified just after the opening of the dura. In posteriorly located tumors, all the spinal nerves and the denticulate ligament are displaced anteriorly and visualized after removal of the tumor. In few patients, the tumor has both anterior and posterior components. In such cases, the anterior component (identified as tumors located anterior to denticulate ligament) can be removed by working in between the nerve rootlets. The C1 and C2 nerve rootlets can be sacrificed safely in case it is required for resection. After removal of the tumor, the dural attachment is coagulated and the thecal sac is closed.

14.6.2 Far Lateral Approach

This is essentially the lateral extension of the suboccipital approach. The far lateral approach was popularized by Heros in the late twentieth century.[29] Various modifications have been introduced to the original description, however, the basic principle involves removal of the lateral rim of the FM towards the condylar fossa along with the part of C1 posterior arch which provides a more inferolateral view to the midclivus without need of brainstem retraction. Need of condyle resection is the most controversial topic in this approach, however, in particular to the FM meningiomas, most of the surgeons agree that condyle resection is not really necessary for the removal of ventral meningiomas.[27,30,31,32,33,34,35]

For a far lateral approach, multiple patient positions have been described including lateral, park bench, and sitting positions. Lateral and park bench positions are mostly used based on surgeon's preference. Sitting positions are preferred by few surgeons as it provides a more anatomical view along with a blood less field. However, complications inherent to sitting positions like air embolism and deep vein thrombosis, makes it less favorable. Irrespective of the position used, it is important to avoid gross manipulation of the craniovertebral junction, especially head flexion, as it may compromise the brainstem which is already compressed by the tumor. Intraoperative monitoring helps identifying any adverse event related to brainstem compression both during positioning and surgery. Most of the surgeons prefer an inverted J-shaped incision with the horizontal arm lying in the midline and the horizontal arm curving below the inion laterally up to the base of mastoid. Alternatively, a curvilinear lazy S incision similar to the incision used for retrosigmoid approaches can also be used, which is also the authors' preferred incision (▶ Fig. 14.1d). After careful soft tissue and muscle dissection, the FM is exposed laterally up to the medial border of the condylar fossa. Similarly, the posterior arch of atlas (and the axis in cases) is exposed laterally up to the tip of the lateral mass. The VA is carefully identified along the upper border of the C1 arch when it curves posteriorly after arising from the C1 foramen. In some cases, the VA groove on the upper surface of C1 arch is ossified and converted into a canal. In such cases, it is very difficult to mobilize the VA and requires careful drilling of the canal. Significant venous bleeding from perivertebral venous plexus is a possible complication during dissection of VA. Therefore, it is advisable to develop a subperiosteal dissection without violating the periarterial soft tissue sheath. Mobilization of the VA from the C1 groove is enough in most of the cases, however, some cases may require more lateral approach and needs complete mobilization of the vertebral artery from the C1 foramen. In such cases, the foramen can be opened with drilling of the posterior ramus. A subperiosteal dissection usually takes the artery out of the foramen. Excision of the lateral mass of the C1 can be done if required for a more lateral exposure and to provide more surgical freedom. This medial transposition of the VA gives more exposure and improves the surgical freedom. Though not considered as a routine in far lateral exposures, medial transposition of the VA is considered essential for extreme lateral approaches. Another important consideration at this point is to identify any possible developmental anomaly of the VA or presence of any aberrant course.

A suboccipital craniotomy is performed similar to standard retrosigmoid approach exposing the junction of the sigmoid and transverse sinuses. However, a more caudal and lateral craniotomy is added by removing the condylar fossa, which is the main bony structure that needs to be removed to achieve a significant lateral exposure. Often termed as "condylar fossa approach", this technique actually gives a significant preliminary exposure to the

petroclival region and midclivus.[15] The condylar fossa contains the condylar vein in its depth which is a tributary of sigmoid sinus and can be easily controlled with coagulation. However, in some patients, the condylar vein is of significant size and needs careful control. Just lateral to the condylar fossa lies the occipital condyle. The occipital condyle is an important landmark in the far lateral approach and is subject to many controversies regarding its need of removal. From an anatomic point of view, occipital condyles occupy the anterolateral quadrant of the FM and should obstruct view of the midclivus while looking from a posterolateral aspect. However, in FM meningiomas, because of significant amount of brain shift, an unrestricted view to the anterior FM can be easily obtained, even in the presence of the condyles (▶ Fig. 14.2 a and b). Many anatomical studies have been carried out to define the significance of condyles in far lateral approaches.[13,36,37] In a subset of patients in whom the occipital condyles are prominent and significantly bulge into the FM can become problematic and can hide a significant proportion of the tumor, even in the presence of brain shift. These factors should be taken into consideration during presurgical planning, and therefore needs careful observation of the bony anatomy in preoperative CT scans. When there is a need of condylar resection, the VA should be carefully mobilized and its dural entry point is ensured. The joint capsule is identified and opened. The posterior lips of the occipital condyles are carefully drilled. The important landmark to the limit of posterior one-third of occipital condyle resection is the hypoglossal canal. The bone can be drilled till cortical bone lining of the hypoglossal canal is reached which is considered to be the maximal safe limit. The orientation of the intradural part of hypoglossal nerve should be observed to

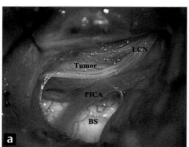
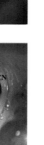
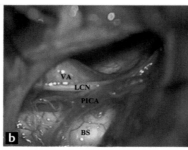
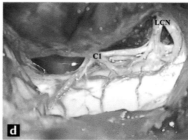

Fig. 14.2 Intraoperative images.
(a) Exposure after far lateral approach showing the tumor in the ventral foramen of magnum, posterior inferior cerebellar artery and the lower cranial nerves.
(b) Image after complete resection of the tumor. (c) Intraoperative images in a craniospinal tumor in the anterolateral location showing relation of the tumor to the lower cranial nerves and the C1 nerve root. (d) Image after complete resection of the tumor.

avoid injury. The lateral extension to the craniotomy can be obtained by doing a more supracondylar drilling which can reach up to the jugular tubercle. By this time, a sufficient exposure of the anterior aspect of medulla and pons is usually obtained to safely perform tumor resection, even in purely ventral tumors with contralateral extension. After sufficient bony work, the dura is opened parallel to the sigmoid sinus that curves around the cuff of VA and extends down to the cervical dura. With lateral retraction of the dura and rostromedial retraction of the cerebellum, the whole of the anterolateral cisterns around the brainstem including the mid and lower clivus can be visualized. At this point, the cranial nerves serve as the main obstacle for dissection. The trigeminal nerve and the VII-VIII nerve complex lie anterolaterally and the lower cranial nerves lie laterally forming a transverse neural barrier. For this reason, the anterior dissection and tumor removal should proceed working in the corridors between the nerves. For posteriorly located tumors, it hardly ever creates problem, because the nerve complex are shifted anteriorly and are seen beneath the arachnoid later in the course. Even with an excellent exposure it is possible to miss some part of the tumor that lies to the contralateral side behind the brainstem because of obstructing line of vision. Therefore, for FM meningiomas with significant contralateral extension, it is important to access the completeness of the tumor removal by looking towards these blind points.

14.6.3 Extreme Lateral Approach

This is the most lateral and direct approach to the anterior FM and clivus. This approach was initially described by Sen and Sekhar and is mostly directed towards extradural lesions at the region of the clivus.[38] In contrast to the far lateral approach, this approach utilizes dissection anterior to the sternocleidomastoid muscle and posterior to the internal jugular vein and provides the shortest route to occipital condyles which needs to be removed to access the anterior clivus.[39] In addition, as the lateral mass of C1 vertebra is encountered en route, the vertebral artery mobilization is usually essential to gain access of the condyles. In comparison to far lateral approach, this approach is technically more demanding and requires extensive mobilization of vascular structures. This approach is rarely used for FM meningiomas and is most useful in en plaque tumors with significant contralateral and extradural extension.

In the extreme lateral approach, the patient is positioned lateral and a skin incision is made anterior to the sternocleidomastoid muscle that extends superiorly to the base of mastoid. After the skin incision, the sternocleidomastoid muscle is divided at its attachment to mastoid leaving a cuff behind for closure. At this point, the accessory nerve should be identified and preserved. One important guide is to identify the nerve at around

3.5 cm below the tip of mastoid. With further dissection, the tip of the transverse process of atlas is identified in the suboccipital triangle. The vertebral artery is identified in the transverse foramen of C1 and is mobilized by drilling its posterior ramus. The transverse process is then removed completely after detaching all its muscular attachments. With continued bone work, the lateral aspect of the occipital condyles with the superior articular facet of atlas are encountered. With further removal of the joint, a direct anterior view of the FM with the dens is obtained.

14.7 Controversies in Surgical Approaches

14.7.1 Need for Condyle Resection

Many of the authors would agree that most of the FM meningiomas can be removed without a condylar resection or at most need a partial resection in cases with significant contralateral extension.[27,30,31,33,34,35] Many studies have quantitatively measured the exposure gained by resection of condyle in far lateral approach.[14,15,16,17,33] In our previous cadaveric study on far lateral approach, we have estimated that the mean degree of visibility gained by resection of one-third of condyle and one-half of condyle were $15.9 \pm 2°$ and $19.9 \pm 2.7°$, respectively.[33] Anhua et al in their study have compared the transcondylar approach (with resection of condyle) with the condylar fossa approach (without resection of condyle) and found that the resection of condyle only slightly improves the exposure of the petroclival region and lower brainstem, however, it does improve the angle of attack to the vertebral artery-posterior inferior cerebellar artery junction.[15] In another study, Spektor et al separately measured the petroclival exposure and the surgical freedom with successive steps of bony removal. In their observation, partial condylectomy only insignificantly improves the exposure, but significantly improved the surgical freedom.[16] Similarly, total condylectomy does not add any significant exposure but carries significant risk of instability. The most important bony landmark that has significant effect on exposure is the jugular tubercle. As expected, this small piece of bony prominence hinders significant portion of the midclivus in the region of VA-BA junction. However, need for resection of jugular tubercle is rare in routine practice.

The second important aspect that has attracted much attention is the maximal extent of condyle resection that can be safely tolerated. As discussed previously, resection of more than one third of the condyle is not associated with any gain in exposure. This mostly corresponds to the level of the hypoglossal canal intraoperatively. However, in certain cases in which the condylar bulge into the foramen of magnum is significant, some surgeons advocate more condylar resection to achieve a better exposure. For extradural lesions located anteriorly in the foramen of magnum, sometimes a more aggressive resection of the condyle is needed.[40,41,42,43,44,45] Condylar resection is almost a part of the extreme lateral approach. Many authors have claimed that, resection of more than a third of the condyle is associated with instability of the cervico-occipital junction and therefore needs instrumentation and fusion. The stability of the occipitocervical junction is governed by many anatomical structures apart from the joint itself.[46,47] These include the alar ligaments, the apical ligament, the posterior and anterior longitudinal ligaments, the tectorial membrane, and atlanto-occipital membrane. During a far lateral approach and transcondylar exposure, many of these ligamentous structures are disrupted which may include the posterior atlanto-occipital membrane, ipsilateral alar ligaments, etc. So, extensive dissection along with opening of the joint have theoretical but definite risk of instability. There are not many studies available in the literature that have compared the true biomechanical stability with different extent of condylar resection. Vishteh et al in 1999 published their findings of biomechanical study on stability of the craniovertebral junction after sequential condylar resection.[48] They found that the flexon-extension movement which is the primary movement of atlanto-occipital joint, is most affected by condylar resection. A significant instability could be observed even with a 25% condylar resection on both OC-C1 and C1-C2 joints. They recommended occipitocervical fusion after a 50% or more of condylar resection. Based on the current evidences, many authors would agree and fuse the occipitocervical junction when there is a resection of more than half of condyle.

14.7.2 Need for C1 Laminectomy

Resection of the posterior arch of atlas provides a more decent exposure of the dura over the craniocervical junction and is used by many of the surgeons during performing a suboccipital craniotomy. A limited posterior laminectomy is a routine for FM meningiomas extending to the cervical spine that needs opening of the cervical canal (▶ Fig. 14.2 c and d). However, the lateral extent of C1 hemilaminectomy is not defined. Excision of the lateral hemilamina provides a more angled view of the petroclival area from an inferolateral aspect. Removal of the bony obstacle in addition provides a great degree of surgical freedom in this area. However, mobilization and excision of the lateral part of C1 posterior arch is not without complications because of the presence of vertebral venous plexus and the VA itself. Careful mobilization of the VA is needed to avoid injury or thrombosis. The most lateral extent of the C1 bony removal is the resection of the lateral mass. It is an essential part during an extreme lateral approach, however, it is not frequently used for a far lateral approach unless there is a need for complete mobilization of the VA.

14.7.3 Need of Vertebral Artery Mobilization

VA mobilization is needed when there is a need for condylar resection and the artery just lies in front of the joint capsule. Secondly, freeing the artery from its bony and dural attachment provides another degree of freedom for instrument manipulation. The artery is usually fixed to the bony canals at the C2 and C1 vertebral foramens and requires the drilling of their posterior ramus to clear it off the foramen. Further mobilization requires a subperiosteal dissection from the vertebral groove on the upper surface of the C1 posterior arch. Finally, the dural entry point of the VA is identified and is divided with a cuff of dura around it. It is important to understand that in few cases, the dural sleeve for the vertebral artery can be really long and may be adhered with the posterior spinal artery, spinal accessory nerve, first cervical nerve, and dentate ligament. Therefore, it is important to identify these structures before completely dividing the dural sleeve. After dural opening, the whole arterial loop of VA can be medially and caudally retracted giving an excellent view to the lower brainstem and petroclival region.[10,44,49,50,51,52] However, the dangers of VA manipulation with risk of injury and development pseudoaneurysm, arteriovenous fistula should be carefully weighed with the need of exposure in this area.[38,41,43,53,54] Bassioni et al in their series did not favor dissection or mobilization of VA.[30] Da li et al in their recent publication have used the VA mobilization only in their patients with epidural invasion along the course of the VA, however, they have cautioned about their use only with experienced hands. They performed resection of the involved VA segment in 4 out of their 71 patients.[51] For most of the FM meningiomas, we feel, complete mobilization of the VA is not required and only separation of the artery from the upper surface of the C1 arch should provide adequate exposure.

14.8 Choosing the Right Approach

The suitable approach for a particular case of FM meningioma depends upon many factors including the size and extent of the tumor, the bony anatomy of the FM especially the morphometry of the occipital condyle, the patient factors like age and comorbidities, and ultimately, the surgeon's preference. In approximately 90% of the cases, the tumor can be removed with a limited posterolateral retrocondylar approach without need of an aggressive resection of condyles. A great number of clinical studies including our personal case series have witnessed the successful removal of tumors without condyle removal.[30,31,32,33,34,35] However, several studies claim its necessity for complete removal of the tumor.[40,41,42,43,44,45] In most of the cases, the contralateral extension of the

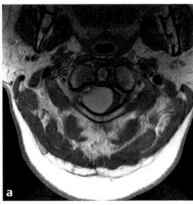 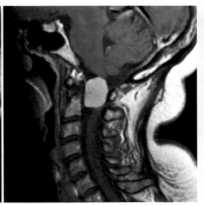

Preoperative Images

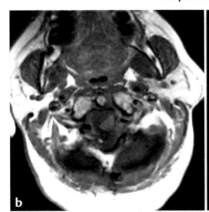 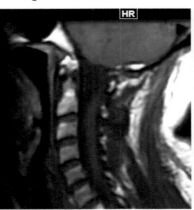

Postoperative Images

Fig. 14.3 54-year-old female with a meningioma at the foramen magnum in the ventrolateral location. Preoperative images **(a)** showing significant brainstem compression with a wide corridor for tumor dissection. Far lateral approach was taken and tumor excision was done without the need of condyle resection. Postoperative images **(b)** showing gross total resection.

tumor dictates the need of more lateral extension of the craniotomy by condyle removal. However, especially for intradural lesions like meninigiomas, a great degree of associated brainstem shift opens up a natural corridor which obviates the need of aggressive bony resection (▶ Fig. 14.3 and ▶ Fig. 14.4). As discussed previously, condylectomy, even if it is partial, has a significant risk of instability and may require additional fusion procedures. In older patients or in patients with significant comorbidities, such extensive resection with additional procedures may prove more harmful than the incomplete removal itself. With recent improvements in the stereotactic radiosurgery, many of the surgeons are favoring a less than total resection to avoid the complications of more aggressive approaches. Overall, the degree of lateral extension of the approach should be tailored individually based on the tumor extension and preference of the surgeon.

14.9 Complications

Surgical morbidity following surgical resection of FM meningiomas have consistently been reported to be high ranging from 40 to more than 70%.[55] The most common complication reported is the lower cranial nerve palsy leading to dysphagia and aspiration and has been reported in almost half of the patients.[49,50] Most of the patients present with swallowing difficulty that improve over time. Permanent deficits requiring tracheostomy are rare. In a series of 64 patients, Talachi et al have reported lower cranial nerve and hypoglossal nerve palsy in 44 and 33% of patients, respectively, with improvement in the deficits occurring in almost 66% of patients.[50] The other important complications are neurological deficits like hemiparesis, hemianesthesia, gait ataxia, etc. All these neurological symptoms including the cranial nerve deficits are related to the degree of manipulation and retraction of the cranial nerves and the brainstem. Direct injury to the brainstem is possible during tumor dissection when there is a breach in the separating arachnoid layer. Similarly, vascular injury of the brainstem perforators, VA branches can lead to ischemic infarction of the brainstem. Increasing the working angle by more bony work that avoids the retraction of neural structures seem to be rational; however, with current perspective of adjuvant radiosurgery, subtotal resection can be another viable option to preserve the quality of life. Some of the factors that have been correlated with poor surgical

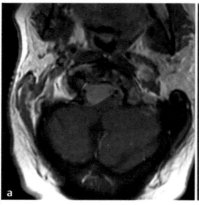
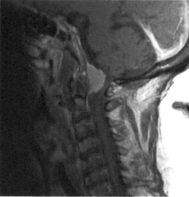

Fig. 14.4 62-year-old female with a meningioma at the foramen magnum. (a) In the ventrolateral location. **(b)** The tumor could be completely resected without the need of condyle drilling.

Preoperative Images

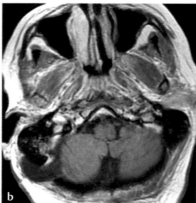
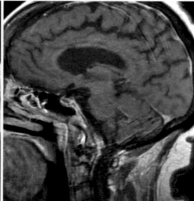

Postoperative Images

outcome include the ventral location of the tumor, tumor extending to lower clivus, encasement of the VA, and recurrent tumors with adhesions.[26,30,34,56]

Non-neurological complications with surgery for FM meningioma include CSF leak, wound infection, pseudomeningocele, and craniospinal instability. CSF leak can be observed in as many as 20% of the patients and are related to inadequate dural closure, hydrocephalus, and prior radiation, etc.[30,57,58] With proper care, most of these complications are preventable and can also be appropriately treated should it occur in the postoperative period. Another important feared complication that is rarely observed is the craniospinal instability which is expected with more than 50% condylar resection. Many authors recommend fusion in such cases, however, cases have also been reported without complications even with total condylar resection.[51,59,60]

The mortality after surgery for meningiomas in the FM region was high in older series ranging from 10 to 25%.[26,32,38,61,62] However, with recent improvements, the surgical mortality has dropped down significantly to less than 3%.[18,26,31,41,45,50,56,57,58] The common causes leading to mortality after surgery include respiratory failure due to brainstem dysfunction or aspiration pneumonia, brainstem infarction due to vascular injury, etc.

14.10 Outcome

There have been a great diversity in the reporting of overall outcome in patients of FM meningiomas over decades because of variability of the patient cohorts. The gross total resection (GTR) rate reported by most of the studies are between 70 and 95%. In a large patient cohort of 114 patients, Zhen wu et al have reported a GTR rate of 86%.[58] Similar rate was observed in another large series by Bruneau et al with 107 patients.[26] In a meta-analysis by Komator et al, the GTR rate observed after a far lateral approach or their variations was 93.2%.[63] Recently, Da li et al have compared their own earlier series of 114 patients with later series of 71 patients and have observed a decrease in the rate of GTR from 86 to 79%.[49] This finding suggests towards a more conservative strategy observed by these authors which have reflected in the decrease of their morbidity rate from 49 to 32% and mortality rate from 2.6 to 0%.

The recurrence rate after surgery have been reported from 0 to 12% in most series. [2,20,26,32,40,49,53,55,56] A GTR is expected to produce low recurrence or progression of tumor over time. With a high GTR rate of 94% and 96%, George et al,[52] and Bassioni et al[30] could achieve a 0% recurrence rate, respectively. However, lower recurrence rates have also been observed with less GTR rates.[49,58] Da li et al have analyzed the adverse factors leading to higher recurrence rates to include type C2 lesions (tumors with partial or total VA encasement with extradural growth), subtotal resections, and pathological mitoses.[49]

The overall quality of life is the current focus as the determinant of outcome. Majority of the patients (up to 80–95%) are reported to be improved and could return to normal productive life after surgery. Surgical morbidity due to aggressive resection, prior comorbidities with poor preoperative Karnofsky's performance score have been correlated with poor quality of life. However, on the other hand, subtotal resections with recurrences may affect the quality of life in long term. Therefore, early surgical intervention with GTR provides the best outcome on a long run. However, a subset of patients with small tumors and calcifications can be considered as candidates for conservative management with a regular follow-up.

14.11 Role of Radiosurgery

Radiosurgery has revolutionized the treatment protocol of primary brain tumors, especially the skull base meningiomas. With excellent reports of gamma knife radiosurgery, the optimal treatment for skull base meningiomas especially at the critical locations have changed towards a more conservative resection. However, for FM meningiomas literature on radiosurgery are sparse and are limited to short case series. The earliest report on success of radiosurgery in FM meningiomas was given by Muthukumar et al in 1999 who treated 5 patients, in which 3 patients were treated with primary radiosurgery and 2 patients for recurrence after surgery.[64] After a mean follow-up of 3 years, 4 patients had stable tumor size. Similarly, Starke et al in 2010 published their experience with 5 patients, in which all patients had either stable disease or reduction of tumor size over a mean follow-up of 6 years.[65] One of their patients had increase in size after initial treatment but became stable after second treatment. To date, the largest series of radiosurgery in FM meningiomas has been published by Zenonos et al, who treated 24 patients out of which 17 patients were managed primarily with radiosurgery.[66] A clinical follow-up data was available in 21 patients and at a median follow-up of nearly 4 years, 10 patients had more than 25% tumor regression and 11 patients had stable tumor size. Although, the current evidences are not robust enough for a definite recommendation, it is quite logical to opt radiosurgery as a primary treatment option when the tumor size is small and is not acutely symptomatic. The indications may extend to patients who are poor candidates for surgery or with recurrent disease. The role of prophylactic radiosurgery after subtotal resections are yet to be defined, but presently, this is a common practice by many of the surgeons. The primary hindrance for radiosurgery at this location is the presence of medulla in the close vicinity of the tumor which limits higher dosing. In patients with already compressed brainstem, post radiosurgery tumor edema is a possible catastrophe. However, adverse effects after radiosurgery at this location have not been reported yet.

14.12 Personal Experience

The authors have treated a total of 30 patients of FM meningioma over a period of 20 years. Out of them, clinical follow-up is available for 25 patients. The authors earlier published a series of 10 patients along with an anatomical description of condyle drilling in cadavers.[33] The average age presentation in a patient cohort was 56 years (range 26 to 79 years). The male to female ratio was 1:4. The most common presentation was headache occurring in 70% of the patients. Two patients were completely asymptomatic and were diagnosed during imaging for other purposes. The other common presentations included spastic hemiparesis in 4, quadriparesis in 8, quadriplegia in 1, and weakness of sternocleidomastoid in 2 patients. 4 of the patients had gait ataxia without pyramidal symptoms. On imaging, 16 patients had tumors in the anterior or anterolateral region of the FM and the other 9 patients had tumors at posterior or posterolateral location. Significant cranial extension up to the midclivus was present in 4 patients. Similarly, significant caudal extension beyond the level of C2 was present in 2 patients.

All the patients were treated primarily with microsurgery. The preferred approach was the far lateral approach with variable lateral extension. However, four of the tumors could be resected using simple posterior suboccipital approach. In the series, the authors never used extreme lateral approach for these meningiomas. Surgery is performed in lateral position with a lazy-S curvilinear incision as described above. Resection of the posterior arch of C1 is routine practice for far lateral approaches, however, in none of the patients the authors needed complete excision up to the transverse process of C1. Vertebral artery mobilization is not a routine practice but was required in 6 patients. In most of the cases, the mobilization of the artery from the C1 groove served the purpose. An excellent exposure for a safe total resection without resection of the condyles, could be achieved in most of the patients (▶ Fig. 14.2, ▶ Fig. 14.3, and ▶ Fig. 14.4). However, a variable degree of condyle resection was required in 6 patients with meningiomas at anterior location extending to the contralateral side. However, in all these patients the extent of condyle resection was less than one-third and therefore an additional fusion procedure was not required. Less degree of brainstem shift was observed in these patients, which mandated a more lateral exposure. The rate of gross total excision, near total resection, and subtotal resection were 87, 8, and 5%, respectively. The rate of postoperative morbidity was 32% which included postoperative dysphagia in 10 patients and worsening of the neurological deficits in 5 patients. However, the neurological deficits were transient and improved in all patients during follow-up. In an average follow-up of 52 months (range 8–82 months), all patients had excellent outcome and had significant improvement in their neurological status as compared to preoperative

state. One patient died after 2 years of surgery but the death was unrelated to the meningioma.

None of the patients had recurrence or progression of the residual tumor in the follow-up period. However, one patient with a significant residual tumor was treated with stereotactic radiosurgery 1 year after the surgery (▶ Fig. 14.5).[67] The tumor has been stable after 3 years of radiosurgery and did not require any further management.

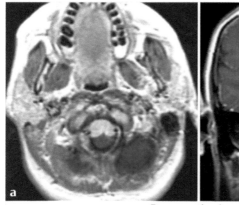
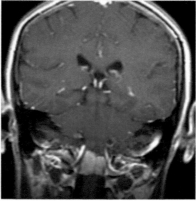

Preoperative Images

Fig. 14.5 59-year-old female with a foramen magnum meningioma at the ventral location. (a) With significant contralateral extension. **(b)** A subtotal excision was done using a far lateral approach without condyle drilling. **(c)** The residual lesion was subjected to gamma knife radiosurgery. The tumor is stable at 3 years of follow-up without any symptoms.

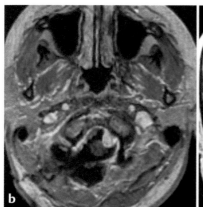
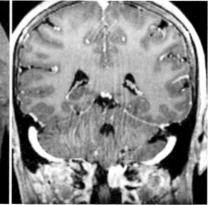

Postoperative Images

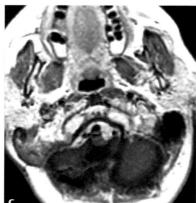
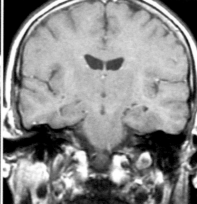

Post SRS after 3 years

14.13 Conclusion

Meningiomas at the FM are complex lesions at a critical location and are difficult to approach. Most of the lesions are slow growing and present late with significant brain stem compression with neurological deficits. Surgical excision is the treatment of choice for a possible cure. Surgical approaches are guided by the location of the tumor with respect to the horizontal plane. Most of the posterior or posterolateral tumors can be easily excised using a standard suboccipital approach. However, tumors at ventral location require a far lateral approach. Need of condylectomy is a controversial topic during a far lateral approach and current evidences suggest that most of the tumors could be easily excised without a condylar resection. However, tumors extending to the contralateral side with minimal brainstem shift may require a more lateral approach with possible condylectomy. Complications after surgery have been significant but in most of the cases are transient. Recurrence after gross total excision is rare and therefore should be the goal of surgery. Definite role of stereotactic radiosurgery as a primary treatment in FM meningiomas have not been consolidated, but many surgeons prefer it as an adjuvant therapy after a subtotal resection. In general, surgery provides the best chance of cure and should be provided to all large or symptomatic patients.

References

[1] Michael C, Ahmed F, Youjin C, Wilson L. Foramen magnum meningiomas. In: Al-Mefty O, DeMonte F, McDermott M, eds. Al-Mefty's Meningioma. 2nd ed. New York, NY: Thieme; 2011

[2] Flores BC, Boudreaux BP, Klinger DR, Mickey BE, Barnett SL. The far-lateral approach for foramen magnum meningiomas. Neurosurg Focus. 2013; 35(6):E12

[3] Hallopeau H. Note sur deux faits de tumeur de mesocephale; communiqués à la Société de Biologie. Gaz Med (Paris) 1874;3 (2):111–112

[4] Frazier CH, Spiller WG. An analysis of fourteen consecutive cases of spinal cord tumor. Arch Neurol Psychiatry. 1922; 8(5):455–501

[5] Elsberg C, Strauss I. Tumors of the spinal cord which project into the posterior cranial fossa. Report of a case in which a growth was removed from the ventral and lateral aspects of the medulla oblongata and upper cervical cord. Arch Neurol Psychiatry. 1929(21): 261–273

[6] Yasargil M, Mortara R, Curic M. Meningiomas of basal posterior cranial fossa. In: H K, ed. Advances and Technical Standards in Neurosurgery. Vienna: Springer-Verlag; 1980: 1–115

[7] George B, Lot G, Velut S, Gelbert F, Mourier KL. [French language Society of Neurosurgery. 44th Annual Congress. Brussels, 8–12 June 1993. Tumors of the foramen magnum]. Neurochirurgie. 1993; 39 Suppl 1:1–89

[8] Heros RC. Lateral suboccipital approach for vertebral and vertebrobasilar artery lesions. J Neurosurg. 1986; 64(4):559–562

[9] Wen HT, Rhoton AL, Jr, Katsuta T, de Oliveira E. Microsurgical anatomy of the transcondylar, supracondylar, and paracondylar extensions of the far-lateral approach. J Neurosurg. 1997; 87(4): 555–585

[10] Safavi-Abbasi S, de Oliveira JG, Deshmukh P, et al. The craniocaudal extension of posterolateral approaches and their combination: a quantitative anatomic and clinical analysis. Neurosurgery. 2010; 66(3) Suppl Operative:54–64

[11] Cavallo LM, Cappabianca P, Messina A, et al. The extended endoscopic endonasal approach to the clivus and cranio-vertebral junction: anatomical study. Childs Nerv Syst. 2007; 23(6):665–671

[12] Kim YD, Mendes GA, Seoane P, et al. Quantitative anatomical study of tailored far-lateral approach for the VA-PICA regions. J Neurol Surg B Skull Base. 2015; 76(1):57–65

[13] Muthukumar N, Swaminathan R, Venkatesh G, Bhanumathy SP. A morphometric analysis of the foramen magnum region as it relates to the transcondylar approach. Acta Neurochir (Wien). 2005; 147(8): 889–895

[14] Açikbaş SC, Tuncer R, Demirez I, et al. The effect of condylectomy on extreme lateral transcondylar approach to the anterior foramen magnum. Acta Neurochir (Wien). 1997; 139(6):546–550

[15] Wu A, Zabramski JM, Jittapiromsak P, Wallace RC, Spetzler RF, Preul MC. Quantitative analysis of variants of the far-lateral approach: condylar fossa and transcondylar exposures. Neurosurgery. 2010; 66 (6) Suppl Operative:191–198, discussion 198

[16] Spektor S, Anderson GJ, McMenomey SO, Horgan MA, Kellogg JX, Delashaw JB, Jr. Quantitative description of the far-lateral transcondylar transtubercular approach to the foramen magnum and clivus. J Neurosurg. 2000; 92(5):824–831

[17] Wanebo JE, Chicoine MR. Quantitative analysis of the transcondylar approach to the foramen magnum. Neurosurgery. 2001; 49(4):934–941, discussion 941–943

[18] George B, Lot G. Foramen magnum meningiomas: a review from personal experience of 37 cases and from a cooperative study of 106 cases. Neurosurg Q. 1995(5):149–167

[19] Yasuoka S, Okazaki H, Daube JR, MacCarty CS. Foramen magnum tumors. Analysis of 57 cases of benign extramedullary tumors. J Neurosurg. 1978; 49(6):828–838

[20] Athanasiou A, Magras I, Sarlis P, Spyridopoulos E, Polyzoidis K. Anterolateral meningioma of the foramen magnum and high cervical spine presenting intradural and extradural growth in a child: case report and literature review. Childs Nerv Syst. 2015; 31(12): 2345–2351

[21] Menezes AH. Craniovertebral junction neoplasms in the pediatric population. Childs Nerv Syst. 2008; 24(10):1173–1186

[22] Pamir MN, Ozduman K. Foramen Magnum Meningiomas. In: Pamir MN, Black PM, Fahlbusch R, eds. Meningiomas: A Comprehensive Text. Philadelphia, PA: Elsevier; 2010: 543–557

[23] Meyer FB, Ebersold MJ, Reese DF. Benign tumors of the foramen magnum. J Neurosurg. 1984; 61(1):136–142

[24] Stein BM, Leeds NE, Taveras JM, Pool JL. Meningiomas of the foramen magnum. J Neurosurg. 1963; 20:740–751

[25] Cushing H, Eisenhardt L. Meningiomas: their classification, regional behaviour, life history, and surgical end results. Springfield, IL: Charles C Thomas Limited; 1938

[26] Bruneau M, George B. Foramen magnum meningiomas: detailed surgical approaches and technical aspects at Lariboisière Hospital and review of the literature. Neurosurg Rev. 2008; 31(1):19–32, discussion 32–33

[27] Gupta SK, Khosla VK, Chhabra R, Mukherjee KK. Posterior midline approach for large anterior/anterolateral foramen magnum tumours. Br J Neurosurg. 2004; 18(2):164–167

[28] Goel A, Desai K, Muzumdar D. Surgery on anterior foramen magnum meningiomas using a conventional posterior suboccipital approach: a report on an experience with 17 cases. Neurosurgery. 2001; 49(1): 102–106, discussion 106–107

[29] Heros RC. Lateral suboccipital approach for vertebral and vertebrobasilar artery lesions. J Neurosurg. 1986; 64(4):559–562

[30] Bassiouni H, Ntoukas V, Asgari S, Sandalcioglu EI, Stolke D, Seifert V. Foramen magnum meningiomas: clinical outcome after microsurgical resection via a posterolateral suboccipital retrocondylar approach. Neurosurgery. 2006; 59(6):1177–1185, discussion 1185–1187

[31] Boulton MR, Cusimano MD. Foramen magnum meningiomas: concepts, classifications, and nuances. Neurosurg Focus. 2003; 14(6):e10

[32] Kratimenos GP, Crockard HA. The far lateral approach for ventrally placed foramen magnum and upper cervical spine tumours. Br J Neurosurg. 1993; 7(2):129–140

[33] Nanda A, Vincent DA, Vannemreddy PS, Baskaya MK, Chanda A. Far-lateral approach to intradural lesions of the foramen magnum without resection of the occipital condyle. J Neurosurg. 2002; 96(2):302–309

[34] Roberti F, Sekhar LN, Kalavakonda C, Wright DC. Posterior fossa meningiomas: surgical experience in 161 cases. Surg Neurol. 2001; 56(1):8–20, discussion 20–21

[35] Sharma BS, Gupta SK, Khosla VK, et al. Midline and far lateral approaches to foramen magnum lesions. Neurol India. 1999; 47(4):268–271

[36] Kalthur SG, Padmashali S, Gupta C, Dsouza AS. Anatomic study of the occipital condyle and its surgical implications in transcondylar approach. J Craniovertebr Junction Spine. 2014; 5(2):71–77

[37] Verma R, Kumar S, Rai AM, Mansoor I, Mehra RD. The anatomical perspective of human occipital condyle in relation to the hypoglossal canal, condylar canal, and jugular foramen and its surgical significance. J Craniovertebr Junction Spine. 2016; 7(4):243–249

[38] Sen CN, Sekhar LN. An extreme lateral approach to intradural lesions of the cervical spine and foramen magnum. Neurosurgery. 1990; 27(2):197–204

[39] Kawashima M, Tanriover N, Rhoton AL, Jr, Ulm AJ, Matsushima T. Comparison of the far lateral and extreme lateral variants of the atlanto-occipital transarticular approach to anterior extradural lesions of the craniovertebral junction. Neurosurgery. 2003; 53(3):662–674, discussion 674–675

[40] Arnautović KI, Al-Mefty O, Husain M. Ventral foramen magnum meninigiomas. J Neurosurg. 2000; 92(1) Suppl:71–80

[41] Bertalanffy H, Gilsbach JM, Mayfrank L, Klein HM, Kawase T, Seeger W. Microsurgical management of ventral and ventrolateral foramen magnum meningiomas. Acta Neurochir Suppl (Wien). 1996; 65:82–85

[42] Marin Sanabria EA, Ehara K, Tamaki N. Surgical experience with skull base approaches for foramen magnum meningioma. Neurol Med Chir (Tokyo). 2002; 42(11):472–478, discussion 479–480

[43] Salas E, Sekhar LN, Ziyal IM, Caputy AJ, Wright DC. Variations of the extreme-lateral craniocervical approach: anatomical study and clinical analysis of 69 patients. J Neurosurg. 1999; 90(2) Suppl:206–219

[44] Samii M, Klekamp J, Carvalho G. Surgical results for meningiomas of the craniocervical junction. Neurosurgery. 1996; 39(6):1086–1094, discussion 1094–1095

[45] Sekhar LN, Babu RP, Wright DC. Surgical resection of cranial base meningiomas. Neurosurg Clin N Am. 1994; 5(2):299–330

[46] Harris MB, Duval MJ, Davis JA, Jr, Bernini PM. Anatomical and roentgenographic features of atlantooccipital instability. J Spinal Disord. 1993; 6(1):5–10

[47] Panjabi M, Dvorak J, Crisco J, III, Oda T, Hilibrand A, Grob D. Flexion, extension, and lateral bending of the upper cervical spine in response to alar ligament transections. J Spinal Disord. 1991; 4(2):157–167

[48] Vishteh AG, Crawford NR, Melton MS, Spetzler RF, Sonntag VK, Dickman CA. Stability of the craniovertebral junction after unilateral occipital condyle resection: a biomechanical study. J Neurosurg. 1999; 90(1) Suppl:91–98

[49] Li D, Wu Z, Ren C, et al. Foramen magnum meningiomas: surgical results and risks predicting poor outcomes based on a modified classification. J Neurosurg. 2017; 126(3):661–676

[50] Talacchi A, Biroli A, Soda C, Masotto B, Bricolo A. Surgical management of ventral and ventrolateral foramen magnum meningiomas: report on a 64-case series and review of the literature. Neurosurg Rev. 2012; 35(3):359–367, discussion 367–368

[51] Gilsbach JM. Extreme lateral approach to intradural lesions of the cervical spine and foramen magnum. Neurosurgery. 1991; 28(5):779

[52] George B, Lot G, Boissonnet H. Meningioma of the foramen magnum: a series of 40 cases. Surg Neurol. 1997; 47(4):371–379

[53] Margalit NS, Lesser JB, Singer M, Sen C. Lateral approach to anterolateral tumors at the foramen magnum: factors determining surgical procedure. Neurosurgery. 2005; 56(2) Suppl:324–336, discussion 324–336

[54] Pirotte BJ, Brotchi J, DeWitte O. Management of anterolateral foramen magnum meningiomas: surgical vs conservative decision making. Neurosurgery. 2010; 67(3) Suppl Operative:ons58–ons70, discussion ons70

[55] Bydon M, Ma TM, Xu R, et al. Surgical outcomes of craniocervial junction meningiomas: a series of 22 consecutive patients. Clin Neurol Neurosurg. 2014; 117:71–79

[56] Kano T, Kawase T, Horiguchi T, Yoshida K. Meningiomas of the ventral foramen magnum and lower clivus: factors influencing surgical morbidity, the extent of tumour resection, and tumour recurrence. Acta Neurochir (Wien). 2010; 152(1):79–86, discussion 86

[57] Pamir MN, Kiliç T, Ozduman K, Türe U. Experience of a single institution treating foramen magnum meningiomas. J Clin Neurosci. 2004; 11(8):863–867

[58] Wu Z, Hao S, Zhang J, et al. Foramen magnum meningiomas: experiences in 114 patients at a single institute over 15 years. Surg Neurol. 2009; 72(4):376–382, discussion 382

[59] Suhardja A, Agur AM, Cusimano MD. Anatomical basis of approaches to foramen magnum and lower clival meningiomas: comparison of retrosigmoid and transcondylar approaches. Neurosurg Focus. 2003; 14(6):e9

[60] Sanai N, McDermott MW. A modified far-lateral approach for large or giant meningiomas of the posterior fossa. J Neurosurg. 2010; 112(5):907–912

[61] Crockard HA, Sen CN. The transoral approach for the management of intradural lesions at the craniovertebral junction: review of 7 cases. Neurosurgery. 1991; 28(1):88–97, discussion 97–98

[62] Guidetti B, Spallone A. Benign extramedullary tumors of the foramen magnum. Adv Tech Stand Neurosurg. 1988; 16:83–120

[63] Komotar RJ, Zacharia BE, McGovern RA, Sisti MB, Bruce JN, D'Ambrosio AL. Approaches to anterior and anterolateral foramen magnum lesions: A critical review. J Craniovertebr Junction Spine. 2010; 1(2):86–99

[64] Muthukumar N, Kondziolka D, Lunsford LD, Flickinger JC. Stereotactic radiosurgery for anterior foramen magnum meningiomas. Surg Neurol. 1999; 51(3):268–273

[65] Starke RM, Nguyen JH, Reames DL, Rainey J, Sheehan JP. Gamma knife radiosurgery of meningiomas involving the foramen magnum. J Craniovertebr Junction Spine. 2010; 1(1):23–28

[66] Zenonos G, Kondziolka D, Flickinger JC, Gardner P, Lunsford LD. Gamma Knife surgery in the treatment paradigm for foramen magnum meningiomas. J Neurosurg. 2012; 117(5):864–873

[67] Konar S, Bir SC, Maiti TK, Kalakoti P, Nanda A. Mirror meningioma at foramen magnum: a management challenge. World Neurosurg. 2016; 85:364.e1–364.e4

15 Tuberculum Sellae/Planum Meningiomas

Luigi Maria Cavallo, Norberto Andaluz, Alberto Di Somma, Domenico Solari, Paolo Cappabianca

Abstract

Planum sphenoidale and tuberculum sellae meningiomas require special surgical attention due to their close proximity to important neurovascular and endocrine structures. Surgical treatment of these anterior cranial base neoplasms has resembled the dramatic advances in neurosurgery over the past century. Being the open transcranial surgical approaches, the well-defined routes for such kind of pathologies, and the recent interest for minimally invasive techniques, has opened a new chapter in the surgical treatment options. The improvement of intraoperative visualization together with refined instrumentation, allowed the evolution of microneurosurgical techniques, and among those, the supraorbital keyhole approach has been used and validated over the last few years for the surgical management of such kind of tumors. On the other hand, recently, expanded endonasal approaches have been developed with the aim of reducing brain retraction and optic chiasm manipulation and improving ophthalmological outcomes by approaching the tumors with a below-to-above trajectory.

Based on these concepts, this chapter will discuss the advantages and limitations of the endoscopic endonasal and supraorbital routes offering an opposite perspective to access the tuberculum sellae and planum sphenoidale meningiomas.

Keywords: tuberculum sellae meningiomas, planum sphenoidale meningiomas, endoscopic skull base surgery, minimally invasive surgery, supraorbital approach

15.1 Introduction

Meningiomas of the anterior cranial fossa are challenging lesions due their mostly close relationship to neurovascular structures and the difficulty of approaching them easily.

In particular tuberculum sellae, comprising 3 to 10% of all intracranial meningiomas, arise from the limbus sphenoidale, chiasmatic sulcus, and tuberculum sellae. They typically present slowly progressive visual deterioration and other symptoms, including seizures, endocrine, or behavioral symptoms as related to tumor size and the eventual perilesional edema. Accordingly, indications for treatment relate exclusively to mass effect and associated symptoms.

Planum sphenoidale meningiomas, accounting for 8 to 18% of intracranial meningiomas together with the olfactory groove, are based at the anterior skull base, in the midline, i.e., at the area of the frontosphenoidal suture. These lesions usually are diagnosed at later stages of the growth, as larger masses, with frontal lobe compression-related symptoms (apraxia, executive dysfunction, behavioral changes) or seizures; larger tumors may present also with optic nerve compression.[1]

In these terms, it is worth reminding that tuberculum sellae meningiomas displace the optic apparatus superiorly and laterally, whereas planum sphenoidale, as well as, olfactory groove meningiomas displace the optic apparatus posteriorly. This represents a very important factor to be recognized during the operative planning for dural-based tumors in this region.

Given the benign nature of such neoplasm, the goal of surgery is complete removal of the tumor, dural attachment, and eventual "infected" bone. Major aims of the resection of these tumors can decompress the optic nerves and prevent further deterioration, or, eventually, reverse damage,[2,3] but subtotal resection followed by radiation therapy may also be reasonable depending on the age of the patient and tumor location.

Open transcranial surgical approaches have been well-defined for such kind of pathologies, and surgical outcome has been improving over the last decades.[4]

In most recent years, the improvement of intraoperative visualization, together with refined instrumentation, allowed the evolution of microneurosurgical techniques. Among those, the supraorbital eyebrow approach is a minimally invasive keyhole technique that is currently used to access lesions located at the anterior skull base.[5,6,7,8,9,10]

The supraorbital route has been a frequently employed surgical resource for the treatment of anterior cranial base meningiomas.[11] Several iterations occurred since its introduction. The most remarkable includes Dandy's "hypophyseal" approach, with a skin incision concealed behind the hairline. Dandy's frontolateral pterional approach was refined with the microsurgical techniques of Yasargil et al[12] in 1975, with drilling of the sphenoid ridge, constituting what has become perhaps the most popular approach in neurosurgery, i.e., the pterional. The landmark description of the supraorbital approach, which sparked an increasing interest in its application was that of Jane in 1982. Ever since this report, and based on the speed, versatility and results reported with the supraorbital/subfrontal route, a series of modifications followed, ranging from larger approaches popularized in the 80 s with the explosion of skull base techniques (i.e., the orbitocranial approach of Al-Mefty[13]), to minimally invasive techniques, as popularized by Perneczky through the keyhole concept.[14,15] With increasing experience in skull base and keyhole techniques, the supraorbital route epitomized the reconciliation of both concepts, benefiting from the tenets of minimal, efficacious access of keyhole approaches, and those of maximal, effective, atraumatic to the brain exposures from skull base. In consequence, a series of modifications that serves as targetable options for approach followed, i.e., the supraorbital eyebrow incision approach, the mini-supraorbital keyhole craniotomy, the transciliary approach, the eyelid approach, and the endoscope-assisted supraorbital approach and its variants.

Recently, expanded endonasal approaches have been developed in an attempt of reducing brain retraction and optic chiasm manipulation and improving ophthalmological outcomes by approaching the tumors from an anteromedial and inferior trajectory.[16,17,18,19,20,21,22,23,24,25,26,27,28,29,30,31,32,33,34,35,36,37] Despite initial discussion about the possibility of accessing the anterior skull base, and eventually dealing with lesions involving this area via the nose, the pure endoscopic endonasal approach (EEA) extended to the suprasellar area and anterior cranial fossa has proved to be both effective and safe.[38]

In regards to the management of planum sphenoidale and tuberculum sellae meningiomas, the advantages of the endonasal approaches are early devascularization of the tumor, removal of all involved bone, lack of brain retraction, and easier dissection of the tumor from the optic nerves and chiasm which are not surgically manipulated. Furthermore, improved visualization of the medial portion of the optic canal can be obtained. However, major drawbacks are, difficult skull base reconstruction, leading to an increased risk for cerebrospinal fluid (CSF) and possible loss of olfaction and other nasal complications. Since the endonasal is a midline pathway, it may limit the access to the lateral extent of the meningioma.[39,40,41,42,43,44,45] For such reason, transcranial approaches are more suitable for tumors that extend lateral to the carotid artery or optic nerve as well as those that may encase the vasculature, providing a wider view of the lateral extent of the tumor. This chapter will focus on the management of tuberculum sellae and planum sphenoidale meningiomas via the endoscopic endonasal and supraorbital approaches which are someway complementary routes, thus overcoming their respective limitations.

15.2 Preoperative Definition of Lesion Features

Preoperative workup includes MRI and CT with two-dimensional reconstructions to assess the relationship of the tumor with the optic nerves and paranasal sinuses, visual acuity and visual field exams, and a vascular anatomy study to establish the relationship of the internal carotid arteries and its branches with the tumor. Our choice of vascular study is CT-angiography. Hence, preoperative evaluation of tumor position, extent, and relationship with critical neurovascular structures is mandatory (▸ Fig. 15.1). Additionally, careful evaluation of the relationship of the tumor with the optic canals and

patterns of optic nerve compression are paramount to deciding the best approach route.

Preoperative tumor embolization in this region is not recommended due to the risk of ischemic injury to the optic apparatus. Careful study of the anterior skull base and paranasal sinuses anatomy is mandatory. Patterns of hyperostosis, pneumatization of the paranasal sinuses in anticipation to planning for the approach and consideration for repair techniques is recommended.

Especially for the endonasal route, the configuration of the sphenoid sinus should be evaluated as well as the conformation of the tuberculum sellae, namely the suprasellar notch.[46] This preoperative analysis is crucial to tailor the bony opening to gain access to the suprasellar area. Particularly, it has to be stressed that acute angle of the suprasellar notch (type I, i.e., angle < 118°) is the most troublesome to deal with during an endoscopic endonasal transtuberculum transplanum approach.[46] Lastly, image guidance protocols, mandatory for neuronavigation systems, may be helpful in selected cases, i.e., in the presence of a conchal-type sphenoid sinus, certain cases of recurrences with a previous history of transsphenoidal surgery, and patients with large lesions involving the para-suprasellar areas. It has to be highlighted that neuronavigation system is useful for surgical planning as it helps in determine the position of the tumor in relation with the key neurovascular structures surrounding it.

On the other hand, when selecting a supraorbital eyebrow approach, care should be taken to the size and lateral extent of the frontal sinus that dictates the placement of the supraorbital craniotomy. A large lateral extension of the frontal sinus may discourage one from using the supraorbital approach, but in general, this is only an issue in a minority of cases.

The location and extent of the tumor also dictates the likelihood of success with a supraorbital approach and the potential need for a larger alternative craniotomy. Axial and coronal MRI sequences should be closely studied to determine the lateral extent of the lesion. The use of image-based frameless stereotaxy is helpful and allows the surgeon to assess the available surgical trajectory prior to making the skin incision.

15.3 Surgical Indications

Which lesions of the planum sphenoidale and/or the tuberculum sellae should be resected transcranially and which should be approached from below, i.e., transphenoidally, remains yet a debate.[3,45,47] Surgeon's technical experience and appropriate patient selection yields excellent extent of resection and reduced complications.[3] The ideal surgical approach should provide enough exposure of the tumor, including its dural attachment, to interrupt its blood supply as early as possible in the procedure. In addition, brain retraction and manipulation of critical neurovascular structures should be minimized in order to

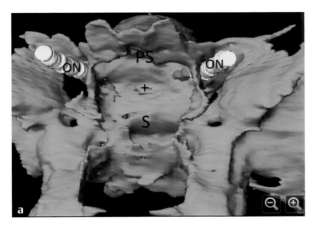
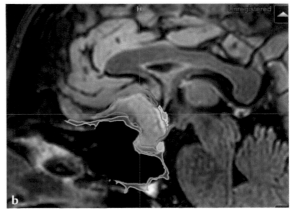
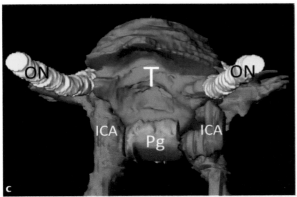
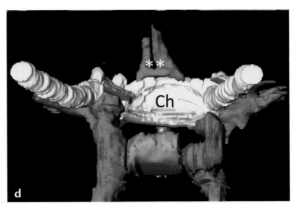

Fig. 15.1 **(a)** Three-dimensional volume-rendered reconstruction as seen from an endonasal perspective, **(b)** sagittal fluid-attenuated inversion recovery (FLAIR) MRI scans showing a tuberculum-planum sphenoidale meningioma. The tumor as well as the main neurovascular structures surrounding it have been highlighted with different color. **(c)** The tumor, as seen via the endonasal pathway, can be appreciated after removing the sphenoid bone. **(d)** The neurovascular structures after virtual tumor removal can be seen as well. These imaging has been obtained using the BrainLAB navigation system (BrainLab Curve, Feldkirchen, Germany). ON, optic nerve; PS, planum sphenoidale; S, sella; T, tumor; ICA, internal carotid artery; Pg, pituitary gland; Ch, optic chiasm; *pituitary stalk; **anterior cerebral-communicating artery complex; +, tuberculum sellae.

avoid procedure-related morbidity. Finally, in choosing the optimal surgical approach, the anatomic limits of each surgical route must be carefully considered.

Generally, the decision to approach these tumors by endonasal, supraorbital, or other wider craniotomies should be based on tumor features, extension, growth pattern, size, and, last but not least, the extent of the surgeon's experience with both transcranial and transnasal cranial base surgery (▶ Table 15.1).

15.3.1 Indications for the Endoscopic Endonasal Approach

Key considerations for endoscopic endonasal surgery of anterior cranial base meningiomas include sphenoid sinus and tuberculum sellae (also called suprasellar notch) anatomy,[46] as well as parasellar extension of the tumor or encasement of neurovascular structures.

Although involvement of the optic canals was initially thought to be a limitation for endoscopic endonasal surgery, adequate and safe opening of the optic canals with resection of the intracanalicular part of the meningiomas has been demonstrated. Hence, it has to be outlined that

Table 15.1 Main factors influencing endonasal or supraorbital approach selection for tuberculum sellae and planum sphenoidale meningiomas

Factors influencing approach selection	
Supraorbital eyebrow	Endoscopic endonasal transtuberculum transplanum
Lateral tumor extension	Midline lesion
Conchal type of sphenoid sinus	Sellar type of sphenoid sinus
Encasement of neurovascular structures	Intrasellar tumor extension

endonasal approach would be difficult in case of conchal sella, "kissing" internal carotid arteries, too-lateral extension, main vessel encasement, large size, or asymmetric shape.

Generally, the most amenable lesions to be selected for endoscopic endonasal management are those that are mostly midline, maintain their arachnoid plane intact as evidenced by a lack of peritumoral edema, do not encase neurovascular structures.

15.3.2 Indications for the Supraorbital Approach

The supraorbital approach is an effective window for the surgical management of planum sphenoidale and tuberculum sellae meningiomas. In cases where tuberculum sellae meningioma has a large extension over the planum sphenoidale with large dural implant in the coronal plane, the supraorbital route offers greater microsurgical control on the tumor borders. On the contrary, meningiomas entering the sellar region and growing below the optic chiasm may be difficult to manage from a transcranial perspective. However, in cases where the tumor extends lateral to one or both of the optic nerves or lateral to the supraclinoid carotid arteries, the supraorbital approach is generally preferred. Regarding optic canal decompression, the supraorbital approach allows both optic nerves to be decompressed from above (superiorly) whereas the endonasal approach allows both optic nerves to be decompressed inferomedially. Thus, tumor location relative to the optic nerves and canals should dictate whether an endonasal or transcranial approach is best suited to allow effective optic nerve decompression.

15.4 Surgical Techniques

15.4.1 Endoscopic Endonasal Approach

For endoscopic endonasal transtuberculum transplanum approach, the patient is placed supine and head is slightly extended in order to optimize the access to the anterior cranial base. The face is turned 5 to 10° toward the surgeon. After induction of general anesthesia, if required, frameless neuronavigation is registered by using CT and/or MRI. Routine nasal mucosal preparation is used: cottonoids, soaked with diluted adrenaline and lidocaine, are inserted in both nostrils between the middle turbinate and the nasal septum and left in place for about 5 minutes. Further, suitable donor sites (fascia lata and/or periumbelical fat) are prepped and draped in order to allow material harvesting.

The nasal phase of the surgical procedure begins with middle turbinate laterally displaced on one side and unilateral middle turbinectomy with removal of the posterior ethmoidal cells, generally performed in the same

cavity where the Hadad-Bassagasteguy nasoseptal flap will be raised. As already highlighted elsewhere,[48,49] elevation of the flap is realized at the end of the procedure, in order to reduce the nasal bleeding during surgery and eventually avoid the ischemia of the flap due to the twisting of its pedicle and, at the same time, increase the adhesive property of the same flap that is lifted from the septum and immediately placed on the osteo-dural defect.

Afterwards, the posterior aspect of the nasal septum is removed minding to not extend anteriorly to the head of the contralateral middle turbinate.

A wide sphenoidotomy is performed with complete removal of the rostrum and flattening of the floor of the sphenoid and intrasinus septae also to aid the placement of the nasoseptal flap at the end of tumor removal.

A high-speed drill with a round diamond bit is used to remove bone over the anterosuperior sella, just below the superior intercavernous sinus, extending up to the tuberculum, lateral to the medial opticocarotid recesses and anteriorly along the planum up to the anterior extent of the tumor attachment.

Therefore, bone removal over the uninvolved pituitary gland is minimized unless the tumor extends into the sella. If optic canal invasion has been identified on preoperative imaging, the medial optic canals should be drilled away to reach the anterior extent of the tumor within the canals (▶ Fig. 15.2).

In cases of tuberculum sellae and planum sphenoidale meningiomas, the coagulation of the dural attachment is achieved immediately after bone opening, so that early tumor devascularization can be obtained. The tumor is then debulked safely and its capsule finally dissected from the surrounding microvascular structures via an extra-arachnoidal route, without or with minimal manipulation of the optic pathways.

In cases of planum sphenoidal meningiomas, the bone opening has to be extended more anterior and laterally above the orbital roof and should include also the isolation of the posterior ethmoidal artery in order to identify the cleavage plane between the lesion and the brain (▶ Fig. 15.3).

After tumor removal, hemostasis is achieved and the large osteodural opening should be sealed. A variety of reconstruction methods and materials are currently available and used. We rather prefer to use the so-called "sandwich technique": the surgical cavity is filled with fat graft sutured to three layers of dural substitute: the first two layers are positioned intradurally and the third one extradurally, wedged in between the dura and bone. At the end, pedicled nasoseptal flap is used to cover the skull base defect (▶ Fig. 15.4).

15.4.2 Supraorbital Eyebrow Approach

The patient is typically placed in the supine position, with the head hyperextended and rotated contralaterally no

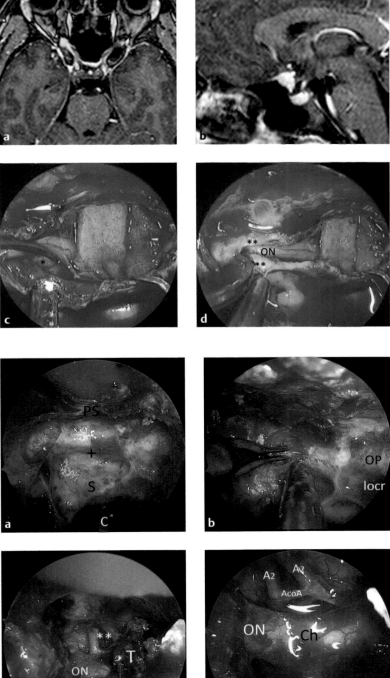

Fig. 15.2 **(a)** Preoperative axial and **(b)** sagittal MRI scans showing a tuberculum sellae extending into the right optic canal. **(c)** The tumor has been removed via an endoscopic endonasal transtuberculum transplanum approach. The optic canal on the right side has been opened thus showing the meningioma below the optic nerve and above the ophthalmic artery. **(d)** The optic nerve sheath has been opened up to the annulus of Zinn. ON, optic nerve. *tumor; **optic nerve sheath.

Fig. 15.3 Endoscopic endonasal transtuberculum transplanum approach for the tuberculum sellae meningioma showed in ▶ Fig. 15.1. **(a)** The posterior wall of the sphenoid sinus is reached and the main anatomic landmarks can be appreciated. **(b)** The dural attachment is coagulated before opening the dura. **(c)** Dissection of the tumor from the surrounding main neurovascular structures and **(d)** close-up view of the surgical cavity after total tumor removal. A1, pre-communicating segment of the anterior cerebral artery; A2, postcommunicating segment of the anterior cerebral artery; ACoA: anterior communicating artery; C: clivus; locr, lateral opto-carotid recess; ON, optic nerve; OP, optic protuberance; Pg, pituitary gland; Ps, pituitary stalk; PS, planum sphenoidale; S, sella; T, tumor. +tuberculum sellae; **anterior cerebral-communicating artery complex.

more than 25°. Anesthetic techniques for appropriate brain relaxation are employed (mild hyperventilation, osmotic therapy). In younger patients, a high-volume spinal tap could also be used to assist with brain relaxation in the initial stages of extradural dissection. Several incisions could be used for the supraorbital approach; an incision behind the hairline, an incision immediately above the eyebrow, or in one of the skin creases in the forehead, or an eyelid incision if incorporation of the roof of the orbit is planned as part of the approach. If an eyebrow incision is chosen, a trajectory lateral to the supraorbital nerve and above the eyebrow is preferred to avoid supraorbital numbness and eyebrow alopecia. If an eyelid incision is chosen, the orbicularis muscle fibers are

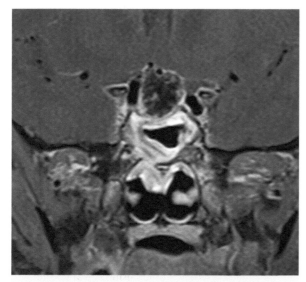

Fig. 15.4 Coronal T1-weighted with fat suppression postoperative MRI scans of the same case presented in ▶ Fig. 15.1. Total removal is shown in these 3-months postoperative scans; the surgical cavity has been filled with reconstruction materials, mainly autologous fat. Note the pedicle nasoseptal flap used to cover the skull base defect.

sectioned along their course to favor anatomic healing, and the orbital septum and periorbital should be preserved.

Careful planning is required for the supraorbital approach regarding the design of the bone cuts in relation to the frontal paranasal sinus (▶ Fig. 15.5). Sinus penetration must be avoided, and some authors consider profuse pneumatization of the frontal sinus extending into the path of the craniotomy as a relative contraindication. In the event of frontal sinus penetration, surgical measures to isolate the frontal sinus from the craniotomy should be undertaken to prevent postoperative CSF leak, pneumocephalus, or mucoceles. The supraorbital notch serves as a reliable landmark to indicate the lateral extension of the ipsilateral frontal sinus. If the decision is made to use intraoperative neuronavigation, this could also be used as an aid to maximize the medial craniotomy extension while preserving the frontal sinus cavity.

Once the incision is made, the deep temporalis fascia is elevated, and a small incision in the superior temporal line at its most frontal attachment is made, leaving a fascial cuff for reconstruction. The temporalis muscle is detached from the superior temporal line and subperiosteally dissected posteriorly, leaving a small opening in the superior to the frontosphenoidal suture for the creation of a Dandy keyhole burr hole.

Using a high-speed drill, a Dandy keyhole is created, to be left hidden completely under the temporalis muscle, leaving enough bone for the application of a cranial plate at the time of closure. The dura is dissected free from the endocranial surface, and the anterior cranial base above the orbit should be exposed through this burr hole. Subsequently, using a protected side-cutting drill bit, an oval-shaped craniotomy is elevated in the frontal bone with extreme care to remain as close to the anterior skull base as possible without penetration of the frontal sinus. The bone flap is elevated with extreme care to preserve the frontal dura and saved in a sterile container with antibiotic solution until the time of closure.

At this point, the basal dura is elevated with a dissector. Using a retractor or a dissector to protect the frontobasal

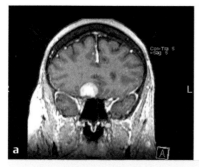
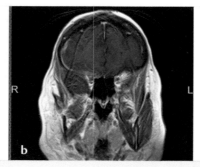
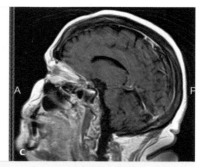

Fig. 15.5 (a) Pre- and (b, c) postoperative MRI images of a 58-year-old woman with history of multiple meningiomas treated with gamma knife. Follow-up after 2 years documented progressive enlargement of planum meningioma after new-onset seizures. Postoperative MRI 6 months after surgery shows gross total resection. Patient remains seizure-free after surgery after discontinuation of seizure prophylaxis postoperatively.

dura, an unguarded side-cutting burr is used to shave the endocranial surface of the orbital roof, to eliminate any irregularities on the surface that may hinder visualization of the basal dura. This step is very important, and drilling should extend beyond the level of the apex of the orbital dome into the endocranial surface, leaving a soft layer of bone covering the circumference of the orbit. During this step, hyperostotic attachments to the tumor based are eliminated. Additionally, branches from the ethmoidal and anterior meningeal arteries that usually provide blood supply to the tumor are eliminated with bipolar cautery. At this stage into the exposure, tumor resection is taking place in an extradural fashion by elevating the tumor from its skull base attachment and eliminating its blood supply. Extradural basal dissection continues until it is felt safe or the attachments of the tumor are removed. The purpose of this approach is to convert a more complex, skull base tumor into a convexity meningioma. Additionally, in cases of optic canal involvement, extradural optic nerve decompression is carried out with a diamond tip burr under constant irrigation to reduce heat applied to the nerve or using an ultrasonic bone curette.

Once the extradural dissection is complete, the dura is opened in a semicircular fashion with an inferior base over the orbital rim and tacked up with stay sutures, the brain is protected with cottonoids and CSF is drained. At this stage, microsurgical dissection is carried out to separate the tumor preserving the arachnoid plane. Sequential debulking with an ultrasonic aspirator or microinstruments will be an aid to reducing the need for brain retraction. Gross total resection should be pursued, including the dural base attachment. In those efforts, care should be exerted at preserving the integrity of the bony base of the skull to prevent postoperative CSF leak. Judicious use of cautery is recommended in proximity of the optic nerve. If needed, in cases where some retraction of the optic nerve is necessary, complete unroofing of the optic canal and section of the falciform ligament are recommended.

Upon completion of the microsurgical resection portion of the procedure, the dura is approximated in a water-tight fashion. The bone flap is reapplied with low profile titanium mini plates and screws using a three-point fixation technique, using a burr hole cover to be covered by the temporalis muscle. Gaps in the bone edges of the craniotomy are filled with a hydroxyapatite cement to ensure cosmetic closure. The incision is closed in layers. A subgaleal drain may be left in patients with hairline incisions, a plastic closure with reabsorbable sutures and skin glue is used for eyebrow incisions. No drains are used for those patients (▶ Fig. 15.6).

Variants to the supraorbital approach frequently used for the treatment of anterior cranial base meningiomas include the addition of an orbital roof osteotomy, lateral orbitotomy, and endoscope-assisted supraorbital approach.

The endoscope-assisted approach follows the same principles as described above. The addition of the endoscope aids with visualization in deeper parts of the surgical field. Angled endoscopes are particularly helpful to visualize beyond the cone of vision provided by the microscope or loupe magnification to ensure tumor resection or to verify integrity of critical structures. Lateral orbitotomies are seldom necessary for tuberculum sellae or planum sphenoidale meningiomas, but they are useful adjuncts in cases where anterior fossa meningiomas extend into the mesial temporal fossa or into the orbit.

The addition of an orbital roof osteotomy is a known maneuver to improve basal exposure, reduce the need for brain retraction, and increase rostral visualization in the surgical plane. Previous studies using the mid-point of the anterior communicating artery as a target documented an average 10° increase in exposure, which translated in more than 50% increased angular exposure when

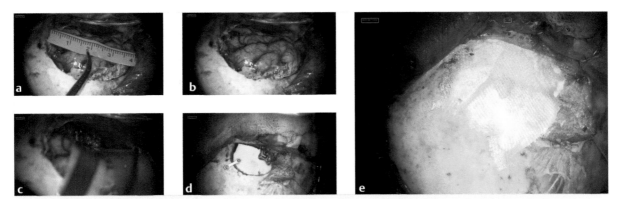

Fig. 15.6 Intraoperative pictures depicting supraorbital craniotomy steps during craniotomy and resection. (a) Craniotomy following durotomy. (b) Notice frontobasal exposure without retraction at the expense of anterior cranial fossa drilling. Microscopic view of planum sphenoidale tumor after initial approach placing a retractor. (c) Notice exposure of the basal dura and tumor attachment. (d) Closure with titanium miniplates. Notice burr hole cover to be hidden under temporalis muscle flap. (e) Cosmetic completion of closure by filling craniotomy gaps with hydroxyapatite cement, covered with oxidase cellulose polymer stamps.

compared with supraorbital approaches. An additional benefit of the orbital osteotomy includes a shortening of the distance to the depth of the surgical filed by bringing the edge of the craniotomy at a lower point (approximately 10 mm on average) by removing the orbital rim. For those tumors extending cranially into midline, a transorbital roof craniotomy may prove beneficial to increase maneuverability and reduce brain retraction. A study evaluating parameters to determine indications for the addition of an orbital osteotomy determined that, for those patients whose orbital heights (i.e., a line adjoining the highest point of each orbit relative to the distance of the latter to the midline in the frontoethmoidal suture as measured in the coronal plane) measuring 11 mm or more would benefit from an orbital roof osteotomy.

Initial steps preceding an orbital roof addition are like those used for a supraorbital craniotomy. Once the skull is exposed, the periosteum above the orbital rim is sectioned along its lateral edge past the point where it is adjoined by the orbital septum. This periosteum is continuous with the periorbita, which is detached subperiosteally from the roof of the orbit extending laterally from the supraorbital notch laterally into the lateral wall of the orbit past the frontosphenoidal suture. If a lateral orbitotomy is planned, dissection should extend towards the inferior orbital fissure. Once exposure is completed, a McCarty burr hole, centered on the frontosphenoidal suture, will expose two halves as separated by the orbital roof; the posterosuperior represented by the anterior fossa dura, and an anteroinferior half into the orbit. From the McCarty burr hole, a supraorbital craniotomy can be elevated as previously described, leaving the orbital roof to be cut from the McCarty burr hole towards the medial cut at an anteroposterior distance no larger than 25 mm to reduce the risk of optic nerve damage. If a one-piece is preferred, the frontal cut with a side-cutting bur extends into the roof of the orbit lateral to the supraorbital nerve and is extended across the orbital bar with an unguarded bit. From the McCarty burr hole, while protecting the orbital contents, a lateral cut extends through the lateral wall into the lateral orbital rim at the height desired. Finally, using an osteotome or a reciprocating saw, the roof of the orbit can be sectioned to elevate the bone flap as one piece. The anesthesiologist should be warned of the possibility of bradycardia due to trigeminal-cardiac reflex that may result from retraction of the orbit. The dura is elevated inferiorly and tack up sutures are used to retract the orbital contents inferiorly. Tumor resection carries on as previously described. Once completed, the dura is closed in a watertight fashion and the closure is completed using the strategies described above.

15.5 Complications

A number of possible complications may be detected after meningiomas removal either via endonasal or through supraorbital path.[50,51,52,53,54,55] During the EEA, each step of the procedure can have different complications. Carotid artery injury is one of the most feared complications during endoscopic endonasal surgery, while accomplishing bone removal; the use of microDoppler probe and neuronavigation system, help surgeons avoiding that.

When performing tumor capsule dissection, it is mandatory to prevent damaging to the blood supply to the optic system, and/or to anterior cerebral arteries complex resulting in tremendous hemorrhage and/or stroke.

Hence, postoperative CSF leak, due to inadequate skull base reconstruction is one of the most troublesome complications. Finally, the endocrine complications can occur as a consequence of pituitary stalk manipulation and can involve both posterior and anterior pituitary insufficiency (hypopituitarism and diabetes insipidus). Hydroelectrolytic disturbances as well as syndrome of inappropriate secretion of antidiuretic hormone (SIADH) or cerebral salt wasting syndrome have to be detected and properly managed. Transient or permanent diabetes insipidus has to be discovered and treated accordingly. Regarding the supraorbital approach, it has to be stressed that it carries little approach-related morbidity but it is associated with a unique set of potential complications. Transient forehead numbness from injury to the supraorbital nerve is a common event in the early postoperative period but is rarely permanent. Transient frontalis weakness from injury or stretching of the frontalis branch of the facial nerve can be seen immediately after surgery but lasting frontalis paresis has been reported in few patients. Both of these complications may be avoided by careful planning of the incision and meticulous soft tissue dissection. The supraorbital nerve is readily identifiable as it courses from the orbit through the supraorbital notch at the medial aspect of the eyebrow incision. CSF rhinorrhea may occur if the frontal sinus is violated and inadequately repaired. This complication can be avoided by carefully planning the craniotomy lateral to the lateral-most edge of the frontal sinus. However, if the sinus is entered it should meticulously have repaired. In all cases, the medial aspect of the craniotomy should be carefully inspected to determine if there is sinus entry. As mentioned above, a small frontal sinus breach may be repaired with bone wax with an overlay of collagen sponge. Larger frontal sinus breaches may require packing with fat or muscle as well as with a pericranial flap and collagen sponge reinforcement.

Overall, because the supraorbital approach utilizes a small incision and involves minimal temporalis dissection, scalp pain, temporalis atrophy, and difficulty with mastication are rarely observed. Briefly, craniotomy-related complications can be avoided through careful preoperative study and planning, including: unsightly scars, skull deformity, skull hardware failure, frontal sinus penetration, mucocele, CSF leak, pneumocephalus, enophthalmos, diplopia, retrobulbar hematoma. Technique related complications include blindness, stroke, intracerebral hemorrhage, venous infarction, anosmia, infection, malignant brain edema, incomplete tumor resection. Systemic complications and seizures may also complicate the postoperative course of these patients.

In a recent comparative series published in the pertinent literature,[3] significantly more patients experienced seizures after transcranial surgery than after EEA. On the other hand, the most common complication in the latter group was CSF leakage while few cases of patients treated via the transcranial route experienced a subarachnoid hemorrhage or stroke.

15.6 Surgical Results

15.6.1 Endoscopic Endonasal Surgery

Improvement or even normalization of vision after removal of meningioma via EEA can be reached in about 85% of cases, particularly in case of tuberculum sellae meningiomas. A Simpson grade I can be achieved in more than 80% of cases.

Regarding complication, the most common was postoperative CSF leaks, which can occur in up to 25.3%, based on a recent surgical series. However, it is important to notice the decrease of this rate in recent years after the routine use of the vascularized nasoseptal flap for skull base reconstruction. The overall rate of postoperative meningitis following CSF leak has been calculated to be 5.3%. Postoperative hydrocephalus requiring ventriculoperitoneal shunt placement has been described as well. Other medical complications include SIADH secretion, pulmonary embolism, respiratory failure, and hypopituitarism.

Recurrence rate was found to be 5.3%, according to most recent data shown in the literature.[44,56]

15.6.2 Supraorbital Surgery

Select large case series in the modern era report, without details on case characteristics distribution, gross total resection rates (Simpson grade I or II) ranging from 84 to 100% and recurrence rates ranging from 0 to 8%. Complications included: CSF leak (range 1–7%), anosmia (5–6%), hemorrhage (2–10%), infection (2–4%), stroke (1–2%), vascular injury (0–6%), and death (1–3%). Transient diabetes insipidus occurred in 0 to 3% of patients and 0% of patients experienced anterior pituitary dysfunction. Postoperatively, vision improved in 64 to 74% of patients, remained stable in 16 to 26% of patients, and worsened in 8 to 12% of patients.

Without uniform criteria for reporting across series, no clear conclusions can be drawn.

15.7 Early- and Long-term Postoperative Management

Lesions treated via an EEA require an intensive and watchful postoperative care.

The patient should rest in bed just for the day of the surgery not supine but with the trunk 30 to 45° raised. Additionally, patients are asked to adopt postoperative habits in order to prevent any intracranial pressure increase and the eventual displacement of skull base reconstruction. It is preferable to cough and/or sneeze with the mouth open, assume as early as possible a stand-up position and start walking, avoid bending over or squatting, and to assume stool softeners.

CT scan is performed routinely at POD#1 in order to evaluate any neurosurgical complication and/or the amount of pneumocephalus. According to a recent contribution, frontal and intraventricular pneumocephalus is not necessarily associated with a postoperative CSF leak; on the other hand, a "suspicious" pattern of air, namely pneumocephalus in the convexity, interhemispheric fissure, and sella, parasellar, or perimesencephalic locations, may be significantly associated with a postoperative CSF leak occurrence, and for such reason, these patients require closer observation.[57]

Based on our experience, we noticed that the sudden onset of patient temperature starting from the POD#2 could be suggestive of a not yet visible leakage. The endoscopic endonasal inspection of the surgical site can be easily performed at patient's bed with the portable Tele pack X Led (Karl Storz GmbH, Tuttlingen) to check the status of the surgical wound and the resiliency of the reconstruction.

In these terms, patients with minimal postoperative CSF leak can be managed without reoperation. If necessary, repeated endoscope-guided fibrin glue injections at the bedside or in the outpatient ward, i.e., according to the so-called "awake sealant technique", can be performed.[58]

However, in cases of severe CSF leak, displacement of the reconstruction materials, and/or evident communication of the sphenoid sinus with the intradural compartment, immediate transsphenoidal reoperation is needed.

Finally, it has to be highlighted that long-term follow-up by means of neuroradiologic evaluation and periodic visual assessment is mandatory to early detect meningioma recurrence. In these terms, patients that presented with recurrence can be treated with radiotherapy, unless there was mass effect on the optic nerve requiring repeat decompression.

After supraorbital approach, early postoperative management includes homeostatic support measures, seizure prevention, osmotic therapy, and prevention of infection.

Long-term management includes any rehabilitation measure required in case of residual effects after treatment, and periodic imaging surveillance according to the degree of tumor resection. For those patients with incomplete tumor resection, the role of repeat resection and that of adjuvant radiation therapy should be determined.

15.8 Conclusion

Tuberculum sellae and planum sphenoidale meningiomas pose a surgical challenge for skull base surgeons because of their critical location and adherence to neurovascular structures and eventual dense consistency. These challenges have resulted in nearly a century of controversy regarding the optimal approach for successful removal. The endonasal and supraorbital keyhole approaches provide similar minimally invasive surgical techniques to access meningiomas of the suprasellar region. The ideal approach for the patient should be selected taking into account the tumor anatomy with special attention to size, lateral extension, and surgeon's experience with both surgical approaches. Ideally, the neurosurgeon should be familiar with both surgical techniques to select the ideal approach for each patient based on the patient's anatomy and surgeon's preference. With increased experience and a prompt learning curve, today skull base neurosurgeons are able to approach more challenging diseases using both of these minimally invasive techniques.

References

[1] Komotar RJ, Starke RM, Raper DM, Anand VK, Schwartz TH. Endoscopic endonasal versus open transcranial resection of anterior midline skull base meningiomas. World Neurosurg. 2012; 77(5–6): 713–724

[2] Clark AJ, Jahangiri A, Garcia RM, et al. Endoscopic surgery for tuberculum sellae meningiomas: a systematic review and meta-analysis. Neurosurg Rev. 2013; 36(3):349–359

[3] Bander ED, Singh H, Ogilvie CB, et al. Endoscopic endonasal versus transcranial approach to tuberculum sellae and planum sphenoidale meningiomas in a similar cohort of patients. J Neurosurg. 2018; 128 (1):40–48

[4] Morales-Valero SF, Van Gompel JJ, Loumiotis I, Lanzino G. Craniotomy for anterior cranial fossa meningiomas: historical overview. Neurosurg Focus. 2014; 36(4):E14

[5] Hickmann AK, Gaida BJ, Reisch R. How I do it: The expanded trans/supraorbital approach for large space-occupying lesions of the anterior fossa. Acta Neurochir (Wien). 2017; 159(5):881–887

[6] Prat-Acín R, Galeano I, Evangelista R, et al. Large suprasellar craniopharyngioma surgery in adults through the trans-eyebrow supraorbital approach. Acta Neurochi (Vienna) 2017:159(8) 1537–1537

[7] Banu MA, Mehta A, Ottenhausen M, et al. Endoscope-assisted endonasal versus supraorbital keyhole resection of olfactory groove meningiomas: comparison and combination of 2 minimally invasive approaches. J Neurosurg. 2016; 124(3):605–620

[8] Dlouhy BJ, Chae MP, Teo C. The supraorbital eyebrow approach in children: clinical outcomes, cosmetic results, and complications. J Neurosurg Pediatr. 2015; 15(1):12–19

[9] Kurbanov A, Sanders-Taylor C, Keller JT, Andaluz N, Zuccarello M. The extended transorbital craniotomy: an anatomic study. Neurosurgery. 2015; 11 Suppl 2:338–344, discussion 344

[10] Reisch R, Marcus HJ, Kockro RA, Ulrich NH. The supraorbital keyhole approach: how I do it. Acta Neurochir (Wien). 2015; 157(6):979–983

[11] Scholz M, Parvin R, Thissen J, Löhnert C, Harders A, Blaeser K. Skull base approaches in neurosurgery. Head Neck Oncol. 2010; 2:16

[12] Yasargil MG, Antic J, Laciga R, Jain KK, Hodosh RM, Smith RD. Microsurgical pterional approach to aneurysms of the basilar bifurcation. Surg Neurol. 1976; 6(2):83–91

[13] Al-Mefty O. Supraorbital-pterional approach to skull base lesions. Neurosurgery. 1987; 21(4):474–477

[14] Reisch R, Perneczky A, Filippi R. Surgical technique of the supraorbital key-hole craniotomy. Surg Neurol. 2003; 59(3):223–227

[15] Reisch R, Perneczky A. Ten-year experience with the supraorbital subfrontal approach through an eyebrow skin incision. Neurosurgery. 2005; 57(4) Suppl:242–255, discussion 242–255

[16] Weiss MH. The transnasal transsphenoidal approach. In: Apuzzo MLJ, ed. Surgery of the Third Ventricle. Baltimore: Williams & Wilkins; 1987:476–494

[17] Mason RB, Nieman LK, Doppman JL, Oldfield EH. Selective excision of adenomas originating in or extending into the pituitary stalk with preservation of pituitary function. J Neurosurg. 1997; 87(3):343–351

[18] Kato T, Sawamura Y, Abe H, Nagashima M. Transsphenoidal-transtuberculum sellae approach for supradiaphragmatic tumours: technical note. Acta Neurochir (Wien). 1998; 140(7):715–718, discussion 719

[19] Kim J, Choe I, Bak K, Kim C, Kim N, Jang Y. Transsphenoidal supradiaphragmatic intradural approach: technical note. Minim Invasive Neurosurg. 2000; 43(1):33–37

[20] Kouri JG, Chen MY, Watson JC, Oldfield EH. Resection of suprasellar tumors by using a modified transsphenoidal approach. Report of four cases. J Neurosurg. 2000; 92(6):1028–1035

[21] Kitano M, Taneda M. Extended transsphenoidal approach with submucosal posterior ethmoidectomy for parasellar tumors. Technical note. J Neurosurg. 2001; 94(6):999–1004

[22] Cook SW, Smith Z, Kelly DF. Endonasal transsphenoidal removal of tuberculum sellae meningiomas: technical note. Neurosurgery. 2004; 55(1):239–244, discussion 244–246

[23] Couldwell WT, Weiss MH, Rabb C, Liu JK, Apfelbaum RI, Fukushima T. Variations on the standard transsphenoidal approach to the sellar region, with emphasis on the extended approaches and parasellar approaches: surgical experience in 105 cases. Neurosurgery. 2004; 55(3):539–547, discussion 547–550

[24] Dusick JR, Esposito F, Kelly DF, et al. The extended direct endonasal transsphenoidal approach for nonadenomatous suprasellar tumors. J Neurosurg. 2005; 102(5):832–841

[25] Laws ER, Kanter AS, Jane JA, Jr, Dumont AS. Extended transsphenoidal approach. J Neurosurg. 2005; 102(5):825–827, discussion 827–828

[26] de Divitiis E, Esposito F, Cappabianca P, Cavallo LM, de Divitiis O. Tuberculum sellae meningiomas: high route or low route? A series of 51 consecutive cases. Neurosurgery. 2008; 62(3):556–563, discussion 556–563

[27] Ditzel Filho LF, Prevedello DM, Jamshidi AO, et al. Endoscopic Endonasal Approach for Removal of Tuberculum Sellae Meningiomas. Neurosurg Clin N Am. 2015; 26(3):349–361

[28] Gardner PA, Kassam AB, Thomas A, et al. Endoscopic endonasal resection of anterior cranial base meningiomas. Neurosurgery. 2008; 63(1):36–52, discussion 52–54

[29] Kasemsiri P, Carrau RL, Ditzel Filho LF, et al. Advantages and limitations of endoscopic endonasal approaches to the skull base. World Neurosurg. 2014; 82(6) Suppl:S12–S21

[30] Prevedello DM, Ditzel Filho LF, Solari D, Carrau RL, Kassam AB. Expanded endonasal approaches to middle cranial fossa and posterior fossa tumors. Neurosurg Clin N Am. 2010; 21(4):621–635, vi

[31] Snyderman CH, Carrau RL, Kassam AB, et al. Endoscopic skull base surgery: principles of endonasal oncological surgery. J Surg Oncol. 2008; 97(8):658–664

[32] Castelnuovo P, Dallan I, Battaglia P, Bignami M. Endoscopic endonasal skull base surgery: past, present and future. Eur Arch Otorhinolaryngol. 2010; 267(5):649–663

[33] Castelnuovo P, Lepera D, Turri-Zanoni M, et al. Quality of life following endoscopic endonasal resection of anterior skull base cancers. J Neurosurg. 2013; 119(6):1401–1409

[34] Frank G, Pasquini E, Mazzatenta D. Extended transsphenoidal approach. J Neurosurg. 2001; 95(5):917–918

[35] Frank G, Pasquini E. Tuberculum sellae meningioma: the extended transsphenoidal approach–for the virtuoso only? World Neurosurg. 2010; 73(6):625–626

[36] Frank G, Pasquini E. The transnasal versus the transcranial approach to the anterior skull base. World Neurosurg. 2013; 80(6):782–783

[37] Cappabianca P, Cavallo LM, Esposito F, De Divitiis O, Messina A, De Divitiis E. Extended endoscopic endonasal approach to the midline skull base: the evolving role of transsphenoidal surgery. Adv Tech Stand Neurosurg. 2008; 33:151–199

[38] Laufer I, Anand VK, Schwartz TH. Endoscopic, endonasal extended transsphenoidal, transplanum transtuberculum approach for resection of suprasellar lesions. J Neurosurg. 2007; 106(3):400–406

[39] Dehdashti AR, Ganna A, Witterick I, Gentili F. Expanded endoscopic endonasal approach for anterior cranial base and suprasellar lesions: indications and limitations. Neurosurgery. 2009; 64(4):677–687, discussion 687–689

[40] Kaptain GJ, Vincent DA, Sheehan JP, Laws ER, Jr. Transsphenoidal approaches for the extracapsular resection of midline suprasellar and anterior cranial base lesions. Neurosurgery. 2008; 62(6) Suppl 3: 1264–1271

[41] Kulwin C, Schwartz TH, Cohen-Gadol AA. Endoscopic extended transsphenoidal resection of tuberculum sellae meningiomas: nuances of neurosurgical technique. Neurosurg Focus. 2013; 35(6):E6

[42] Mascarella MA, Tewfik MA, Aldosari M, Sirhan D, Zeitouni A, Di Maio S. A simple scoring system to predict the resectability of skull base meningiomas via an endoscopic endonasal approach. World Neurosurg. 2016; 91:582–591.e1

[43] Mortazavi MM, Brito da Silva H, Ferreira M, Jr, Barber JK, Pridgeon JS, Sekhar LN. Planum sphenoidale and tuberculum sellae meningiomas: operative nuances of a modern surgical technique with outcome and proposal of a new classification system. World Neurosurg. 2016; 86: 270–286

[44] Ottenhausen M, Banu MA, Placantonakis DG, et al. Endoscopic endonasal resection of suprasellar meningiomas: the importance of case selection and experience in determining extent of resection, visual improvement, and complications. World Neurosurg. 2014; 82(3–4):442–449

[45] Schroeder HW. Indications and limitations of the endoscopic endonasal approach for anterior cranial base meningiomas. World Neurosurg. 2014; 82(6) Suppl:S81–S85

[46] de Notaris M, Solari D, Cavallo LM, et al. The "suprasellar notch," or the tuberculum sellae as seen from below: definition, features, and clinical implications from an endoscopic endonasal perspective. J Neurosurg. 2012; 116(3):622–629

[47] Turel MK, Tsermoulas G, Yassin-Kassab A, et al. Tuberculum sellae meningiomas: a systematic review of transcranial approaches in the endoscopic era. J Neurosurg Sci. 2016

[48] Hadad G, Bassagasteguy L, Carrau RL, et al. A novel reconstructive technique after endoscopic expanded endonasal approaches: vascular pedicle nasoseptal flap. Laryngoscope. 2006; 116(10):1882–1886

[49] Kassam AB, Thomas A, Carrau RL, et al. Endoscopic reconstruction of the cranial base using a pedicled nasoseptal flap. Neurosurgery. 2008; 63(1) Suppl 1:ONS44–ONS52, discussion ONS52–ONS53

[50] Black PM, Zervas NT, Candia GL. Incidence and management of complications of transsphenoidal operation for pituitary adenomas. Neurosurgery. 1987; 20(6):920–924

[51] Cappabianca P, Cavallo LM, Colao A, de Divitiis E. Surgical complications associated with the endoscopic endonasal transsphenoidal approach for pituitary adenomas. J Neurosurg. 2002; 97(2):293–298

[52] Ciric I, Ragin A, Baumgartner C, Pierce D. Complications of transsphenoidal surgery: results of a national survey, review of the literature, and personal experience. Neurosurgery. 1997; 40(2):225–236, discussion 236–237

[53] Kassam AB, Prevedello DM, Carrau RL, et al. Endoscopic endonasal skull base surgery: analysis of complications in the authors' initial 800 patients. J Neurosurg. 2011; 114(6):1544–1568

[54] Iacoangeli M, Nocchi N, Nasi D, et al. Minimally Invasive Supraorbital Key-hole Approach for the Treatment of Anterior Cranial Fossa Meningiomas. Neurol Med Chir (Tokyo). 2016; 56(4):180–185

[55] Thaher F, Hopf N, Hickmann AK, et al. Supraorbital Keyhole Approach to the Skull Base: Evaluation of Complications Related to CSF Fistulas and Opened Frontal Sinus. J Neurol Surg A Cent Eur Neurosurg. 2015; 76(6):433–437

[56] Koutourousiou M, Fernandez-Miranda JC, Stefko ST, Wang EW, Snyderman CH, Gardner PA. Endoscopic endonasal surgery for suprasellar meningiomas: experience with 75 patients. J Neurosurg. 2014; 120(6):1326–1339

[57] Banu MA, Szentirmai O, Mascarenhas L, Salek AA, Anand VK, Schwartz TH. Pneumocephalus patterns following endonasal endoscopic skull base surgery as predictors of postoperative CSF leaks. J Neurosurg. 2014; 121(4):961–975

[58] Cavallo LM, Solari D, Somma T, Savic D, Cappabianca P. The awake endoscope-guided sealant technique with fibrin glue in the treatment of postoperative cerebrospinal fluid leak after extended transsphenoidal surgery: technical note. World Neurosurg. 2014; 82(3–4):e479–e485

16 Cavernous Sinus Meningiomas

Antonio Bernardo, Philip E Stieg

Abstract

Meningiomas involving the cavernous sinus (CS) are some of the most challenging lesions of the skull base due to the dense surrounding neurovasculature, including the internal carotid artery (ICA) and plexus, cranial nerves (CNs) II through VI, and important venous pathways that run deep within this compact region. As such, resection of cavernous sinus meningiomas (CSM) is complicated by their location and high potential for neurovascular injury. This chapter provides an exhaustive review of the diagnosis, management, and treatment of CSMs with an emphasis on microsurgical resection, including a stepwise explanation of the different surgical approaches and techniques available and a detailed description of CS exploration. In an extensive experience with these lesions, the authors believe that the best outcomes are achieved from a multidisciplinary approach from a team of neurosurgeons, neuro-oncologists, and radiation oncologists who can evaluate the patient-specific risks and benefits of different treatment modalities.

Keywords: cavernous sinus, meningiomas, microsurgical resection

16.1 Introduction

Cavernous sinus meningiomas (CSMs) are classified as either primary tumors arising from the meningeal wall of the cavernous sinus (CS) or extensions of extracavernous tumors—often meningiomas of the lesser sphenoid wing, orbit, middle fossa, clivus, or petrous bone.[1,2,3,4] In children, intracranial meningiomas are rare and represent only 1.0–4.2% of central nervous system tumors.[5] Meningiomas arising from the lateral wall of the CS represent less than 1% of all intracranial meningiomas.[6]

16.2 Anatomy

The CS is an anatomical space located on both sides of the sella turcica at the convergence of the anterior fossa, middle fossa, sphenoid ridge, and petroclival ridge (▶ Fig. 16.1). The contents of the CS are contained within a membranous structure. Inferiorly and medially, this membrane is composed of periosteum and is contiguous with the periosteal layer of dura covering the middle fossa and sella turcica. The superior and lateral portion of this outer cavernous membrane is contiguous with the connective tissue sheaths of cranial nerves (CNs) III, IV, and V. The outer cavernous membrane forms the outer boundaries of the CS. CNs III, IV, and V are located within this membrane and are thus within the lateral wall of the CS. This rich venous plexus maintains connections to the ophthalmic veins, pterygoid plexus, superior and inferior petrosal sinuses, basilar venous plexus, and middle and inferior cerebral veins (▶ Fig. 16.1).

The CS can be divided into three distinct venous spaces, namely, the medial compartment between the internal carotid artery (ICA) and the lateral wall of the sella, the anteroinferior compartment which is the space anterior to the ICA, and the posterosuperior compartment which is delimited by the ICA and the posterior portion of the roof of the CS. The CS is approximated by four walls, anterior, posterior, lateral, and medial, as well as by its roof and floor. The anterior wall mostly corresponds to the superior orbital fissure (SOF), which separates the CS from the orbit anteriorly. The medial wall corresponds to the pituitary gland and sella turcica superiorly and sphenoid bone inferiorly. The lateral wall is formed by CNs III, IV, and V—including the Gasserian ganglion—and faces the medial surface of the temporal lobe. The posterior wall separates the CS from the posterior cranial fossa and corresponds to the Dorello's canal inferiorly, Gruber's ligament laterally, and the posterior petroclinoid ligament superiorly. The roof of the CS faces the basal cisterns, extending from the anterior clinoid process (ACP) to the posterior clinoid process (PCP).

The ICA and its branches, accompanied by a sympathetic plexus of nerves, pass through the sinus, along with CN VI on its course to the SOF under the ophthalmic division of CN V (CN V1). The meningohypophyseal trunk (MHT) usually arises from the posterior bend of the intracavernous ICA and has three branches, the tentorial (Bernarconi-Cassinari), dorsal meningeal, and inferior hypophyseal arteries—all of which display some degree of variability. The inferolateral trunk usually arises from the lateral aspect of the ICA as it courses anteriorly. The ICA exits the cavernous at the level of the ACP, piercing the outer cavernous membrane which forms a ring around the vessel, known as the proximal dural ring.

16.3 Development

CSMs can arise from the dura of the CS itself—true CS meningiomas—or from the dura of the sphenoid ridge, clinoid processes, or petroclival region and extend into or infiltrating the CS. CSMs that are not wholly located within the CS can grow to considerable size before becoming symptomatic. Meningiomas originating outside the CS can easily invade the CS through the anatomical openings created by CNs III and IV.

The oculomotor canal is the most common CS entry point for meningiomas arising from the PCP, ACP, lateral portion of the diaphragma sellae, anterior portion of the

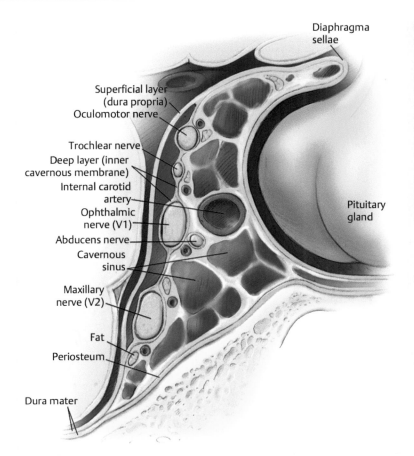

Diaphragma sellae

Superficial layer (dura propria)

Oculomotor nerve

Trochlear nerve

Deep layer (inner cavernous membrane)

Internal carotid artery

Ophthalmic nerve (V1)

Abducens nerve

Cavernous sinus

Maxillary nerve (V2)

Fat

Periosteum

Dura mater

Pituitary gland

Fig. 16.1 Membranous structure of the cavernous sinus. The lateral wall of the cavernous sinus consists of two layers, the superficial layer and deep layer. The superficial layer is the dura propria of the temporal lobe; the deep layer is the inner cavernous membrane that is a fusion of the epineurium of the oculomotor, trochlear, and trigeminal nerves. (Reproduced from Fukuda H., Evins A. I., et al. The meningo-orbital band: microsurgical anatomy and surgical detachment of the membranous structures through a frontotemporal craniotomy with removal of the anterior clinoid process. J Neurol Surg B Skull Base. 2014; 75(2):125–132.)

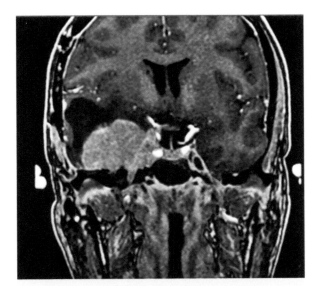

Fig. 16.2 MRI showing a meningioma originating in the perisellar area and invading the cavernous sinus thorough the anatomical openings created by cranial nerves III and IV.

edge of the tentorium, area of the oculomotor trigone, and/or the area of the tuberculum and dorsum sellae. Most meningiomas originating in this perisellar area invade the optic canal when extending anteriorly (▶ Fig. 16.2).

Meningiomas originating from the tentorial edge, posterior to the PCP along the petrous ridge, and from the dura of the clivus can invade the CS along the course of CNs IV and V and through Dorello's canal. These lesions can become large in size but the majority of the tumor grows in the posterior fossa, and thus, it is important to distinguish these lesions from petroclival meningiomas which require a different surgical strategy (▶ Fig. 16.3).

Meningiomas arising in the middle fossa can also invade the CS directly through the lateral wall of the CS. These meningiomas can also become large in size and invade the sella and optic canal before becoming symptomatic.

Meningiomas that extend throughout the entirety of the CS including the superior, anterior, posterior, and inferior compartments, up to the foramen rotundum and foramen ovale, encasing the ICA, CN VI, and the MHT, very likely infiltrate the adventitia of the vessel (▶ Fig. 16.4). These lesions, although benign histologically, pose substantial surgical challenges and should be treated as malignant lesions, with subtotal surgical resection and adjuvant radiotherapy.

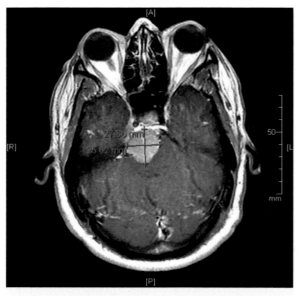

Fig. 16.3 MRI showing a meningioma originating from the tentorial edge at the petrous ridge and invading the cavernous sinus likely along the course of cranial nerves IV and V and through Dorello's canal.

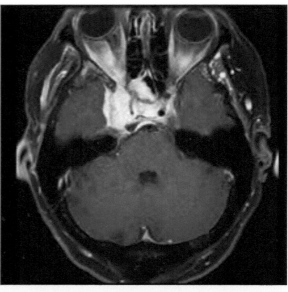

Fig. 16.4 MRI of a meningioma extending through the entire cavernous sinus and encasing the internal carotid artery.

16.4 Symptoms

Symptoms at presentation depend on the specific neurovascular involvement and may often include oculomotor nerve deficits (ptosis, diplopia, anisocoria, ophthalmoplegia), Horner's syndrome, proptosis, sensory loss or pain in one or more trigeminal divisions, visual field deficits, and/or ischemic events due to compression of the ICA. Palsy of CNs III, IV, or VI is extremely common as are trigeminal nerve deficits. Pituitary dysfunction rarely manifests at initial presentation, but can occur and should be considered.[7,8] Assessment of cerebellar function and coordination may provide useful information on tumor extension into the posterior fossa with compression of the brainstem. Differential diagnosis should include other lesions known to invade the CS, including metastatic lesions, pituitary adenomas, perineural spread of head and neck malignancies, hemangiomas, and other neurogenic tumors. Additionally, non-neoplastic pathologies, such as thrombophlebitis, infections, vascular lesions including ICA aneurysms, carotid-cavernous fistulas, dural arteriovenous shunts, and inflammatory lesions (Tolosa-Hunt syndrome, inflammatory pseudotumor) should be considered.[8]

16.5 Diagnosis

CSM often present radiologically as hypointense to isointense lesions with enlargement of the CS, thickening of the lateral wall of the CS, and homogeneous contrast enhancement with nonspecific dural tail sign (▶ Fig. 16.2). Calcifications may be seen as hypointense regions within the tumor and CT may also demonstrate associated hyperostosis. In cases where CSMs invade the walls of the sphenoid sinus, it is most often the unique results of bony thickening rather than destructions.[9] Magnetic resonance angiography often provides useful information about vascular relationships and involvement without the risks of conventional angiography. In patients with extensive lesions who are at high risk for ICA involvement, conventional angiography should be considered with assessment of the collateral circulation by a balloon occlusion test. Patents with poor collateral circulation are good candidates for vascular bypass.

16.6 Treatment

Treatment of CSMs has considerably evolved over the past three decades. Initially, CSM were not considered surgically, however, the emergence of microneurosurgical techniques, coupled with a better understanding of CS anatomy and increasing microsurgical experience, opened the door for surgical management. Currently, there are three main options for the management of CSMs: observation, microsurgical resection, and/or stereotactic radiosurgery (SRS). Patients with asymptomatic or minimally symptomatic CSMs without observed growth may be candidates for observation.[7] However, up to 25% of conservatively managed meningiomas described in the literature show some degree of growth.

Hashimoto et al reported that skull base meningiomas have slower growth rates compared with non-skull base meningiomas, with growth around 0.67–1.2 cm³/year.[4,10,11] Different attempts at pharmacological treatment, including hydroxyurea, mifepristone, or tamoxifen regimens, have all failed to sufficiently treat meningiomas.[7] Intervention, either microsurgical resection or SRS, is indicated in patients with progressively worsening symptoms or demonstrated growth on serial imaging.[7] In general, large symptomatic, or increasingly symptomatic, lesions or those that demonstrate early growth are often surgically resected with or without SRS.

A number of reports have demonstrated significant postoperative neurological deficits, the difficulty of achieving gross-total resections, and the continued need for follow-up due to the possibility of recurrence. Many surgeons opt for a more conservative approach that involves removal of the tumor from the lateral aspect of the CS without entering the sinus proper, due to the high potential for postoperative morbidity.[6]

In 1999, Levine et al proposed the so-called Levine-Sekhar grading system to predict the resectability and prognosis of skull base meningiomas,[12] and a 2016 study by Nanda and colleagues confirmed this to be a good predictor of surgical resectability in finding that ICA encasement significantly reduced complete resection rates.[1,13] Additionally, Nanda et al found that tumor recurrence was significantly lower in patients who underwent adjuvant SRS.[1] Despite the growing body of data, there remains no consensus on an optimal treatment strategy for CSMs, and some authors have even advocated for Gamma Knife radiosurgery as the first line treatment.[14]

It is our belief that tumors with significant extracavernous components that demonstrate brainstem compression and hydrocephalus necessitate surgical intervention. Tumors compressing the optic nerve or chiasm should also be considered prime candidates for resection in order to avoid the risk of radiation-induced optic neuropathy. Although aggressive resection of CSMs has not proven to be the optimal treatment option, it must be considered for tumors greater than 3.0–3.5 cm in diameter and are not ideal candidates for SRS.

We believe that the best outcomes in patients with CSMs are achieved from a multidisciplinary approach from a team of neurosurgeons, neuro-oncologists, and radiation oncologists who can evaluate the patient-specific risks and benefits of different treatment modalities.

16.7 Surgical Approaches

Several different surgical approaches have been described for the resection of lesions involving the middle fossa. In tumors that extend significantly into the CS from adjacent areas, the addition of an orbitozygomatic osteotomy to a standard pterional approach may be required to improve surgical exposure and to provide vascular control of the ICA (► Fig. 16.5). When lesions are confined to the lower compartment of the CS, a pterional approach with removal of the zygomatic arch may be sufficient to expose the posterior and inferior compartments of the CS (► Fig. 16.6), however, with poor visualization of the more distal compartments. For lesions involving the CS, parasellar region, upper clivus, and adjacent neurovascular structures, we prefer to use a fronto-orbitozygomatic approach—a pterional approach with removal of the zygomatic arch and lateral wall and roof of the orbit—to achieve a wide angle of surgical exposure.

16.7.1 Preoperative Preparation

Mild hypocapnia is recommended, however, profound hypocapnia should not be induced unless indicated for

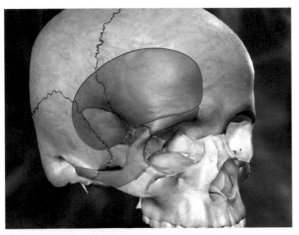

Fig. 16.5 The orbitozygomatic osteotomy. A pterional craniotomy is extended by removing the zygomatic arch and the lateral wall and roof of the orbit.

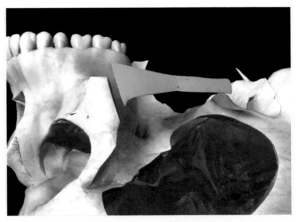

Fig. 16.6 A fronto-temporo-zygomatic craniotomy. This consists of a pterional approach with additional removal of the zygomatic arch to reach lesions confined to the lower compartments of the cavernous sinus.

control of edema or increased surgical exposure. Intraoperative somatosensory evoked potential, motor evoked potential, and electroencephalography monitoring is recommended. As a precaution, a lumbar drain should be placed, but should remain closed for the entire extradural portion of the approach, and in most cases is not needed at all throughout the procedure.

16.7.2 Positioning and Incision

Initial patient positioning is the same as that used in the pterional approach, wherein the head is extended, rotated 25–35° away from the lesion, oriented with the vertex slightly downwards. A curvilinear incision should be planned beginning just anterior to the tragus, at the level of the inferior margin of the zygomatic arch, up to the superior temporal line, curving to terminate at the hairline superior to the contralateral midpupillary line (▶ Fig. 16.7). A narrow strip of hair along the planned incision should be shaved and the skin prepped. During the incision, care should be taken to preserve the superficial temporal artery in the event that intracranial bypass is needed.

Following the incision, the skin flap can be elevated, and the underlying temporalis fascia exposed. The fascia can then be sharply incised along the margin of the superior temporal line and elevated separately to perform a subfascial dissection. This technique protects the frontal branch of the facial nerve, which lies in the subgaleal fat pad and runs along the superficial surface of this fascial plane. The dissection can then be continued anteriorly to expose the orbital rim, malar eminence, and zygomatic

arch. The temporalis muscle is then raised independently, exposing the root of the zygoma and pterion. The muscle flap is left attached to the cranium at its vascular pedicle in the infratemporal fossa. The skin flap and temporalis muscle are then retracted anteriorly and inferiorly with surgical fish hook retractors attached to a bar (▶ Fig. 16.8).

16.7.3 Fronto-Orbitozygomatic Osteotomy

The cranio-orbital flap can be elevated in two pieces. A pterional craniotomy is fashioned and dural tack-up sutures are placed. The periorbita is detached from the lateral and superior aspects of the orbit using a sharp Penfield no. 1 dissector, completing exposure of the zygoma and entire orbital rim (▶ Fig. 16.9). The supraorbital nerve is then freed from its bony canal using a small chisel or diamond drill.

The orbital and zygomatic osteotomies can then be performed by fashioning six cuts using a reciprocating saw (▶ Fig. 16.10). The first cut is placed through the root of the zygomatic process. Care should be taken to avoid violation of the temporomandibular joint capsule. The second and third cuts divide the zygomatic bone just above the level of the malar eminence. The fourth cut divides the superior orbital rim and roof. The last two cuts free the lateral wall of the orbit by connecting the inferior orbital fissure (IOF) and SOF. The IOF should be identified by direct visualization or by palpating the infratemporal fossa with a no. 4 Penfield dissector. The fifth cut is a short cut made from the IOF to the temporal fossa and the sixth and final cut is placed from the lateral margin of the SOF to join the fifth cut from the inferior orbital fissure. The orbitozygomatic bone flap is now free and can be gently elevated (▶ Fig. 16.11).

In order to decrease the need for temporal retraction and provide a more basal viewing angle that increases

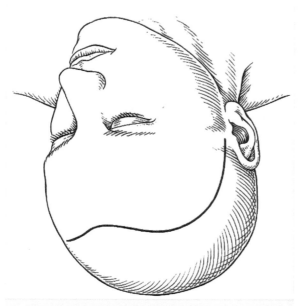

Fig. 16.7 Patient positioning and incision. The head is extended, rotated 25 to 35° to the contralateral side, and the vertex is angled slightly down. The incision extends from the tragus to the contralateral midpupillary line

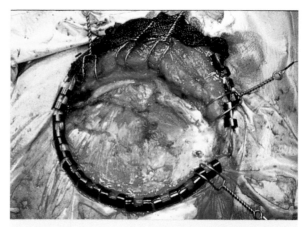

Fig. 16.8 The orbital rim, malar eminence, and zygomatic arch are exposed following elevation of the skin flap and interfascial fat pad.

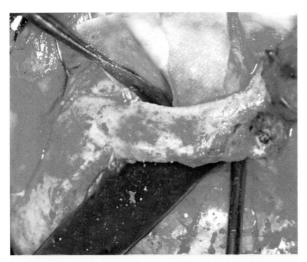

Fig. 16.9 The periorbita is carefully detached from the lateral and superior aspects of the orbit using a sharp Penfield no. 1 dissector. (Reproduced from Bernardo A. and Stieg P. E. Orbitocranial Zygomatic Approach for Upper Basilar Artery Aneurysms. In: Macdonald, Loch, eds. Neurosurgical Operative Atlas. Georg Thieme Verlag KG Stuttgart. 2009.)

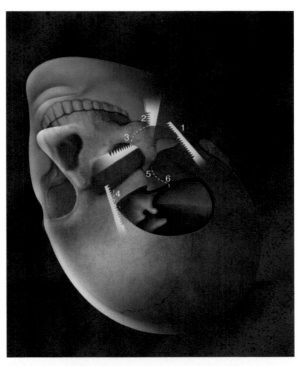

Fig. 16.10 Orbitozygomatic bone cuts. Following the pterional craniotomy, six bone cuts are placed for the orbital and zygomatic osteotomies. (Reproduced from Bernardo A. and Stieg P. E. Orbitocranial Zygomatic Approach for Upper Basilar Artery Aneurysms. In: Macdonald, Loch, eds. Neurosurgical Operative Atlas. Georg Thieme Verlag KG Stuttgart. 2009.)

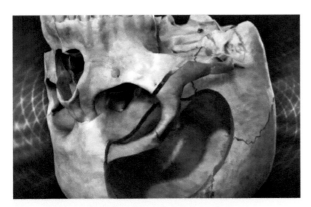

Fig. 16.11 Graphical depiction of elevation of the orbitozygomatic bone flap.

the field of view at the deep end of the surgical corridor, the temporal cranial opening should be drilled so that it is flush with the floor of the middle fossa.

16.7.4 Drilling of the Sphenoid Ridge

Medial exposure of the CS and exposure of the cavernous ICA is obtained by drilling the sphenoid ridge and remainder of the roof of the orbit, removal of the ACP and optic strut, and unroofing of the optic nerve. To begin, the dura is elevated from the floor of the anterior fossa and sphenoid ridge. Using a high-speed drill, the sphenoid ridge is progressively flattened until the most lateral aspect

of the lesser wing of the sphenoid and base of the ACP are reached. In a similar fashion, the bony striations of the orbital roof are then drilled. With the orbit now exposed, electromyographic electrodes can be placed directly onto the superior oblique, superior rectus, and lateral rectus muscles to monitor CNs III, IV, and VI function.

16.7.5 Identification and Dissection of the Meningoorbital Band

On the lateral side of the SOF, between the greater and the lesser wings of the sphenoid, the periosteum of the orbit is continuous with the periosteal dura of the middle fossa forming a 3 to 4 mm dural bridge known as the meningo-orbital band (▶ Fig. 16.12). This band houses the meningo-ophthalmic artery and needs to be cut in order to allow for sufficient retraction of the temporal tip dura and thus improved exposure of the ACP, SOF, and anterior portion of the CS. Once the lateral wall of the SOF is partially removed, the lateral periosteal dura can be carefully incised using microscissors or a scalpel to fully detach the meningo-orbital band from the periorbita and the dura propria of the temporal lobe can then be peeled from the inner cavernous membrane (▶ Fig. 16.13).

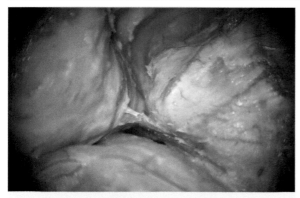

Fig. 16.12 The meningo-orbital band is located lateral to the superior orbital fissure, between the greater and the lesser wings of the sphenoid, and is continuous with the periosteum of the orbit.

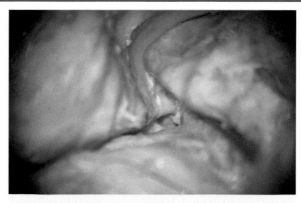

Fig. 16.13 Following cutting of the meningo-orbital band, the dura of the temporal lobe can be gently detached form the superior orbital fissure to expose the most anterior portion of the cavernous sinus.

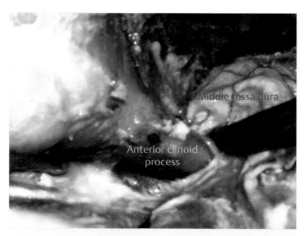

Fig. 16.14 The anterior clinoid process is exposed by detaching the dura overlying its superior and inferior surfaces.

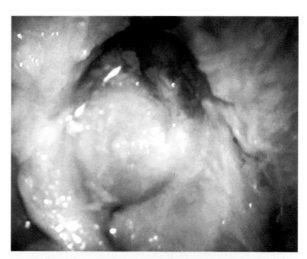

Fig. 16.15 The clinoid internal carotid artery and the proximal and distal dural rings are visible after removal of the anterior clinoid process.

16.7.6 Anterior Clinoidectomy

Removal of the ACP—located between the SOF laterally and optic canal medially—exposes the infraclinoid ICA, which is both extradural and extracavernous, and provides distal control of the artery. To begin, the dura overlying the superior and inferior surfaces of the ACP is gently detached from the bony surface and the ACP is removed piecemeal in order to avoid injury to the surrounding neurovasculature (▸ Fig. 16.14). A small diamond burr is placed at the center of the ACP and the ACP is hollowed and a small shell of cortical bone is left in place. Once drilling is complete, the small shell of bone can be fractured into small little pieces and removed using a blunt dissector. It is important to be conscious of the immediate surrounding structures. CN II is located just medially, CN III covered by dura, is located just

laterally, and the clinoid ICA is located just interiorly inside the clinoidal triangle. Once the ACP has been completely removed, the clinoid ICA becomes visible and the optic canal becomes open on its lateral side (▸ Fig. 16.15). Bleeding in the clinoid space following removal of the ACP is not common but can be easily managed with Surgicel. At this point, the optic strut, which connects the ACP with the lateral aspect of the body of the sphenoid bone, needs to be carefully removed.[15]

16.7.7 Unroofing the Optic Nerve

The optic canal, which marks the medial border of the clinoid space, can now be unroofed to expose and mobilize the optic nerve. To accomplish this, the dura is further gently elevated from the floor of the anterior cranial fossa toward the tuberculum sellae until the point where the optic nerve exits the optic canal. The bony roof of the optic canal is then drilled using a diamond burr until only a thin depressible shell of bone remains on top of the nerve. Care should be taken to avoid entering the ethmoid sinus, which is medial to the optic canal, and copious irrigation should be used to avoid thermal injury to the underlying optic nerve. This shell can then be fractured and completely removed with a small dissector to allow for medial mobilization of the nerve (▸ Fig. 16.16). This is essential to avoid injury to the optic nerve during subsequent dissection. By this point, it will be possible to identify the proximal and distal dural rings.

16.7.8 Extradural Exposure of the Cavernous Sinus

Accurate extradural exposure is essential whether as initial preparation for a combined intra-extradural approach or as the main avenue of surgical exposure. Thorough knowledge of the CS meningeal architecture helps minimize troublesome bleeding while exposing the lateral wall of the CS (▸ Fig. 16.17 and ▸ Fig. 16.18). The intracranial dura consists of two layers: the periosteal dura and dura propria. At the foramen or fissure where cranial nerves and/or vessels exit the skull, the periosteal dura folds back along the bone and exits with the structure to

become extracranial periosteum, whereas the dura propria remains intracranial. At the point of exit from the foramen or fissure, in some cases, there is a space filled with loose connective tissue between the dura propria and epineurium of the cranial nerves. The CS venous plexuses

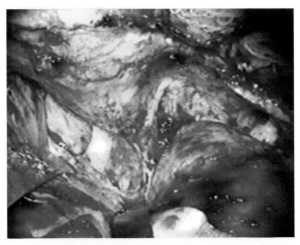

Fig. 16.16 Cranial nerve II is freed and mobilized by carefully removing the roof of the optic canal with a diamond drill under copious irrigation to avoid thermal injury.

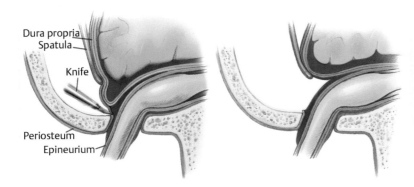

Fig. 16.17 Using sharp dissection, the dura propria of the temporal lobe can be separated from the periosteal layer of the middle fossa and, using the inner reticular layer as a cleavage plane, is elevated off of the epineurium of trigeminal nerve. (Reproduced from Fukuda H., Evins A. I., et al. The meningo-orbital band: microsurgical anatomy and surgical detachment of the membranous structures through a frontotemporal craniotomy with removal of the anterior clinoid process. J Neurol Surg B Skull Base. 2014; 75(2):125–132.)

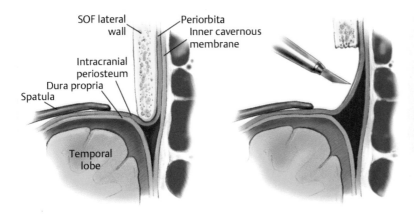

Fig. 16.18 The dura propria can be further retracted and elevated from the inner cavernous membrane with sharp cuts using a #15 blade or microscissors. (Reproduced from Fukuda H., Evins A. I., et al. The meningo-orbital band: microsurgical anatomy and surgical detachment of the membranous structures through a frontotemporal craniotomy with removal of the anterior clinoid process. J Neurol Surg B Skull Base. 2014; 75(2):125–132.)

leave the sinus attached to and within the periosteal layer and exit the foramen rotundum and foramen ovale as they course into the pterygopalatine and infratemporal fossae. The two dural layers usually attach at the level of the foramina where the cranial nerves exit the intradural space.

Extradural exposure of the CS can begin at the SOF, foramen ovale, or foramen rotundum. Using sharp dissection, the two dural layers can be separated and, using the inner reticular layer as a cleavage plane, the dura propria can be elevated off of the epineurium (▶ Fig. 16.17 and ▶ Fig. 16.18). This maneuver is crucial in order to minimize the troublesome and discouraging venous bleeding that happens to all surgeons at the beginning of CS exposure. This reduced venous bleeding can be easily controlled with Surgicel and cottonoid patties. The inner cavernous membrane, formed by the epineurium of the CNs III, IV, V1, V2, and V3, should come into view. Loose connections between the two layers can be peeled of and the dura propria can be further retracted and elevated from the inner cavernous membrane with sharp cuts using a number 15 blade or microscissors (▶ Fig. 16.17 and ▶ Fig. 16.18).

The dura of the middle fossa can then be elevated in an anterior to posterior direction from the middle fossa until the CNs V2 and V3 are identified exiting their respective

foramina (▶ Fig. 16.19). The middle meningeal artery should be identified and cut. The greater superficial petrosal nerve can be identified emerging from the facial hiatus and should be dissected free of the dura. The intrapetrous ICA can be exposed in the Glasscock triangle between the facial hiatus, anterior margin of foramen ovale, and the intersection of the greater superficial petrosal nerve and lateral aspect of CN V3 (▶ Fig. 16.20a). This segment of the intrapetrous ICA, between the cochlea posteriorly and posterior aspect of CN V3 anteriorly, can be used for temporary occlusion or proximal control if needed or as a donor site for intracranial vascular bypass, should the need to sacrifice a diseased portion of the intracavernous ICA arise (▶ Fig. 16.20b). The temporal lobe dura should be gently detached and elevated and the lateral wall of the CS entirely exposed (▶ Fig. 16.21). While elevating the temporal lobe dura, cutting of the loose connections and separating the two layers should proceed uniformly in all directions to avoid stretching of CNs III and IV at the paraclinoid space which can lead to inadvertent iatrogenic injury. Venous bleeding through inner cavernous membrane can be easily controlled with Surgicel.

16.7.9 Cavernous Sinus Exploration

Once exposed, the CS can be accessed through several entry points defined as CS triangles. The anatomical triangles of the CS are organized into ten main triangular windows, which all have their own surgical significance. The CS triangles define regions or corridors bounded by dura, bone, nerve, or vessel and can be divided into three main subregions: parasellar (clinoidal, oculomotor, supratrochlear, and infratrochlear triangles), paraclival (inferomedial and inferolateral triangles), and middle fossa (anterolateral, lateral, posterolateral, and posteromedial triangles) (▶ Fig. 16.22).

The infratrochlear (Parkinson's) triangle is the main extradural surgical window into the CS. It is anatomically situated between CN IV and CN V1 and can be enlarged by depressing the CN VI and elevating CN V1. To minimize the use of the spatula and potential consequent nerve injury, the Parkinson's triangle can be enlarged by freeing CN IV from the periorbita just distal to the SOF (▶ Fig. 16.23). Inferior displacement of CN V1 exposes CN VI (▶ Fig. 16.24). The posterior-superior, anterior-inferior,

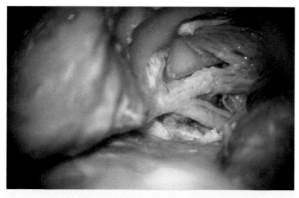

Fig. 16.19 The dura of the middle fossa is elevated from the superior orbital fissure and from the lateral wall of the cavernous sinus in an anterior to posterior direction until cranial nerve V2 is identified exiting foramen rotundum.

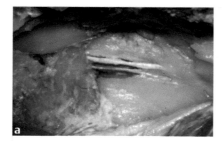

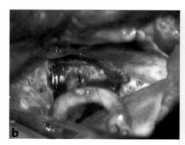

Fig. 16.20 (a) The intrapetrous internal carotid artery (ICA) is exposed in the Glasscock triangle between the facial hiatus, anterior margin of foramen ovale, and the intersection of the greater superficial petrosal nerve, and lateral aspect of cranial nerve V3. (b) High flow bypass between the right intrapetrous and supraclinoid ICA to bypass an intracavernous portion of the ICA completely encased and infiltrated by tumor.

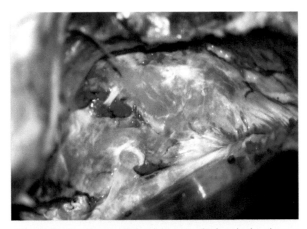

Fig. 16.21 The temporal lobe dura is gently detached and elevated, and the lateral wall of the cavernous sinus is entirely exposed. Care should be taken to avoid tension on cranial nerves III and IV while elevating the dura from the Gasserian ganglion.

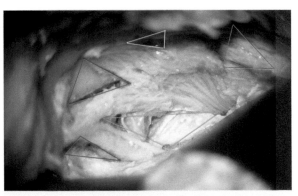

Fig. 16.22 The lateral wall of the cavernous sinus can be entered through several corridors based on the location of the intracavernous lesion. The infratrochlear corridor is the main extradural surgical window into the cavernous sinus. It is anatomically situated between cranial nerves (CNs) IV and V1, and can be enlarged by depressing the CN VI and elevating CN V1.

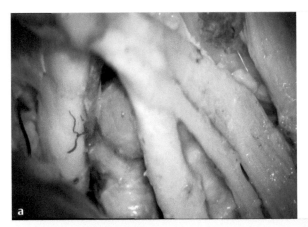

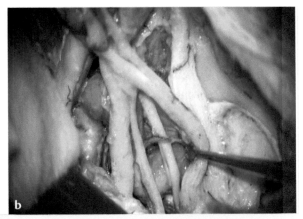

Fig. 16.23 (a and b) Unlocking of the structures in the superior orbital fissure and freeing cranial nerve IV and V1 from the periorbita allows for enlargement of the Parkinson's triangle and minimal spatula retraction.

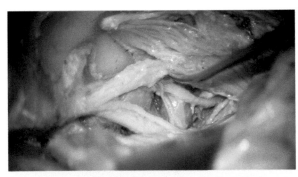

Fig. 16.24 Inferior displacement of cranial nerve (CN) V1 exposes CN VI and the sympathetic bundle.

and lateral venous spaces as well as the lateral surface of the clinoid and ophthalmic segments of the ICA can be well exposed through this surgical window (▶ Fig. 16.25). In cases of large tumors mainly involving the inferior venous compartments, the inferior access corridors (inferomedial and inferolateral triangles) can be enhanced by skeletonizing the foramen rotundum and foramen ovale and displacing CNs V2 and V3.

Typically, venous bleeding from the cavernous space is not a problem when dealing with intracavernous meningiomas, as the venous space is obliterated by the lesion itself. Bleeding can occur as tumor is debulked and adjacent intracavernous venous channels become decompressed, but if encountered, this can be controlled by elevating the patient's head and packing the sinus with Surgicel or fibrin glue.

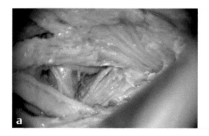
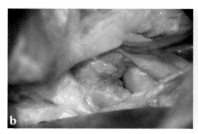

Fig. 16.25 (a) The posterior-superior, anterior-inferior, and lateral venous spaces can be seen through the Parkinson's triangle. (b) The lateral surface of the clinoid and ophthalmic segments of the internal carotid artery can be best exposed through the supratrochlear and oculomotor triangles above cranial nerve III.

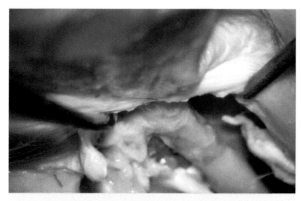

Fig. 16.26 The porus oculomotoris can be opened and dissected anteriorly until the superior orbital fissure in order to free and displace cranial nerve III, and facilitates intradural access through the roof of the cavernous sinus.

Early identification of intracavernous structures, especially CN VI at its exit from Dorello's canal and the sympathetic fibers traveling through the posterolateral fibrous ring of the ICA at the level of the foramen lacerum, is crucial to avoid the deleterious complications of CS surgery. Capsular arteries are usually protected by the ICA in their medial location, however, it is important to identify them early along with origins on the ICA. Additionally, careful attempts should be made to identify CN VI, the MHT, and entire course of the intracavernous ICA. Once these intracavernous structures are identified, complete excision of the tumor can be easily accomplished. Dissection within the CS should be performed carefully using microdissectors and microscissors. Sharp dissection is necessary in most instances in order to avoid traction on any intracavernous cranial nerves or arteries.

If a tumor originates in the intradural parasellar space and only involves the superior venous compartments, the CS can be entered through its roof intradurally in the space between the CN III laterally and the supraclinoid ICA medially after debulking the intradural component of the tumor. In order to enhance the surgical corridor, the supraclinoid ICA can be freed and displaced medially by cutting the distal dural ring, and the oculomotor nerve can be freed by opening the porus oculomotoris (▶ Fig. 16.26). CN III can be freed until its entry into the SOF and mobilized laterally, and the CS can be entered

through its roof/superior compartment. In these cases, the extradural exposure stage is unnecessary and the tumor can be controlled from an intradural approach.

If the tumor is originating from within the CS and enters the orbit through the SOF, the annulus of Zinn (annular tendon) must be opened and the intra-annular structures safely exposed (▶ Fig. 16.27). The pattern of tumor growth in these cases can vary and can thus displace the intra-annual structures medially or laterally. After the tumor is initially debulked in the CS, the extra-annular structures can be dissected along the lateral edge of V1 and displaced medially. The annulus of Zinn is then exposed and opened, the orbit is entered, and the remaining tumor is removed. Care must be taken not to damage the ophthalmic artery (▶ Fig. 16.27).

If the tumor involves the optic canal and the paraclinoid space, surgical exposure can be enhanced by cutting the distal dural ring and displacing the ICA from the body of the sphenoid bone. Cases in which the tumor originates from the sellar floor and extends extradurally to the CS, the tumor should first be debulked intracavernously and can then be followed into the sella extradurally in the space between the roof of the CS and the paraclinoid dura, after removal of the ACP.

If the tumor involves the perisellar space intradurally and extends through the entire CS, a combined intra- and extradural exposure is necessary. In cases of meningiomas originating from the tentorial edge at the petrous ridge, or at the dorsum sellae with intradural perisellar and significant CS extension, the anterior petrosal approach can be combined with intra- and extradural exposure of the CS to provide access to the entire lesion. In cases of large petroclival meningiomas with minimal but symptomatic cavernous extension, a combined perilabyrinthine subtemporal transtentorial approach can be used to access the petroclival component and the CS can be entered through its posterior wall in the space between CN V and the lateral edge of the dorsum sellae—superior and medial to Dorello's canal. Conversely, if the meningioma originates from the CS and extends minimally into the petroclival space, the lesion can be initially debulked from within the CS and then followed into the petroclival space by opening the dura of the posterior wall of the sinus from an anterior perspective. This surgical window exposes the midportion of the clivus from just below the PCP to the area in which the anterior

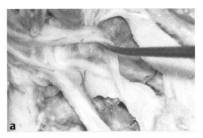
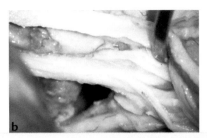
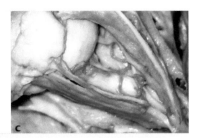

Fig. 16.27 (a) The extra-annular structures can be dissected along the lateral edge of cranial nerve (CN) V1 and can be displaced medially to expose the annulus of Zinn. (b) The annulus of Zinn is exposed and opened along the medial aspect of CN III to enter the orbit. (c) Care is taken to avoid damage to the ophthalmic artery.

inferior cerebellar artery originates—which is almost always visible.

If the meningioma occupies the entire CS and completely surrounds the ICA, the vessel wall is likely to be infiltrated by the tumor and thus would lack a clear cleavage plane, complicating separation of CN VI from the tumor. In these cases, complete resection is not possible without iatrogenic damage to both the vessel and nerve, and thus it is wise to leave a small layer of tumor attached to the ICA which can be treated postoperatively with radiosurgery. Alternatively, intracranial bypass between the intrapetrous and supraclinoid segments of the ICA (▶ Fig. 16.20b) could be performed to allow for complete resection and decrease the potential for morbidity from cranial nerve injury—a dreaded complication following CSM resection. Existing preoperative cranial nerve deficits rarely resolve or improve postoperatively, whereas new postoperative onset deficits tend to resolve.

The main goals of reconstruction, following a fronto-orbitozygomatic approach, are to prevent CSF leakage and achieve a satisfactory cosmetic outcome. Any inadvertent opening of the paranasal sinuses should be managed by packing with fat, fascia, and/or fibrin glue. If the frontal sinus is entered, the mucosa should be completely stripped and the sinus should be packed with fat to prevent CSF leak. Watertight dural closure is preferable but incomplete closure can be supplemented with autologous fascia and dural substitute. The orbitozygomatic bone flap is placed in situ and secured with titanium plates and screws. Any excessive bone defect must be reconstructed to prevent postoperative enophthalmos. Dural tack-up sutures are placed around the edge of the petrional bone flap to eliminate dead space and mitigate the risk of postoperative epidural hematomas. The temporalis muscle is reflected back to the temporalis fossa, and the periosteum is accurately reconstructed. The scalp is then finally closed in layers.

Safe surgical exploration of the CS and its various compartments is possible when following a purposeful and logical sequence of surgical maneuvers that avoids unnecessary exploration of critical spaces. The CS must not be treated like any other intracranial space wherein minimal exposure is sufficient. A meticulous and well-planned extradural preparation can enlarge surgical corridors and minimize the need for retraction in this very confined microsurgical space. The potential for severe iatrogenic injury in CS surgery is enormous, however, CS surgery is possible and should only be undertaken by surgeons who truly master the anatomy of this region and who possess a realistic appreciation of their own capabilities.

16.8 Surgery and Radiosurgery

Previous studies have shown no significant relationship between tumor extension and recurrence or progression.[16] Additionally, previous surgery or radiation has been shown to have no significant relationship with surgical resectability.[16,17] A 2010 meta-analysis compared the efficacy of gross total resection, subtotal resection, and SRS alone in 2,065 patients with CSMs, and found that SRS resulted in a significantly reduced recurrence rate as well as a reduced rate of postoperative nerve deficits, with no statistically significant differences between gross total and subtotal resection.[18]

Fractioned radiotherapy is also a viable treatment option but has been shown to have less long-term tumor control compared to SRS, thus, should be reserved for very large lesions that would be less likely to respond to SRS.[14]

There remains an ongoing debate as to the optimal intervention and time of intervention for CSMs. Better designed large population studies are necessary to achieve greater consensus on the management of these tumors. We believe, based on our extensive experience with these tumors, that most symptomatic cases or cases with documented radiological progression warrant intervention. Small (< 20–30 cm³) primarily intracavernous lesions are ideal candidates for SRS. Large meningiomas, either intracavernous or extracavernous, require surgical resection or debulking with postoperative SRS, especially if there is recurrence or symptomatic progression.

16.9 Acknowledgments

The authors would like to sincerely thank Dr Alexander I Evins for his contributions and assistance with this chapter.

References

[1] Nanda A, Thakur JD, Sonig A, Missios S. Microsurgical resectability, outcomes, and tumor control in meningiomas occupying the cavernous sinus. J Neurosurg. 2016; 125(2):378–392

[2] Sekhar LN, Althschuler EM. Meningiomas of the cavernous sinus. In: Al-Mefty O, ed. Meningiomas. New York, NY: Raven Press; 1991

[3] Oya S, Kim SH, Sade B, Lee JH. The natural history of intracranial meningiomas. J Neurosurg. 2011; 114(5):1250–1256

[4] Bindal R, Goodman JM, Kawasaki A, Purvin V, Kuzma B. The natural history of untreated skull base meningiomas. Surg Neurol. 2003; 59 (2):87–92, discussion 92

[5] Erşahin Y, Ozdamar N, Demirtaş E, Karabiyikoğlu M. Meningioma of the cavernous sinus in a child. Childs Nerv Syst. 1999; 15(1):8–10

[6] Klinger DR, Flores BC, Lewis JJ, Barnett SL. The treatment of cavernous sinus meningiomas: evolution of a modern approach. Neurosurg Focus. 2013; 35(6):E8

[7] Heth JA, Al-Mefty O. Cavernous sinus meningiomas. Neurosurg Focus. 2003; 14(6):e3

[8] Lee JH, Lee HK, Park JK, Choi CG, Suh DC. Cavernous sinus syndrome: clinical features and differential diagnosis with MR imaging. AJR Am J Roentgenol. 2003; 181(2):583–590

[9] Cattin F. Cavernous sinus meningioma. In: Bonneville JF, Bonneville F, Cattin F, Nagi S, eds. MRI of the Pituitary Gland. Cham, Switzerland: Springer; 2016

[10] Walsh MT, Couldwell WT. Management options for cavernous sinus meningiomas. J Neurooncol. 2009; 92(3):307–316

[11] Hashimoto N, Rabo CS, Okita Y, et al. Slower growth of skull base meningiomas compared with non-skull base meningiomas based on volumetric and biological studies. J Neurosurg. 2012; 116(3):574–580

[12] Levine ZT, Buchanan RI, Sekhar LN, Rosen CL, Wright DC. Proposed grading system to predict the extent of resection and outcomes for cranial base meningiomas. Neurosurgery. 1999; 45(2):221–230

[13] Spiegelmann R, Cohen ZR, Nissim O, Alezra D, Pfeffer R. Cavernous sinus meningiomas: a large LINAC radiosurgery series. J Neurooncol. 2010; 98(2):195–202

[14] Nicolato A, Foroni R, Alessandrini F, Maluta S, Bricolo A, Gerosa M. The role of Gamma Knife radiosurgery in the management of cavernous sinus meningiomas. Int J Radiat Oncol Biol Phys. 2002; 53 (4):992–1000

[15] Fukuda H, Evins AI, Burrell JC, Iwasaki K, Stieg PE, Bernardo A. The meningo-orbital band: microsurgical anatomy and surgical detachment of the membranous structures through a frontotemporal craniotomy with removal of the anterior clinoid process. J Neurol Surg B Skull Base. 2014; 75(2):125–132

[16] De Jesús O, Sekhar LN, Parikh HK, Wright DC, Wagner DP. Long-term follow-up of patients with meningiomas involving the cavernous sinus: recurrence, progression, and quality of life. Neurosurgery. 1996; 39(5):915–919, discussion 919–920

[17] Pichierri A, Santoro A, Raco A, Paolini S, Cantore G, Delfini R. Cavernous sinus meningiomas: retrospective analysis and proposal of a treatment algorithm. Neurosurgery. 2009; 64(6):1090–1099, discussion 1099–1101

[18] Sughrue ME, Rutkowski MJ, Aranda D, Barani IJ, McDermott MW, Parsa AT. Factors affecting outcome following treatment of patients with cavernous sinus meningiomas. J Neurosurg. 2010; 113(5): 1087–1092

17 Reconstruction of the Skull Base

Sebastien Froelich, Domenico Solari, Moujahed Labidi, Shunya Hanakita, Anne Laure Bernat, Philippe Herman, Paolo Cappabianca

Abstract

Skull base surgery represents a continuously evolving field of neurosurgery.

In recent years, a variety of innovative skull base craniofacial approaches including anterior, anterolateral, and posterolateral routes have been developed to access skull base meningiomas. Recently, technical advances and scientific progress have led to a progressive reduction of the invasiveness of these approaches and the possibility to access different areas of the skull base.

In these terms, it should be noticed that the reconstruction segment of any surgical procedure at the level of the skull base represents one of the most important steps of this kind of surgery; indeed, the development of reliable reconstructive materials/techniques has definitely proceeded throughout the evolution of skull base surgery. Moreover, the constant refinements of reconstruction techniques have also improved aesthetic outcomes, thus improving patients' satisfaction.

An effective watertight closure is mandatory to restore the natural intra- and extradural compartments and to prevent postoperative cerebrospinal fluid (CSF) leakage. Failure to create adequate reconstruction may lead to significant complications, such as meningitis, brain herniation, and tension pneumocephalus.

In the present manuscript, the materials used and nuances of techniques of reconstruction of skull base are presented and discussed, also in regard to the surgical approaches for skull base meningiomas.

Keywords: CSF leak, skull base reconstruction, dural substitute, osteodural breach, multilayer reconstruction, vascularized flap, cranioplasty

17.1 Introduction

Skull base surgery represents a highly specialized discipline that gathers the expertise of different specialties, that is, ENT surgeons, neurosurgeons, radiotherapists, oncologists. In the last decades, it has been rapidly evolving, thanks to developments in surgical technique, technological advancements, and, accordingly, expanded surgical indications. A variety of innovative skull base craniofacial approaches including anterior, anterolateral, and posterolateral routes have been developed over the past years to reach deep-seated lesion, while reducing the need for brain retraction.[1,2,3,4,5,6,7,8,9,10,11,12,13,14,15,16,17] Recently, technological advances (endoscopy, neuronavigation, monitoring, intraoperative imaging) have led to a progressive reduction in the invasiveness of these approaches and the possibility to access deep lesions at the skull base through small opening, together with improved visualization and control of critical neurovascular structures.

As with any surgical procedure, closure and reconstruction in the skull base is one of the most important steps of the surgery. With the increasing use of expanded approaches and more radical tumor resections, the need for more complex reconstructions has arose. Conversely, the development of more reliable reconstructive materials/techniques has definitely participated in the renewal and expanding of certain surgical corridors (i.e., the endonasal route following the popularization of the Hadad flap).[18,19,20] Moreover, the constant refinements of reconstruction techniques have also improved aesthetic outcomes, thus improving patients' satisfaction.

To achieve a successful reconstruction after skull base surgery, the following points should be addressed: (1) isolation of the intradural compartment; (2) water and airtight closure to prevent CSF leak, pneumocephalus, ascending meningitis, and other intracranial infections; (3) obliteration of dead space; (4) coverage of critical extradural structure to avoid infection; (5) promotion of the healing process; (6) preservation and rehabilitation of function and cosmesis; (7) management of risk factors of increased intracranial pressure (ICP).[21]

Accordingly, the reconstruction of the surgical pathways can be performed choosing different suitable, autologous, or heterologous materials that can be used in various methods, individually or combined according to the pathology targeted and the route chosen to approach it.[22] In this chapter, we will review the materials used and discuss nuances of techniques of reconstruction, in regard to the surgical approaches for skull base meningiomas.

17.2 Reconstruction Techniques and Materials

Reconstruction of the skull base after tumor removal should be devised in a way that recreates the anatomical and functional integrity of each of the compartments transgressed. The choice and planning of the approach for tumor resection should also take into account the expected skull base defect and materials and tissues that will be available to achieve an adequate reconstruction. In fact, reconstruction of defect begins during the opening stage of the surgery. An adequate skin incision, careful dissection of the soft tissues, along with temporalis muscle, and preservation of neurovascular pedicles can make closure at the end of the surgery much simpler. Avoiding overly aggressive and unnecessarily wide exposures is an important general principle. The bigger the opening, the bigger the closure!

Skull base defects can be broadly divided into extradural and transdural, the latter implying a transgression of the intradural compartment and, frequently, opening of the subarachnoid spaces. The level of intraoperative CSF leak can then be subdivided into low- and high-flow CSF leaks, depending if the communication also involves multiple subarachnoid cisterns or a ventricle.

At least three levels of interest are encountered and needs to be addressed during closure: the intradural space, the osteodural defect, and the extracranial tissues.

Prior to the repair, the surgical site to be reconstructed needs to be prepared to receive the grafts, flaps, and/or any other reconstruction material. In order to favor integration, especially of free or pedicled fascial and/or myofascial flaps, the target site should be ridden of any residual nonviable or interposed tissue (mucosa, necrotic, infected material, etc.).

Several factors should be considered when reconstructing a skull base:

- Size and location of the bony and dural defects.
- High- versus low-flow CSF leaks.
- Prior radiation therapy or scheduled postoperative radiotherapy.
- Previous surgery.
- Presence of comorbidities or imaging findings that may be associated with high ventricular pressure: morbid obesity, dilated ventricles, empty sella, or dilated optic nerves.

Current options available to reconstruct the skull base bone and dura can be divided in heterologous and autologous, the latter can then be subdivided in free or vascularized grafts. Autologous grafts represent the most valuable materials as they are easily harvested from the main surgical site or eventually from distant donor sites. Above all, the ability of such tissues to rapidly interact with the surrounding physiological structures quickens the recovery of the anatomical barrier and reduces the potential for infectious complications. On the other side, the development of new materials either heterologous and/or synthetic has provided a wide array of alternative solutions that help avoid morbidity related to the second surgical site. These materials can be used in various ways, individually or in combination in a multilayer fashion.[21,22]

17.2.1 Free Autografts

Use of autologous materials is the ideal choice for reconstruction; they are perfectly biocompatible, do not provoke any immune or inflammatory response, and integrate quickly. However, they often require additional incision(s) and approach(es), are associated with potential morbidities, and, in some cases, increase postoperative pain or discomfort.

Free autografting indicates the harvesting of tissue from an autologous donor site, thereafter transferred and implanted in a recipient site. Free tissue grafts do not have their own blood supply, they thus require a well-vascularized recipient bed to allow integration.

Free autografts most often used in neurosurgical reconstruction procedures include muscle fascia (i.e., fascia lata and/or temporalis fascia), the galea capitis and/or periosteal layers, cartilage/bone and fat.

The abdominal fat is usually harvested from the periumbilical or pelvic areas and can be useful alone or as adjunct to other materials to fill the surgical cavity, dead spaces, and/or any gap created by extensive bone removal (e.g., mastoidectomy, orbital roof removal, frontal sinus opening) (▶ Fig. 17.1, ▶ Fig. 17.2).

Free abdominal fat may also serve as a radiological spacer to enable contrast between the soft tissues used in reconstruction and the tumor bed postoperatively. This improves the ability of the radiation oncologist to target any residual tumor and to minimize collateral radiation injury to adjacent organs at risk.[21] In a recent study, fat graft showed signs of progressive reabsorption. The evolution of its magnetic resonance (MR) characteristics was found to be easily misdiagnosed as residual or recurrent tumor. Besides, fat evolves into a strong scar and generates fibrosis, eventually hindering the identification and dissection of neurovascular structures.[21] This fact should be taken into consideration when dealing with pathology that has the propensity to recur and may need (multiple) reoperation(s), in high-grade meningiomas for instance. Fascia lata is a valid and versatile graft for dural substitution, which was adopted for various reconstructive procedures, thanks to its resilience and resistance. Anatomically, the fascia lata is constituted by the deep fascia covering the thigh muscle, forming the outer limit of its fascial compartments. Usually, it is thickened at its most

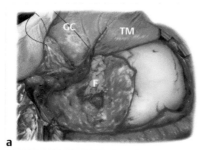
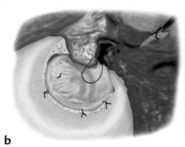

Fig. 17.1 Fat graft used to fill the osteodural gap and the mastoid cells after a combined petrosal approach. A temporal craniotomy and a mastoidectomy are previously performed. The temporalis muscle has been overturned and the galea capitis has been preserved during the approach. **(a)** Artistic drawing. **(b)** Intraoperative picture. F, fat; GC, galea capitis; TM, temporalis muscle.

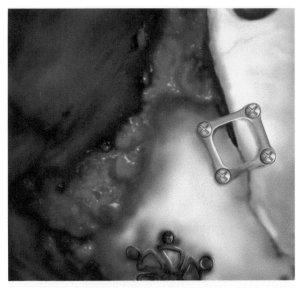

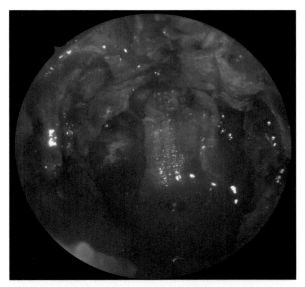

Fig. 17.2 Osteodural defect filled by the fat graft after the repositioning of the bone flap. The bone is fixed to the cranium by screw and miniplates.

Fig. 17.3 Middle turbinate mucoperichondrium covering the osteodural defect after endoscopic endonasal transsphenoidal approach.

lateral aspect, where it defines the iliotibial tract, a structure that runs to the tibia serving as site of muscle attachment. Care should be taken when harvesting the fascia lata as procedural errors can result in delayed donor site morbidity. Most commonly, injury to the lateral femoral cutaneous nerve can cause neuropathic pain or resection of an overly large portion of the fascia can cause muscle prolapse.[23]

For transcranial open approaches, temporalis fascia is a strong dural substitute comparable to the fascia lata. It is thicker and stronger than the pericranium. It can be harvested together with the fat located between the superficial and deep temporalis fascia. Care should be taken to preserve the frontalis branch of the facial nerve. The muscle fibers are preserved and the temporalis muscle innervation and vascularization is not impaired.

When an endoscopic endonasal approach has been performed, free autografts can be harvested from the structures encountered during nasal exposure. A bony-cartilaginous buttress can be created from the vomer and/or perpendicular plate of the ethmoid for instance. This solid barrier, used in conjunction with other materials, can be very useful in cases in which a wide craniectomy has been created or in patients with increased ICP (e.g., obese patients, suffering of sleep apnea) to prevent the occurrence of an encephalocele or meningocele. On the other side, it is worth remembering that bone autografts can undergo radiation necrosis and that they are not recommended when adjuvant radiotherapy is expected. Similarly, in cases where the middle turbinate has been removed to get more space inside one nostril, its mucoperichondrium can be used to cover the skull base defect (▶ Fig. 17.3).

17.2.2 Nonautologous Materials

The use of nonautologous materials, either heterologous or synthetic, for reconstruction of skull base defects is a viable alternative in cases when autologous grafts are either unavailable or not suitable for the defect. Moreover, they have the advantage of being readily available and avoid the donor site morbidity altogether. The ideal biomaterial should be safe in terms of infectious disease transmission, present a high biocompatibility, provide adequate bolstering, be malleable and easy to handle, in order to be molded into the specifically tailored shape. Moreover, nonautologous materials intended to be used as dural substitutes should be impermeable to ensure a watertight closure. Most contemporary grafts do not create severe adhesion with the surrounding tissues, which is helpful to maintain distinct anatomical planes.

Different materials, for example, collagen matrix, bovine and/or porcine pericardium, equine tendon, are currently available and widely adopted in reconstruction after skull base approaches. They can be used either as replacement for the dura or as supplemental layer over a primary closure of the dura mater.

In the vast majority of the procedures, the craniotomy flap can be positioned back in place to restore skull continuity and preserve from aesthetic deformities.[24,25,26,27,28] A variety of options are available for bone flap fixation, including nonabsorbable sutures, plates and screws, clamps, etc. (▶ Fig. 17.2). Low-profile plating systems are probably preferable in the frontal, pterional, or orbitozygomatic region. In some cases, when the tumor has invaded or eroded the bone or after some skull base approaches, an artificial material for cranial bone reconstruction is required.[29,30,31] There are many options for calvarial bone substitution, including titanium, polyetheretherketone (PEEK), hydroxyapatite, polymethyl methacrylate (PMMA).[32,33,34,35] With some materials, the implant can be molded during the surgery, while others are custom made before the surgery based on a volumetric computed tomography (CT) scan with 1- to 2-mm slices. To determine which implant is best suited, a variety of factors should be taken into account, including the size, location, and shape of the defect, as well as the indication and cost/availability of the cranioplasty implant.[29,36,37,38,39]

Titanium mesh is a great example of a readily available material that can be molded during the case to fit a variety of small-sized defects. In our practice (S.F.), it is often used to supplement the bone flap in the pterional region in order to avoid hollowing in the keyhole region and compensate for temporalis muscle atrophy. Other options include calcium pyrophosphate putty or PMMA cement to fill the craniotomy lines.

Implants that are prepared before the surgery can be made using different materials, most commonly titanium, PMMA, hydroxyapatite, or PEEK.[32,33] Titanium alloy cranioplasty is easy to prepare and put in place and its use can thus shorten the operative time.[27,33,38] On the other hand, it may be associated with a higher risk of postoperative infection and implant exposure. Moreover, it causes significant artefacts on MRI and CT scanner and should be avoided in tumor cases that need neuroimaging follow-up. Hydroxyapatite has high biocompatibility and a lower risk of infection. It also has osteoconductive properties that may accelerate integration.[40,41] Conversely, it is more expensive and intraoperative positioning is time consuming, as fine adjustments are usually required.[32]

17.2.3 Vascularized Flaps

Over the years, along with the development of different corridors to access multiple areas of the skull base, many local and regional vascularized flaps have also been described to improve the reconstruction phase of the surgical procedure. A thorough knowledge of the surgical anatomy of myofascial and/or mucosa layers with underlying feeding vessels is crucial in order to use these vascularized grafts optimally. More recently, the use of pedicled or free flap for covering osteodural defects has been found effective in reducing the rate of postoperative CSF leakage in endoscopic endonasal surgery.[21] Indeed, intranasal vascularized flaps include posterior pedicled nasoseptal flap, reverse flap, inferior turbinate flap, middle turbinate flap, anteriorly based lateral nasal wall flap, and posteriorly based lateral nasal wall flap. The most popular and widely used is the nasoseptal flap (NSF) (Hadad–Bassagasteguy flap); its main features are a consistent vascular supply, based on a fairly long and robust pedicle made of the branches of the sphenopalatine artery, the ease of harvest, and the possibility of tailoring the mucosa surface according to the size of the defect.[42,43]

Several other flaps have been described usually to increase the surface of the graft or to replace the NSF if it has been compromised. Among these, there is the rescue flap, a modification of the original posterior pedicle NSF,[44] the inferior turbinate flap,[45,46] the vascularized middle turbinate flap,[47,48,49] etc.

On the other side, vascularized flaps which can be used to cover defect in transcranial surgery include transfrontal pericranial flap, transpterygoid temporoparietal fascia flap, occipital galeopericranial flap, facial artery myomucosal (or mucosal) flap, along with tailored galea sheet harvested from the proximity of the approach. In multioperated cases in which an endonasal mucosal flap is no longer available, regional vascularized flaps have been developed (pericranial flap, palatal flap, and temporoparietal fascia flap) and can have good results even in complex reconstruction scenarios (active infection, CSF fistula, postradiation, etc.).

The transfrontal pericranial flap is a regional pedicled flap that can cover defects from the frontal sinus to the sella and from one orbit to the other. It is extremely useful for large anterior skull base defects.[50] This area of pericranium has strong neurovascular supply by both the supraorbital and supratrochlear bundles.

The temporoparietal fascia flap also relies on very consistent vascular support, the anterior branch of the superficial temporal artery. It can be extended to provide a very large coverage surface. It is constituted of a strong fascial layer connecting the overlying fibrous septae of the subcutaneous tissue at the temporoparietal region of the skull.[51]

17.3 Current Reconstruction Techniques

17.3.1 Transcranial Approaches

After tumor removal and meticulous hemostasis have been completed, the repair can be initiated. Reconstruction aims at covering exposed dura, preventing CSF leakage and brain herniation, and replacing surgical dead space with healthy, vascularized tissue. Careful and watertight closure of the dura should be the goal. It is worth reminding that throughout the initial exposure, pericranial, galeal, and/or muscular layers have to be identified, protected, and mobilized as they often are the most adequate tissues for reconstruction. According to the surgical route used, proper maneuvers can facilitate harvesting of these tissues at the end of the case. It is important to ensure their viability all along the procedure by avoiding desiccation and excessive traction. Similarly, carefully positioned osteotomies and bone resection can make closure easier (i.e., placement of flap). Hereafter, we will present specific considerations in reconstruction after most frequently used approaches to different skull base areas.

Anterior Skull Base Reconstruction

Reconstruction starts with careful duraplasty. Small dural defects are sutured, whereas larger defects resulting from intradural tumor involvement are patched either with pericranium and/or temporal fascia. Watertight closure is mandatory and the best primary protection against CSF leak. Lyophilized homograft dura or bovine pericardium layer can also be used to repair larger defects, but pericranium harvested locally over and around the bone flap is a very efficient closure material. The use of thin 5–0 sutures reduce the risk of leakage around the hole needle. Whether suturing is complete or not, the dural closure can by supplemented by fibrin glue on certain occasions (open ventricle, opened frontal sinuses, etc.). After resection of anterior cranial base meningiomas invading the cribriform plate, the floor of anterior fossa also needs to be reconstructed. In these cases, a flap of pericranium, pedicled on the supraorbital and supratrochlear arteries, can be wedged between the cranial floor bone and the overlying dura and secured with sutures through the bone or anchored with fibrin glue.

If the frontal, ethmoid, or sphenoid sinuses are opened during the approach or removed because of involvement with disease, communication between the paranasal sinuses and intradural space must absolutely be prevented. To do so, two main strategies have been employed: sinus "cranialization" and sinus exclusion with maintenance of adequate drainage. The main concern and the objective of both techniques are the occurrence of delayed mucocele, which happens when mucosa is isolated from its drainage path. When doing sinus cranialization, the sinus mucosa must be carefully and totally resected. Drilling of the inner surface of the bony structure of the sinus should be done with a diamond burr to make sure that all the mucosa has been resected. When the sinus has been breached during craniotomy, the mucosa in the bone flap should not be forgotten. The nasofrontal canal mucosa is the infolded and pushed toward the nasal cavity without disrupting it. A piece of temporalis muscle or fascia can be added to secure the occlusion of the nasofrontal pathway. The sinus is then packed with fat and fibrin glue and the pericranial flap is turned over the frontal sinus and extended over any defect in the floor of the anterior fossa. When the sinus is excluded, the drainage path of the sinus must first be explored to ensure that it is free from obstruction. Its

mucosa is then carefully dissected and its edges are then either sutured together or coagulated to create infolding of the mucosa. Additionally, a thin layer of bone wax can then be used to isolate the sinus, but packing of the sinus should be avoided. Whenever applicable, the area of mucosa that is on the side of the bone flap should be removed when the sinus is excluded. Ideally, this should be done during the opening and before durotomy to reduce the risk of intracranial infection.

After dural closure, the bone flap is placed back into its position, usually with low-profile plates. The burr holes should be covered, either with titanium burr hole covers or with commercially available plugs. In the frontal area, craniotomy lines can sometimes be seen under the skin, which is obviously displeasing aesthetically. This phenomenon occurs when adhesions develop between the galea capitis and the dura and retraction ensures. Careful positioning of the bone flap and the use of cement, calcium pyrophosphate, or any other nonabsorbable filling agent is thus encouraged. When removal of the orbital wall and roof was necessary to manage tumor, it can be reconstructed with lyophilized cartilage grafts, collagen sponges, or equine tendon graft (*Tachosil*) (▶ Fig. 17.4). However, in spheno-orbital meningiomas, even when there is extensive exposure of the periorbital after resection of the tumor, when the periorbital is intact, we have not found that patient complain of pulsatile exophthalmos. When the periorbital is opened or disrupted, its reconstruction is mandatory, with the use of thin sutures (6–0) that progressively reapproximate the margins, combined with a layer of equine tendon graft (*Tachosil*).

Pedicled flaps other than the pericranium and free vascularized flaps are usually unnecessary in the reconstruction unless there has been prior radiation therapy and residual tissues have poor vascularity. Moreover, they may preclude detection of early tumor recurrence.

Middle Fossa Reconstruction

Again, a successful reconstruction is based on adequate tumor removal and safe and precise hemostasis. Primary duraplasty is preferred, although it is not always possible in this area, especially in cases of anterior transpetrosal or cavernous sinus surgery. After an anterior transpetrosal, the dura is first reapproximated with sutures and an onlay of pericranium of temporalis fascia is positioned

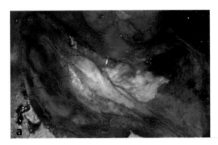
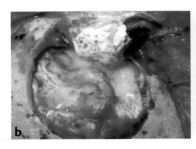

Fig. 17.4 Anterior skull base reconstruction after a cranio-orbital approach. (a) Collagen sponge as a sustainer of the skull base defect. The periorbital fat is visible after the drilling of orbital rim and roof and the opening of the periorbita. **(b)** Collagen sponge is covering the periorbital fat, while fibrin glue is injected on the dura matter.

over the defect and sutured in place. The space left by the bone removal is then filled with fat and fibrin glue. CSF leaks are quite rare after a *Kawase* approach since the temporal lobe falls back into position and helps in completing the reconstruction. When a CSF leak occurs, it is usually because an air cell in the middle fossa was not adequately close. These can be identified on the preoperative CT scans (dehiscent middle ear, zygomatic air cell, large pneumatized mastoid, etc.) and should be carefully closed. Our technique is to first cover the air cell with a thin layer of bone wax, which is then covered by a layer of fascia and fibrin glue.

In some cases, when a defect of the cranial base has created a communication with the infratemporal or sphenopalatine fossae, especially when the sphenoid or maxillary sinuses are breaches, adequate reconstruction must be accomplished. A layer of fascia lata or another dural substitute can be slid along the floor in between dural and the bone and/or, eventually, a pedicled flap of temporalis muscle can be placed when fat is deemed inadequate (sinus opening) (▶ Fig. 17.1). When the breach in a sinus is small, a small piece of muscle can be wedge in the opening. This maneuver, nicknamed the "yo-yo" technique, has been described in cases of opening of a pneumatized optic strut in anterior clinoidectomy.[52] In case of extensive skull base removal, free tissue transfer is preferred. Free rectus abdominis or myocutaneous flaps provide reliable one-stage reconstruction of complex temporal bone defects.

Finally, the bone flap, including eventually orbital rim, is reattached to the cranial vault with plates and screws, and the temporalis muscle is returned to its anatomical position and secured at the bone along the superior temporal line (even if partially used for reconstruction of the floor of the middle fossa) (▶ Fig. 17.2). This can be done either with the use of a muscle cuff or with direct suspension to the bone with sutures or screws.[53,54]

Posterior Skull Base Reconstruction

The dura of the posterior fossa frequently shrinks during surgery and the risk of CSF leak being greater in this location, a dural graft is often necessary to achieve a watertight closure. When the mastoid air cells have been opened, for a retrosigmoid craniotomy for example, reconstruction proceeds in a similar way to the middle fossa, with first a thin layer of bone that does not fill the air cell, followed by a layer of fascia and fibrin glue. In the cerebellopontine angle, after opening of the internal auditory canal, a piece of muscle or fascia and fibrin glue help prevent postoperative CSF leak through the middle ear.

Concerning the bone, whether an occipital craniotomy and/or craniectomy has been made, the flap is repositioned and/or eventually replaced with synthetic compound, molded according to the size and shape of the defect. The splenius capitis, the longus capitis, and the sternocleidomastoid muscles are sutured back in their original position.

After mastoidectomy, the mastoid antrum is first closed with a thin layer of bone wax and then covered with fascia and fibrin glue. The empty space created by the drilling is then filled with autologous fat and fibrin glue. In some cases, a vascularized flap made by either temporalis muscle of parietal pericranium can be used to cover the dura in cases where healing is expected to be inadequate. When exposed, the petrous segment of the internal carotid artery (ICA) should be covered, either with free fat graft of a vascularized flap in order to avoid infection and damage if the patient undergoes postoperative radiation therapy.

17.3.2 Endoscopic Endonasal Approaches

With modern endoscopic techniques and instrumentation, the reach of the endonasal route has expanded to cover all the craniocaudal axis of ventral skull base. A number of lesions, among them carefully selected cases of anterior skull base and posterior fossa meningiomas, can be treated through this corridor.

Meningiomas and other skull base lesions' removal via the endonasal corridor requires a wide osteodural breach, with some case dural resection that extends beyond the craniectomy edges, extensive opening of arachnoid cisterns, and/or sometimes of the third ventricle; a large communication between a sterile intradural compartment, and a septic cavity, that is, the sinonasal compartment is created.

An effectively watertight closure is mandatory to restore the natural intra- and extradural compartments and to prevent postoperative CSF leakage. Failure to create adequate reconstruction may lead to severe complications, such as meningitis, brain herniation, and tension pneumocephalus.[18]

After lesion removal, the reconstruction has to be tailored to the location and size of the defect, and also to the extent of the CSF pathways opening. This can be assessed with Kelly's scale, acting as for grade 3 leakage.[55] A thin layer of fat and fibrin glue (Tisseel, Baxter, Vienna, Austria) is first positioned intradurally. The osteodural defect is then closed, often by means of the so-called "gasket seal" or "grandma's cap" technique. In these techniques, a layer of dural substitute is positioned in the extradural space[56,57] with a tailored foil of resorbable semisolid material overlapped in order to fix the first one in the extradural space. A vascularized Hadad pedicled flap[42,43] and, eventually, a free mucoperichondrium flap can be used to cover the compound along with fibrin glue and oxidized cellulose to hold the material in place.

Nowadays, at the Division of Neurosurgery of the Università degli Studi di Napoli Federico II, the most reliable technique to achieve an adequate reconstruction of the osteodural skull base defect after an extended endoscopic endonasal approach was found to be the so-called "sandwich technique."

The surgical cavity is filled with a fat graft sutured with 6.0 prolene to the inner sheet of a three-layer foil of fascia lata or dural substitute, whose two most inner layers are positioned intradurally, while the outer in the extradural space. The "sandwich" is realized outside the nasal cavity and is then inserted through it. We have developed this technique based on our long-lasting experience of about 30 years with endoscopic endonasal surgeries, both on standard and extended cases[57] (▶ Fig. 17.5, ▶ Fig. 17.6).

A NSF-vascularized flap is used to cover the posterior wall of the sphenoid sinus and then sphenoid sinus is filled with fibrin glue and oxidized cellulose to flatten the mucosa of the flap over the bony surface to favor the rooting (▶ Fig. 17.7). Intensive and watchful postoperative care is mandatory for a proper healing process to take place. CT scan is performed routinely at POD#1 in order to evaluate any neurosurgical complication and/or the amount of pneumocephalus.

The patient should adopt adequate postoperative habits in order to prevent any ICP increase and displacement of the reconstruction. We advise our patient to resume ambulation as early as possible, to avoid bending over or squatting, to avoid sneezing and blowing their nose, and to take stool softeners. Lumbar drainage is not used anymore.

The principles of reconstruction after endonasal endoscopic approach (EEA) may be summarized as follows: (1) Attain a watertight closure that separates the intracranial

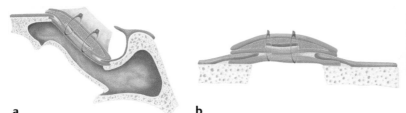

a   b

Fig. 17.5 Artistic drawing of the repair of osteodural defect through "sandwich technique" after an endoscopic endonasal extended approach. **(a)** Sagittal view. **(b)** Coronal view.

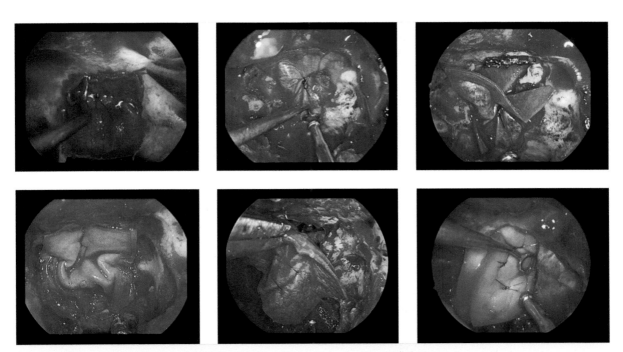

Fig. 17.6 Intraoperative endoscopic phases of skull base reconstruction using "sandwich technique."

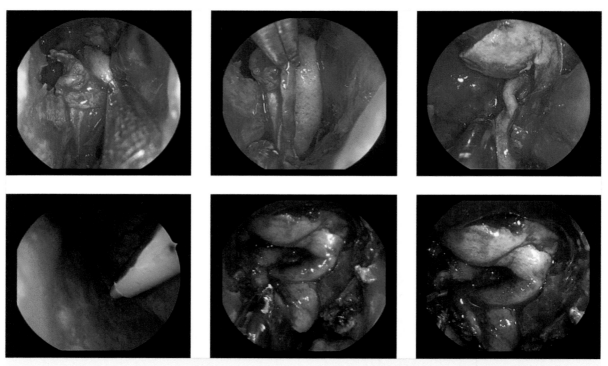

Fig. 17.7 Intraoperative endoscopic phases of preparing and positioning of a pedicle nasoseptal flap to enforce the skull base reconstruction.

space and the sinonasal compartment, thus avoiding infections, prevent airflow into the intracranial space (pneumocephalus); (2) provide adequate strength to support the intracranial contents, thereby preventing brain herniation into the surgical defect; and, finally (3) maintain a functional sinonasal system and respect cosmesis.

17.4 Discussion and Conclusions

Multilayer reconstruction supported in select cases by vascularized mucosal or myofascial flaps offer the most reliable reconstruction of large skull base defects. This ensures the successful isolation of the intracranial space from the external environment, thus preventing complications such as meningitis, intracranial abscesses, encephaloceles, CSF leaks, and tension pneumocephalus. The use of free or pedicled flaps can be useful on some occasions. They are particularly helpful especially when dealing with high-flow CSF leaks, in case of large skull base defects, and/or in patients that will receive radiation therapy (i.e., poor vascularization of the recipient site).

It is mandatory to define and preserve the tissues to be used at the end, during the opening phase of the surgical procedure. Another important aspect is that to achieve a good osteodural reconstruction, the dural and bony planes have to be preserved at least in part.

References

[1] Al-Nashar IS, Carrau RL, Herrera A, Snyderman CH. Endoscopic transnasal transpterygopalatine fossa approach to the lateral recess of the sphenoid sinus. Laryngoscope. 2004; 114(3):528–532

[2] Fahlbusch R, Schott W. Pterional surgery of meningiomas of the tuberculum sellae and planum sphenoidale: surgical results with special consideration of ophthalmological and endocrinological outcomes. J Neurosurg. 2002; 96(2):235–243

[3] Magro F, Solari D, Cavallo LM, et al. The endoscopic endonasal approach to the lateral recess of the sphenoid sinus via the pterygopalatine fossa: comparison of endoscopic and radiological landmarks. Neurosurgery. 2006; 59(4) suppl 2:ONS237–ONS242, discussion ONS242–ONS243

[4] Parkinson D. Extradural neural axis compartment. J Neurosurg. 2000; 92(4):585–588

[5] Prevedello DM, Kassam AB, Snyderman C, et al. Endoscopic cranial base surgery: ready for prime time? Clin Neurosurg. 2007; 54:48–57

[6] Solari D, Magro F, Cappabianca P, et al. Anatomical study of the pterygopalatine fossa using an endoscopic endonasal approach: spatial relations and distances between surgical landmarks. J Neurosurg. 2007; 106(1):157–163

[7] Tschabitscher M, Galzio RJ. Endoscopic anatomy along the transnasal approach to the pituitary gland and the surrounding structures. In: de Divitiis E, Cappabianca P, eds. Endoscopic Endonasal Transsphenoidal Surgery. Vienna, New York: Springer-Verlag; 2003:21–39

[8] Wen HT, Rhoton AL, Jr, Katsuta T, de Oliveira E. Microsurgical anatomy of the transcondylar, supracondylar, and paracondylar extensions of the far-lateral approach. J Neurosurg. 1997; 87(4): 555–585

[9] Javed T, Sekhar LN. Surgical management of clival meningiomas. Acta Neurochir Suppl (Wien). 1991; 53:171–182

[10] Kawase T, Shiobara R, Toya S. Anterior transpetrosal-transtentorial approach for sphenopetroclival meningiomas: surgical method and results in 10 patients. Neurosurgery. 1991; 28(6):869–875, discussion 875–876

[11] Lang DA, Neil-Dwyer G, Iannotti F. The suboccipital transcondylar approach to the clivus and cranio-cervical junction for ventrally placed pathology at and above the foramen magnum. Acta Neurochir (Wien). 1993; 125(1–4):132–137

[12] MacDonald JD, Antonelli P, Day AL. The anterior subtemporal, medial transpetrosal approach to the upper basilar artery and ponto-mesencephalic junction. Neurosurgery. 1998; 43(1):84–89

[13] Miller E, Crockard HA. Transoral transclival removal of anteriorly placed meningiomas at the foramen magnum. Neurosurgery. 1987; 20(6):966–968

[14] Nakamura M, Samii M. Surgical management of a meningioma in the retrosellar region. Acta Neurochir (Wien). 2003; 145(3):215–219, discussion 219–220

[15] Reisch R, Bettag M, Perneczky A. Transoral transclival removal of anteriorly placed cavernous malformations of the brainstem. Surg Neurol. 2001; 56(2):106–115, discussion 115–116

[16] Seifert V, Raabe A, Zimmermann M. Conservative (labyrinth-preserving) transpetrosal approach to the clivus and petroclival region–indications, complications, results and lessons learned. Acta Neurochir (Wien). 2003; 145(8):631–642, discussion 642

[17] Sepehrnia A, Knopp U. The combined subtemporal-suboccipital approach: a modified surgical access to the clivus and petrous apex. Minim Invasive Neurosurg. 2002; 45(2):102–104

[18] Cappabianca P, Solari D. Skull base osteo-dural repair: the Achilles' heel of the extended transsphenoidal skull base approaches. World Neurosurg. 2010; 73(6):627–629

[19] Hachem RA, Elkhatib A, Beer-Furlan A, Prevedello D, Carrau R. Reconstructive techniques in skull base surgery after resection of malignant lesions: a wide array of choices. Curr Opin Otolaryngol Head Neck Surg. 2016; 24(2):91–97

[20] Thorp BD, Sreenath SB, Ebert CS, Zanation AM. Endoscopic skull base reconstruction: a review and clinical case series of 152 vascularized flaps used for surgical skull base defects in the setting of intraoperative cerebrospinal fluid leak. Neurosurg Focus. 2014; 37(4):E4

[21] Campbell RG, Patwa H, Tang IP, Otto BA, Prevedello DM, Carrau RL. Cranial base reconstruction after transcranial and transnasal skull base surgery for median lesions. In: Cappabianca P, Cavallo LM, de Divitiis O, Esposito F, eds. Midline Skull Base Surgery. Switzerland: Springer International Publishing; 2016:333–336

[22] Reyes C, Mason E, Solares CA. Panorama of reconstruction of skull base defects: from traditional open to endonasal endoscopic approaches, from free grafts to microvascular flaps. Int Arch Otorhinolaryngol. 2014; 18 suppl 2:S179–S186

[23] Amit M, Margalit N, Abergel A, Gil Z. Fascia lata for endoscopic reconstruction of high-flow leaks: the champagne cork technique. Otolaryngol Head Neck Surg. 2013; 148(4):697–700

[24] Afifi A, Djohan RS, Hammert W, Papay FA, Barnett AE, Zins JE. Lessons learned reconstructing complex scalp defects using free flaps and a cranioplasty in one stage. J Craniofac Surg. 2010; 21(4):1205–1209

[25] Baumeister S, Peek A, Friedman A, Levin LS, Marcus JR. Management of postneurosurgical bone flap loss caused by infection. Plast Reconstr Surg. 2008; 122(6):e195–e-2-08

[26] Shonka DC, Jr, Potash AE, Jameson MJ, Funk GF. Successful reconstruction of scalp and skull defects: lessons learned from a large series. Laryngoscope. 2011; 121(11):2305–2312

[27] Yano T, Okazaki M, Tanaka K, Iida H. The flap sandwich technique for a safe and aesthetic skull base reconstruction. Ann Plast Surg. 2016; 76(2):193–197

[28] Yano T, Tanaka K, Kishimoto S, Iida H, Okazaki M. Review of skull base reconstruction using locoregional flaps and free flaps in children and adolescents. Skull Base. 2011; 21(6):359–364

[29] Archavlis E, Carvi Y Nievas M. The impact of timing of cranioplasty in patients with large cranial defects after decompressive hemicraniectomy. Acta Neurochir (Wien). 2012; 154(6):1055–1062

[30] Bender A, Heulin S, Röhrer S, et al. Early cranioplasty may improve outcome in neurological patients with decompressive craniectomy. Brain Inj. 2013; 27(9):1073–1079

[31] Chang V, Hartzfeld P, Langlois M, Mahmood A, Seyfried D. Outcomes of cranial repair after craniectomy. J Neurosurg. 2010; 112(5):1120–1124

[32] Lindner D, Schlothofer-Schumann K, Kern BC, Marx O, Müns A, Meixensberger J. Cranioplasty using custom-made hydroxyapatite versus titanium: a randomized clinical trial. J Neurosurg. 2017; 126(1):175–183

[33] Wiggins A, Austerberry R, Morrison D, Ho KM, Honeybul S. Cranioplasty with custom-made titanium plates—14 years experience. Neurosurgery. 2013; 72(2):248–256, discussion 256

[34] Ridwan-Pramana A, Marcián P, Borák L, Narra N, Forouzanfar T, Wolff J. Finite element analysis of 6 large PMMA skull reconstructions: a multi-criteria evaluation approach. PLoS One. 2017; 12(6):e0179325

[35] Jaberi J, Gambrell K, Tiwana P, Madden C, Finn R. Long-term clinical outcome analysis of poly-methyl-methacrylate cranioplasty for large skull defects. J Oral Maxillofac Surg. 2013; 71(2):e81–e88

[36] Huang YH, Lee TC, Yang KY, Liao CC. Is timing of cranioplasty following posttraumatic craniectomy related to neurological outcome? Int J Surg. 2013; 11(9):886–890

[37] Zanaty M, Chalouhi N, Starke RM, et al. Complications following cranioplasty: incidence and predictors in 348 cases. J Neurosurg. 2015; 123(1):182–188

[38] Yano T, Okazaki M, Tanaka K, et al. A new concept for classifying skull base defects for reconstructive surgery. J Neurol Surg B Skull Base. 2012; 73(2):125–131

[39] Archer JB, Sun H, Bonney PA, et al. Extensive traumatic anterior skull base fractures with cerebrospinal fluid leak: classification and repair techniques using combined vascularized tissue flaps. J Neurosurg. 2016; 124(3):647–656

[40] Piitulainen JM, Kauko T, Aitasalo KM, Vuorinen V, Vallittu PK, Posti JP. Outcomes of cranioplasty with synthetic materials and autologous bone grafts. World Neurosurg. 2015; 83(5):708–714

[41] Staffa G, Barbanera A, Faiola A, et al. Custom made bioceramic implants in complex and large cranial reconstruction: a two-year follow-up. J Craniomaxillofac Surg. 2012; 40(3):e65–e70

[42] Hadad G, Bassagasteguy L, Carrau RL, et al. A novel reconstructive technique after endoscopic expanded endonasal approaches: vascular pedicle nasoseptal flap. Laryngoscope. 2006; 116(10):1882–1886

[43] Kassam AB, Thomas A, Carrau RL, et al. Endoscopic reconstruction of the cranial base using a pedicled nasoseptal flap. Neurosurgery. 2008; 63 suppl 1:ONS44–ONS52, discussion ONS52–ONS53

[44] Rivera-Serrano CM, Snyderman CH, Gardner P, et al. Nasoseptal "rescue" flap: a novel modification of the nasoseptal flap technique for pituitary surgery. Laryngoscope. 2011; 121(5):990–993

[45] Harvey RJ, Sheahan PO, Schlosser RJ. Inferior turbinate pedicle flap for endoscopic skull base defect repair. Am J Rhinol Allergy. 2009; 23(5):522–526

[46] Yip J, Macdonald KI, Lee J, et al. The inferior turbinate flap in skull base reconstruction. J Otolaryngol Head Neck Surg. 2013; 42:6

[47] Prevedello DM, Barges-Coll J, Fernandez-Miranda JC, et al. Middle turbinate flap for skull base reconstruction: cadaveric feasibility study. Laryngoscope. 2009; 119(11):2094–2098

[48] Simal Julián JA, Miranda Lloret P, Cárdenas Ruiz-Valdepeñas E, Barges Coll J, Beltrán Giner A, Botella Asunción C. Middle turbinate vascularized flap for skull base reconstruction after an expanded endonasal approach. Acta Neurochir (Wien). 2011; 153(9):1827–1832

[49] Wang X, Zhang X, Hu F, et al. Middle turbinate mucosal flap in endoscopic skull base reconstruction. Turk Neurosurg. 2016; 26(2):200–204

[50] Patel MR, Shah RN, Snyderman CH, et al. Pericranial flap for endoscopic anterior skull-base reconstruction: clinical outcomes and radioanatomic analysis of preoperative planning. Neurosurgery. 2010; 66(3):506–512, discussion 512

[51] Fortes FS, Carrau RL, Snyderman CH, et al. Transpterygoid transposition of a temporoparietal fascia flap: a new method for skull base reconstruction after endoscopic expanded endonasal approaches. Laryngoscope. 2007; 117(6):970–976

[52] Chi JH, Sughrue M, Kunwar S, Lawton MT. The "yo-yo" technique to prevent cerebrospinal fluid rhinorrhea after anterior clinoidectomy for proximal internal carotid artery aneurysms. Neurosurgery. 2006; 59 suppl 1:ONS101–ONS107, discussion ONS101–ONS107

[53] Arnaout O, Al-Mefty O. Combined petrosal approach for petroclival meningioma. Neurosurg Focus. 2017; 43 VideoSuppl2:V6

[54] Abolfotoh M, Dunn IF, Al-Mefty O. Transmastoid retrosigmoid approach to the cerebellopontine angle: surgical technique. Neurosurgery. 2013; 73(1) suppl Operative:ons16–ons23, discussion ons23

[55] Esposito F, Dusick JR, Fatemi N, Kelly DF. Graded repair of cranial base defects and cerebrospinal fluid leaks in transsphenoidal surgery. Neurosurgery. 2007; 60(4) suppl 2:295–303, discussion 303–304

[56] Leng LZ, Brown S, Anand VK, Schwartz TH. "Gasket-seal" watertight closure in minimal-access endoscopic cranial base surgery. Neurosurgery. 2008; 62(5) suppl 2:E342–E343, discussion E343

[57] Cavallo LM, Messina A, Esposito F, et al. Skull base reconstruction in the extended endoscopic transsphenoidal approach for suprasellar lesions. J Neurosurg. 2007; 107(4):713–720

18 Management of Recurrent Skull Base Meningiomas

Sheri K. Palejwala, Garni Barkhoudarian, Walavan Sivakumar, Daniel F. Kelly

Abstract

Skull base meningiomas, due to their frequent investment or encasement of critical neurovascular structures, are challenging to resect in their entirety, both with initial resection and reresection. Up to one-third of such meningiomas will recur or progress after initial surgery. Given their complex and varied spectrum of location and growth pattern, such meningiomas pose a significant management challenge. They are typically best treated with judicious use of maximal surgical reresection, and/or stereotactic radiotherapy (SRT) or radiosurgery (SRS), with the aim of reversing neurological deficits and slowing or stopping tumor progression. While complete surgical excision remains the strongest prognosticator for recurrence free-survival, independent of the frequency of recurrence, SRT and SRS remain key treatment options for many recurrent meningiomas. Depending upon the tumor location, focused radiation with SRS or SRT has shown comparable outcomes to surgery when used alone, and with good tumor control rates when used as an adjuvant, with both subtotal and complete resection, as well as with some high-grade (atypical) and multiply recurrent tumors. Beyond repeat surgery and radiation, multiple chemotherapeutic and hormonal therapies have been trialed, and some demonstrate limited efficacy, but without evidence of lasting regression or remission. Ultimately, recurrent or progressive meningiomas of the skull base are best managed with a team approach that offers multimodality therapies including a combination of traditional and endoscopic keyhole surgical approaches for maximal safe resection, focused radiation treatments with SRS and SRT, and a continued search for effective targeted medical therapies based on tumor genetics and biomarkers.

Keywords: anaplastic, atypical, chemotherapy, endoscopic surgery, meningioma, microsurgery, minimally-invasive, radiosurgery, recurrence, skull base

18.1 Introduction

Meningiomas account for over one-third of all brain tumors, making them the most common primary brain tumor in the United States, with a lifetime risk of approximately 1%. According to the 2016 World Health Organization (WHO) Classification guidelines, roughly 70 to 80% of all meningiomas are WHO grade I, while 20 to 25% are WHO grade II and 1 to 6% WHO grade III. Incidence of meningioma increases steadily with age, with a median presentation age of 65 years, and a 2 to 3-fold increased likelihood in females.[1] Given the overall prevalence of meningiomas, and that up to 30% may be higher grade, the lifetime risk of recurrence after initial treatment is significant. For purposes of this chapter, skull base meningiomas include those of the sella and parasellar spaces, olfactory groove, tuberculum, sphenoid, petrous ridge, and the foramen magnum. Skull base meningiomas are more likely to recur than other subtypes, and their relationship to critical neurovascular structures makes their management more challenging.

18.2 Recurrence

Up to 20% of benign meningiomas and 70% of atypical meningiomas that were initially treated with gross total surgical resection recur.[1,2] Recurrence depends on several variables especially the extent of initial resection, intracranial tumor location, initial tumor histopathology and molecular genetics, the use of upfront adjuvant therapy (before recurrence or treatment failure), and the unique situations of meningiomas associated with radiation or genetic syndromes. Skull base meningiomas, which make up approximately 20 to 30% of meningiomas, are particularly prone to progression and recurrence given that these tumors are invested in and around the critical neurovascular structures of the cranial base making complete resection less feasible.[3]

18.2.1 Presentation

Most recurrent skull base meningiomas are diagnosed with follow-up magnetic resonance imaging (MRI) or computed tomography (CT), as long-term follow-up with serial imaging for distant recurrence surveillance has become common practice.[1,4] In contrast, some patients may present with focal deficit due to compression of neurovascular structures, especially when located along the skull base or causing parenchymal mass effect. This presentation is more likely when the tumor is rapidly growing, such that the surrounding structures do not have adequate time to compensate for the relatively brisk growth rate.

18.2.2 Extent of Resection

Since initially described by Simpson in 1957, extent of resection has been held as the most important indicator of meningioma recurrence, and duration of recurrence-free survival (▶ Table 18.1). The greatest likelihood of recurrence prevention is an initial complete or Simpson grade I–II resection.[5,6,7] However, grade I resection is often not possible to achieve for skull base meningiomas, given the involvement of critical neurovascular structures.

Nevertheless, even achieving grade II or III resection is associated with decreased rates of recurrence and increased rates of recurrence-free survival.[6,7,8] Hence, the likelihood of obtaining a complete, and potentially curative resection is more likely on initial resection than in the setting of recurrence, but should remain the goal of surgical resection if possible, even with multiple recurrences. However, in many recurrent skull base meningiomas, curative resection is not a reasonable goal and instead bony decompression and safe but effective debulking with adjuvant radiotherapy or radiosurgery offer the best treatment options.[9,10,11,12]

18.2.3 Location

Intracranial meningiomas are often divided into skull base lesions and those located along the cranial convexities. Skull base meningiomas are more likely to recur than convexity meningiomas, irrespective of tumor grade, as most atypical and anaplastic meningiomas occur along the cranial convexity. The higher rate of recurrence in cranial base meningiomas is attributable primarily to the challenges of resection in proximity to critical neurovascular structures.[5,6,13] Parasagittal meningiomas, however, should be considered separately than their convexity counterparts, as involvement or frank invasion of the superior sagittal sinus poses similar surgical constraints as those presented by the cranial nerves. This is especially true of falcine and parafalcine meningiomas adjacent to sensorimotor cortex.[1,5] In these cases, complete surgical resection can be unduly morbid, especially in the setting of an otherwise benign disease

process, and Simpson I resection is, by definition, impossible without significant and unwarranted morbidity and even mortality. As a result, skull base and parasagittal meningiomas are associated with significantly higher rates of tumor regrowth, recurrence, and decreased overall survival.[1,2,5,6,13]

18.2.4 Histopathology

The WHO recognizes 15 subtypes of meningiomas and divides them into three cohorts: WHO grade I, WHO grade II (atypical), and WHO grade III (anaplastic) meningiomas, with increasing rates of recurrence and invasion.[1] As a result of the 2016 grading criteria, the subset of atypical, WHO grade II, meningiomas has grown from 6 to 10% of all meningiomas, to 20 to 25%, while the outcomes of WHO grade I meningiomas are improved and more reflective of a benign disease process.[1,6] Tumor histology plays a significant role in the likelihood of tumor recurrence. Although WHO grade III tumors are far less common, they are much more likely to recur in short interval, than their more benign counterparts. When they do occur, they are more aggressive and locally invasive, and in late stages, even present with extracranial metastases. ▶ Table 18.2 outlines an overview of meningioma incidence, survival, and recurrence, stratified by WHO grades. Based on several large studies, skull base meningiomas in general do not appear to have a higher proportion of grade II or III meningiomas relative to other locations.[1,13,14]

Hormone Receptor Status

Estrogen receptors, though seldom expressed in meningiomas, are more likely to be present with WHO grade I meningiomas. Progesterone receptor presence is strongly correlated with grade I meningiomas, and are nearly absent in atypical meningiomas. Progesterone receptor presence, however, has not been shown to be an independent predictor of a more favorable outcome.[1] Some studies have shown a greater Ki-67 in progesterone receptor-negative meningiomas, however, this cannot be used to imply a causative relationship between receptor status and tumor aggression, as receptor status is correlative with a number of confounding variables, the most significant of which is histologic grade.[15]

Table 18.1 Simpson grading of meningioma extent of resection[7]

Simpson grade	Extent of resection
I	Complete macroscopic tumor resection, surrounding bone and dura
II	Complete macroscopic tumor resection, with excision of involved dura, not bone
III	Complete macroscopic tumor resection, without bone or dura resection
IV	Subtotal resection with macroscopic residual
V	Biopsy alone

Table 18.2 Meningioma incidence, progression-free and overall survival, and recurrence rate based on World Health Organization grade

WHO grade	Incidence (%)	Progression-free survival (%)		Overall survival (%)		Recurrence rate* (%)
		5-year	10-year	5-year	10-year	
I	70–80	97.5	87.5	92	81	7–25
II	20–25	48.4	22.6	78.4	53.3	<70
III	1–6	8.4	0	44.0	14.2	50–94

*After gross total resection (Simpson grade I–II).

18.2.5 Radiation-induced Meningiomas

Radiation is the only known environmental risk factor for meningioma formation, and meningiomas are the most common cerebral neoplasms caused by radiation.[1,16] Radiation-induced meningiomas are roughly six times more likely to demonstrate multiplicity, occurring in 5 to 19% of cases. Also, radiation-induced meningiomas are much more likely to be atypical or anaplastic, with a high incidence of nuclear atypia, pleomorphism, cellularity, necrosis, local invasion, and mitoses.[16,17] As expected from these higher-grade tumors, recurrence rates are significantly higher with radiation-induced meningiomas at 25.6% as opposed to 11.4% in sporadic meningiomas, when looking across all subtypes, WHO grades, and variable degrees of resection. Multiple recurrences also occurred in 11.6% of all treated radiation-induced menigniomas.[16,17,18]

The treatment of choice for radiation-induced meningiomas is no different than for their genetic or sporadic counterparts, complete surgical resection. However, due to their local invasiveness and multiplicity, this presents additional challenges. When considering surgical resection, it is important to consider not only prior exposures as well as the devascularized, radiated scalp and soft tissue.[16] In these situations, minimally invasive and endoscopic-assisted techniques could play an essential role in minimizing the surgical impact, optimizing wound healing and expediting recovery. Given that radiation-induced meningiomas are more likely to be higher grade and locally invasive, more aggressive surgical excision with wide dural and bony margins is recommended when possible. Expectedly, skull base and parafalcine radiation-induced meningiomas have higher recurrence rates than those located on the convexity due to the same anatomical constraints on aggressive resection in these locations as with sporadic menigniomas.[16,17] Paradoxically, radiation therapy or radiosurgery may also serve as an important adjunct in the management of these tumors, and has often times been used successfully both as adjuvant therapy or as the sole treatment.[16,18]

18.2.6 Adjuvant Therapy of De Novo Meningiomas

Some groups advocate the use of upfront adjuvant radiosurgery after initial subtotal resection of even WHO grade I tumors or for atypical and higher-grade meningiomas, before evidence of regrowth or recurrence. In cases of tumors invading the cavernous sinus or other critical neurovascular structures of the skull base, treatment might be staged, with the intent of resecting what is safely accessible and using adjuvant radiosurgery for the more invasive and less surgically accessible portions.[19]

Using this paradigm of radiation for anything other than the complete resection of a WHO grade I meningioma, the

recurrence or residual growth rate is 4 to 8%, though a few have a transient growth period.[20] One argument against this practice is the early execution of one of the major tools in the surgeon's armamentarium for the management of tumor recurrence. The premature use of radiosurgery for "disease control" of residual tumor, or radiating the tumor bed of higher-grade tumors can leave the brain vulnerable to adverse radiation effects if future radiation becomes necessary.

18.2.7 Multiple Recurrences

Multiple recurrences are more common in the setting of atypical meningiomas, where the average patient has 3 to 4 instances of tumor recurrence. Initial recurrences (1–3) are strongly correlated with extent of resection whereas subsequent recurrences (≥ 4) are independent of the initial treatment modality (surgery vs. radiation or radiosurgery) as well as extent of resection or radiation dose. Furthermore, initial recurrences are more likely to be local, while subsequent recurrences are progressively peripheral then distant to initial tumor location.[13]

Genetic analysis of patients with more than or equal to three meningiomas showed the same copy of chromosome X was inactivated or the same NF2 mutation was present. This supports the widely-purported hypothesis that multiple meningiomas are still clonal and arise via dural spread.[1] Similarly, pathologic studies have shown evidence of meningothelial cell nests in peritumoral and even distant strips of otherwise unremarkable dura.[21] As mentioned previously, multiple recurrences are more common in the setting of familial syndromes with germline mutations and radiation-induced tumors, essentially, higher-grade meningiomas. It is intuitive that frequency of tumor recurrence is a clear demonstration of tumor aggression and, in turn, increases the likelihood of future recurrence, with progressively shorter intervals between recurrences.

18.3 Management

The management of recurrent or progressive skull base meningiomas present the surgeon, his/her team, and the patient with the same basic options as for management of the initial tumor: surveillance, repeat surgical resection through the same or a different approach, stereotactic radiotherapy (SRT) or radiosurgery (SRS), adjuvant medical therapies, or in many cases, some combination of these therapies. The decision-making process should be individualized based on the patient's age, comorbidities, recurrence location, tumor histology and their prior surgical and nonsurgical treatments. For example, a meningioma with cranial nerve or vascular investment that has been previously debulked without SRT or SRS, and now shows progressive growth, may be best treated with SRS or SRT alone (Case 1). In contrast, a progressively growing previously operated parasellar meningioma (from a lateral approach) with new brainstem compression, may be best treated with endonasal transclival bony decompression and tumor debulking, followed by imaging and/or SRT (Case 3). In some patients with multiple comorbidities and an aggressive, highly invasive skull base meningioma that has already had reasonable surgical debulking and SRS/SRT, more unproven therapies such as chemotherapy or hormonal therapy (e.g., mifepristone) may be considered. It is also important for the patient to understand that while surgical resection and radiation with SRS or SRT are standard and proven effective therapies for managing skull base meningiomas, other therapies such as chemotherapy and hormonal therapies are considered experimental. Setting appropriate expectations is critical in these challenging patients.

18.3.1 Surveillance

Surveillance with serial imaging is always a viable option especially in the setting of small recurrences, low-grade tumors, asymptomatic tumors, high-risk patients, proximity to critical structures, and less readily accessible lesions. This is especially true in the early stages of regrowth when it can be challenging to differentiate tumor recurrence from postsurgical and/or postradiation changes. It is important to note that although a higher proportion of WHO grade II–III meningiomas recur, most meningiomas are WHO grade I, which remain slow-growing tumors that can often be safely followed with serial MRIs, particularly in the elderly patient population or those with significant comorbidities. In most patients with an asymptomatic but slowly enlarging meningioma (particularly in older patients), it is reasonable to perform surveillance MRIs at 6-month intervals. If mass effect or symptoms develop, then reresection, SRS/SRT, or other adjuvant therapies can be considered at that time.

18.3.2 Surgical Resection

A majority of patients with a symptomatic recurrence of a skull base meningioma will be best served by reresection, as will those patients without symptoms but with progressive tumor growth and mass effect seen on serial imaging. Many if not most of these patients will also benefit at some point from subsequent SRS or SRT given that a complete removal will often not be possible, particularly for invasive skull base meningiomas with vascular and/or cranial nerve encasement. As such, these patients should be counseled prior to reresection that such multimodality treatment will likely be needed.

As with the initial resection, the single most important factor in preventing further recurrence and improving both recurrence-free and overall survival is the extent of resection.[13] While some have recommended radical resection, even at the risk of transient morbidity such as

cranial nerve palsies or cerebrospinal fluid (CSF) leak, due to the poor prognosis associated with multiple recurrences,[5] others including our group, advocate for maximal but safe reresection with the primary goal being neurological preservation and restoring or maintaining quality of life.[12]

Goals of Surgery

Surgical goals in the treatment of recurrent skull base meningiomas can vary from maximal resection to decompression of critical neurovascular structures. Early radical resection has been shown to portend a survival benefit in the setting of recurrence. Furthermore, radical Simpson grade I–II resection is particularly advocated for surgically accessible tumors and symptomatic patients.[13] It is important to note that radical reresection is not as effective as initial complete resection, but still remains the greatest predictor of disease-free survival.[5] Conversely, patients' quality of life can be significantly compromised with significant morbidity following overzealous reresection, often without a corresponding survival advantage. As always, the goals of surgery should be a realistic understanding of the feasibility of radical resection weighed against the potential neurologic deficits and/or other complications incurred by such a surgery.

Approach

The optimal surgical approach for a recurrent skull base meningioma is primarily dependent on tumor location, the prior approach used, the recurrence growth pattern, anatomical constraints imposed by cranial nerves and vasculature surrounding the tumor, and if the patient had prior SRS or SRT. Given that many if not most recurrent skull base meningiomas arise in or near the midline, several approach options are often possible including using a traditional lateral skull base approach, a retromastoid approach as well as somewhat newer keyhole approaches that incorporate endoscopy such as the supraorbital eyebrow approach, mini-pterional approach and endonasal endoscopic approach.[11,12,13,22,23]

The aims in selecting a surgical approach is ensuring access to the tumor mass, gaining adequate control of the relevant vasculature, decompressing vital structures, obtaining a wide resection of dural margins when possible, and avoiding unnecessary manipulation of vital neurovascular structures.

Same Approach

Using the same approach as the initial resection is beneficial in the setting of local recurrence that does not extend beyond the previous exposure. However, residual left in the initial resection from limited visualization is likely to be similarly obscured on repeat resection, and the use of endoscopy, for example, might be beneficial. Additionally, there is increased risk to critical neurovascular structures that have been previously manipulated surgically and/or radiated. Anatomical landmarks can also be obscured from fibrosis and scar, which can also increase the likelihood of cranial nerve palsies and vascular injuries. Finally, wound healing can also become troublesome with repeat surgery and previous radiation. This is especially relevant in the setting of radiation-induced meningioma recurrence, where patients may require tissue grafts to ensure adequate scalp closure.[16] With respect to endonasal approaches, reconstruction can be particularly challenging as some autologous local tissue grafts such as naso-septal mucosa may no longer be available, and risk of CSF leak, especially with previous radiation, is higher.

Different Approach

A different approach might be indicated for distant recurrences or regrowth of residual tumor, which was inaccessible with the initial approach. Added benefits of using a different approach, when possible, include avoidance of scar tissue, as clearly demarcated landmarks will allow for reliable identification of critical structures, and may decrease the incidence of complications. Many skull base meningiomas lend themselves to multiple approaches from the offset, including transcranial and/or endoscopic endonasal approaches. An anterior cranial fossa floor or olfactory groove meningioma, for example, could be approached via a subfrontal or expanded endoscopic approach. In these instances, the area of tumor recurrence may have been at the limits of the previous exposure, lending the regrowth to the other approach, or the alternative approach may simply be advantageous due to the avoidance of scar tissue.

Similarly, suprasellar meningiomas can be approached from a transphenoidal or transcranial (pterional/orbitozygomatic) approach. The supraorbital craniotomy to the suprasellar space is an underutilized approach that provides a direct trajectory to the tumor while largely avoiding scar tissue from previous approaches and allowing access for decompression of the optic apparatus. Endoscopy can be added to traditional microsurgical techniques in order to safely maximize tumor removal, in the setting of a less invasive approach (▶ Fig. 18.1). Using an eyebrow incision, the tissue is less likely to be previously radiated, minimizing postoperative wound complications, and CSF leak. McLaughlin et al describe seven patients who underwent the supraorbital approach, with endoscopy, for the resection of meningiomas with recurrence or delayed progression, where all patients had adequate tumor removal and two-thirds had improvement in their visual acuity.[24]

The utility of minimally invasive and keyhole procedures, especially via an endoscopic endonasal approach, is important even in the setting of recurrent skull base meningiomas, where the goals of surgery have typically been complete radical resection. In these instances,

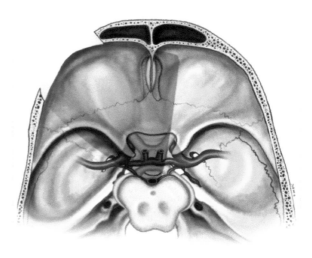

Fig. 18.1 Illustration of surgical access afforded by a supraorbital eyebrow craniotomy with addition of an endoscope.

complete resection may be impossible without significant morbidity, and the plan of care for tumor management instead becomes multimodal. Surgical approaches, especially endoscopic approaches, may be used to achieve bony decompression of critical neurovascular structures, for example the optic apparatus or pituitary gland, such to help protect these structures from radiation with an adequate margin from the tumor, and to prevent bony entrapment if there is edema associated with tumorigenesis or radiation. Surgical decompression via selective tumor removal is more effective than radiation alone in providing symptomatic relief of cranial nerve palsies, such that it should be attempted even if complete resection is not practical.[10] Subtotal surgical resection, in addition to decompressing critical structures, improving the safety of radiation, and providing clinical symptom relief, can also help devascularize any less accessible tumor remnants.

The second stage of tumor management is radiosurgery or fractionated radiation treatment for tumor control. This can be a useful paradigm in the setting of parasellar meningiomas, with cavernous sinus invasion, where the pituitary gland, optic chiasm, and carotid arteries can be decompressed, while tumor invading the cavernous sinus and/or Meckel's cave can be more safely radiated in a second stage.[19] A similar approach can be taken for petroclival, sphenoid wing, or foramen magnum meningiomas, with maximal safe resection, focusing on decompression and creating a safe margin (≥2 mm) between critical, radiosensitive structures, and the residual tumor. The advantage of using endoscopic, keyhole, and other minimally invasive techniques, in this setting, can be to minimize manipulation of already sensitized neurovascular structures, reduce brain manipulation, and decrease the surgical impact, facilitating recovery in these patients who frequently undergo multiple procedures.

Combination of Approaches

Depending on the pattern of recurrence, a combination of approaches might be indicated for complete resection, such as transcranial and endoscopic, transorbital and transcranial, etc. This can be performed concurrently or in a staged fashion and can greatly facilitate maximal safe resection or even complete resection. Again, any residual meningioma can be treated in a staged fashion with postoperative radiation treatment.

Case Examples

Case 1: Radiation Therapy after Supraorbital Approach in Recurrent Tuberculum Sella Meningioma with Optic Nerve Involvement.

A 70-year-old female underwent a right supraorbital eyebrow craniotomy for a tuberculum sella meningioma with displacement of the optic apparatus (▶ Fig. 18.2a and b), with small adherent residual tumor left under the ipsilateral optic nerve (▶ Fig. 18.2c and d). She was followed with serial imaging and 8 months after surgery was found to have regrowth of the residual tumor (▶ Fig. 18.2e and f) without any visual changes or other symptoms. She was then treated with 30 Gy of SRT, without further tumor growth on follow-up serial imaging.

Case 2: Same Approach after Prior Mini-pterional Approach in Recurrent Sphenoid Wing Meningioma.

An 80-year-old female initially presented with monocular vision loss, progressive ptosis and proptosis. MRI demonstrated an invasive spheno-orbital meningioma with infratemporal fossa invasion (▶ Fig. 18.3a and b), for which she underwent a mini-pterional approach for Simpson grade IV resection and orbital decompression in conjunction with a transorbital approach with ophthalmology (▶ Fig. 18.3c and d). Histology confirmed a WHO I meningioma with a Ki-67 of 1%. She had improvement in vision, proptosis, and headaches postoperatively, and did well until 2 years later when she presented with subacute visual loss and slight increase in tumor volume on MRI (▶ Fig. 18.3e and f). She then underwent reresection using the same approach again for removal of the orbital portions of tumor and decompression of the orbital apex (▶ Fig. 18.3g and h). Pathology was again WHO I, and she had mild improvement in her vision postoperatively. Subsequently, she was followed with serial MRI surveillance without evidence of regrowth at early six-month follow-up, but it is anticipated that she will likely need radiotherapy in the future.

Case 3: Endonasal Transclival Approach after Prior Lateral Skull Base Approach in Recurrent Petroclival Meningioma.

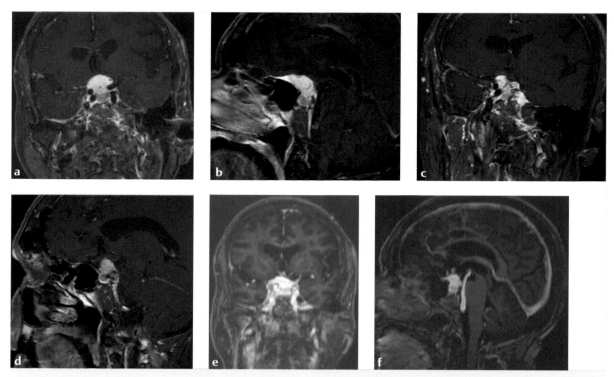

Fig. 18.2 Preoperative **(a)** coronal and **(b)** sagittal T1-weighted, contrast-enhanced MRI demonstrating a tuberculum sella meningioma with upward displacement of the optic apparatus. Postoperative **(c)** coronal and **(d)** sagittal T1-weighted, contrast-enhanced MRI after supraorbital eyebrow craniotomy with small adherent residual tumor left under the right optic nerve. **(e)** Coronal and **(f)** sagittal T1-weighted, contrast-enhanced MRI demonstrating interval regrowth 8 months after surgical resection.

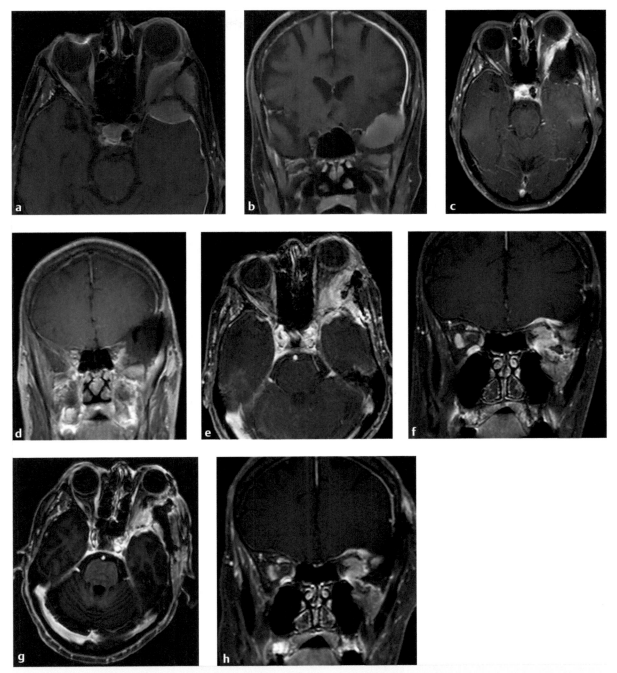

Fig. 18.3 Preoperative **(a)** axial and **(b)** coronal T1-weighted, contrast-enhanced MRI showing a left sphenoid wing meningioma with involvement of the orbit, middle and infratemporal fossae. Postoperative **(c)** axial and **(d)** coronal T1-weighted, contrast-enhanced MRI after meningioma resection via a mini-pterional approach. **(e)** Axial and **(f)** coronal T1-weighted, contrast-enhanced MRI after recurrence. Postoperative **(g)** axial and **(h)** coronal T1-weighted, contrast-enhanced MRI after meningioma reresection via another mini-pterional approach.

A 38-year-old male initially presented with headache and diplopia with an MRI demonstrating a petroclival meningioma. The tumor was resected at an outside institution via a left transpetrosal skull base craniotomy resulting in 60 to 65% resection of his WHO I meningioma. Postoperatively, he had worsened abducens palsy and facial numbness. Ten months after surgery, he was treated with 6 weeks of proton beam surgery. He presented to our institution 8 years after his original surgery with worsened left facial paresthesias. MRI revealed a petroclival meningioma measuring 16 × 26 mm in greatest diameter with brainstem edema (▶ Fig. 18.4a and b). He was treated with a staged extended endonasal endoscopic transclival approach for tumor debulking and reconstruction performed with an autologous fat graft and nasoseptal flap, leaving only residual tumor only where it was adherent to the brainstem (▶ Fig. 18.4c–e).

Case 4: Endonasal Transsellar Transplanum Approach then Supraorbital Approach for Optic Canal Decompression and Suprasellar Tumor Removal in Multiple Recurrent and Radiated Tuberculum Sella Meningioma.

A 64-year-old female with a multiple recurrent left sphenoid wing and parasellar WHO I meningioma, was originally diagnosed at an age of 40 years and treated elsewhere. She first underwent a left frontotemporal craniotomy (Simpson grade IV resection) and then had a repeat resection, 3 years later, via the same approach as well as intentional left optic nerve transection for tumor recurrence. Another 4 years after reresection, MRI demonstrated further tumor progression and she underwent a trans-sphenoidal approach for tumor debulking followed by 30 fractions of SRT. Thirteen years later (and 20 years after original diagnosis), she again had tumor progression treated with hypofractionated CyberKnife (Accuray, Sunnyvale, California) radiosurgery. The residual tumor remained stable for 4 years, until she began experiencing right eye vision loss and presented to our institution for further management, 24 years after

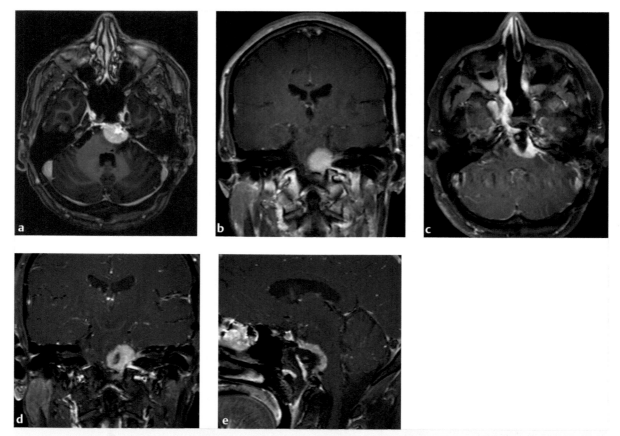

Fig. 18.4 **(a)** Axial and **(b)** coronal T1-weighted, contrast-enhanced MRI before reresection showing a recurrent 12 × 22 × 22 mm petroclival meningioma, previously partially resected via a transpetrosal approach now with interval regrowth and brainstem compression. Postoperative **(c)** axial, **(d)** coronal, and **(e)** sagittal T1-weighted, contrast-enhanced MRI demonstrating central cytoreduction with residual tumor along the brainstem following an expanded endoscopic endonasal approach.

original diagnosis and treatment (▶ Fig. 18.5a–c). Given the multiple recurrent and radiated tumor with progressive tumor growth around her only functioning right optic nerve, realistic expectations were established with a surgical goal of right optic nerve decompression, for vision preservation, and tumor debulking via an endonasal endoscopic transellar transplanum approach. Bony optic canal decompression and intradural tumor resection in the midline and right suprasellar space along the medial right optic nerve were performed, with nasoseptal flap reconstruction. (▶ Fig. 18.5d and e). Pathology returned as a WHO grade I progesterone receptor positive, estrogen receptor negative meningioma with a Ki-67 of 1 to 2%. Postoperatively, she had an improvement in her right eye vision from 20/40 preoperatively to 20/20 after surgery. Her vision remained improved for 3 months with some fluctuation over the next 6 months (▶ Fig. 18.5f–h); however, 9 months later, she had clear tumor progression and returned to the operating room for a right supraorbital eyebrow craniotomy with further tumor resection and optic nerve decompression (▶ Fig. 18.5i–k). Although she had a near complete tumor resection, she had no visual improvement. She was counseled extensively and recommended to pursue medical therapy with mifepristone, octreotide, everolimus, and nivolumbab, but has declined for now. Now 26 years since initial treatment, she continues to be followed with serial MRI without evidence of early recurrence over the past 6 months.

Case 5: Supraorbital Approach after SRS in Recurrent Planum Sphenoidale Meningioma.

A 60-year-old female with a history of breast cancer presented with a meningioma along the planum sphenoidale that was initially treated with 54 Gy of radiation in 30 fractions (▶ Fig. 18.6a and b). Five years after treatment, serial MRI demonstrated interval tumor growth, and her tumor was followed conservatively for another several years until she began to demonstrate peritumoral edema and mass effect (▶ Fig. 18.6c and d). Eight years after initial treatment, the patient underwent resection using an eyebrow approach for a supraorbital craniotomy with endoscopic assistance for gross total resection (▶ Fig. 18.6e and f). Pathology revealed a WHO II meningioma with minimal progesterone-receptor expression, and at 3-month follow-up, the MRI was concerning for minimal but new areas of enhancement which remained stable on 7-month MRI. Options for targeted and hormonal chemotherapies have been discussed with implementation predicated on a more robust tumor recurrence.

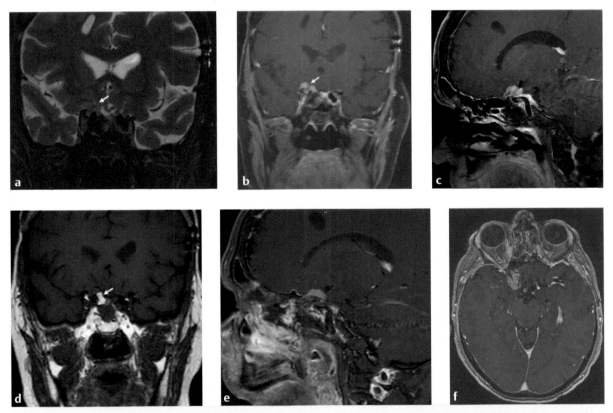

Fig. 18.5 Coronal (a) T2-weighted and (b) T1-weighted, contrast-enhanced MRI with arrow indicating optic nerve entrapment with recurrent tuberculum sella meningioma, as well as (c) sagittal T1-weighted, contrast-enhanced MRI after presentation to our institution. Postoperative (d) coronal T1- weighted MRI, with arrow indicating relative optic nerve decompression, and (e) sagittal T1-weighted contrast-enhanced MRI after endonasal endoscopic transellar transplanum approach for right optic nerve decompression and tumor debulking. (f) Axial, (*Continued*)

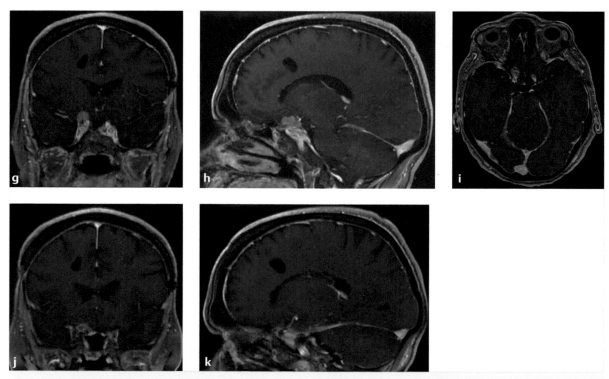

Fig. 18.5 (*Continued*) **(g)** coronal, and **(h)** sagittal T1-weighted, contrast-enhanced MRI demonstrating tumor regrowth around the right optic nerve three months after her last surgical resection. **(i)** Axial, **(j)** coronal, and **(k)** sagittal T1-weighted, contrast-enhanced MRI after right supraorbital eyebrow craniotomy for tumor resection and optic nerve decompression.

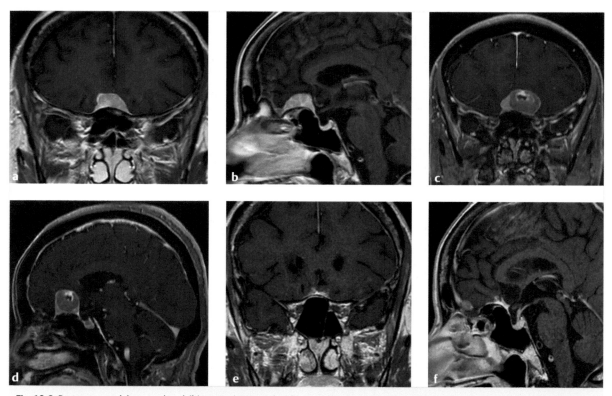

Fig. 18.6 Pretreatment **(a)** coronal and **(b)** sagittal T1-weighted, contrast-enhanced MRI. Preoperative **(c)** coronal and **(d)** sagittal T1-weighted, contrast-enhanced MRI after interval growth. Postoperative **(e)** coronal and **(f)** sagittal T1-weighted, contrast-enhanced MRI after meningioma resection via an eyebrow supraorbital approach.

Case 6: Suboccipital Craniotomy for Tumor Debulking Followed by SRT of Forman Magnum Meningioma.

A 65-year-old male with multiple meningiomas initially presented with new onset seizures and a left frontal parafalcine WHO II atypical meningioma, which was completely resected without incident, followed by SRS for recurrence prevention. Three and a half years later, surveillance postoperative MRI revealed a de novo left ventrolateral foramen magnum meningioma (▶ Fig. 18.7a–c). He then underwent a midline suboccipital craniotomy and C1 laminectomy, the tumor was adherent to the brainstem, vertebral artery, and cranial nerves XI–XII, and small residual was left behind, adherent to these critical structures (▶ Fig. 18.7d–f). Pathology demonstrated a WHO I

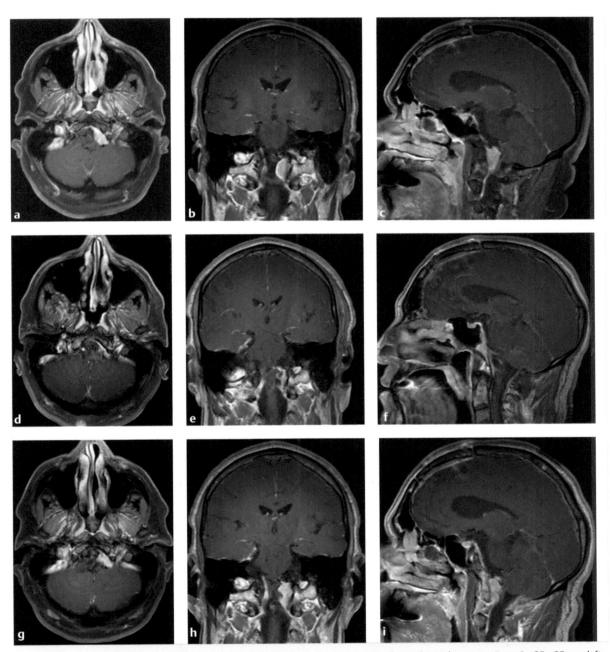

Fig. 18.7 Preoperative **(a)** axial, **(b)** coronal, and **(c)** sagittal T1-weighted, contrast-enhanced MRI demonstrating a 9 × 25 × 25 mm left ventrolateral foramen magnum meningioma. Postoperative **(d)** axial, **(e)** coronal, and **(f)** sagittal T1-weighted, contrast-enhanced MRI after subtotal meningioma resection via a suboccipital craniectomy and C1 laminectomy. Recurrent 13 × 17 × 23 mm foramen magnum meningioma seen in the **(g)** axial, **(h)** coronal, and **(i)** sagittal planes on T1-weighted, contrast-enhanced MRI 4 months after resection.

meningioma (Ki67 3%, with areas of increased mitotic activity up to Ki67 10%). Four months after resection, the residual foramen magnum meningioma was found to have progressed (▶ Fig. 18.7g–i) and he underwent 54 Gy of SRT over 30 fractions. Subsequently, he has been followed with serial MRIs for his meningiomas and his foramen magnum meningioma remains stable, nearly 4 years after SRT.

18.3.3 Radiation

Surgical resection is clearly the standard of care in the management of meningiomas, however, adjunctive radiation therapy has been consistently shown to improve progression-free and recurrence-free survival. For patients who are symptomatic, surgical decompression is more likely to alleviate symptoms and mass effect than radiation alone. Radiation therapy is typically reserved for minimally symptomatic, less accessible, residual, high grade, or recurrent disease.[25]

Radiosurgery and Radiation Therapy

Most authors maintain that microsurgical resection is the mainstay in the management of recurrent meningiomas, however, salvage SRS and SRT have been successfully applied when secondary surgical resection was not practical or feasible.[20] SRS is indicated for small to moderately-sized tumors, especially as adjuvant or staged-therapy with microsurgery.[19]

In the setting of meningioma recurrence, SRS alone, without surgical reresection, has shown 90 to 100% control rates with < 8% incidence of cranial neuropathies.[26] Furthermore, overall survival was more than 90% at 5 years.[27] Similar control rates were achieved with the use of hypofractionated radiosurgery, which is a technique often used to spare cranial nerves and with the treatment of larger tumors.[26] Radiosurgery is often used as an adjuvant therapy with repeat, secondary resection as well.[13] In these instances, the recurrent tumor is managed with maximal safe surgical resection and the tumor bed, including any residual tumor, is then treated with radiation. Similar outcomes are observed when comparing SRS alone and adjuvant radiation in the setting of recurrent meningiomas, however, surgical resection has the added benefit of resampling the tumor, debulking the tumor for more effective radiosurgery, and decompressing critical structures to improve symptoms, reduce mass effect, and decrease the incidence of cranial neuropathies, vascular injuries, and cerebral edema associated with radiation effect.

When single-dose or hypofractionated gamma knife radiosurgery was used for meningioma recurrence after initial surgical resection, failure rates of 6.5% were reported. However, failure rates were lower (3%), following radiosurgery used as the first line therapy for recurrence.[20] This is understandable given that the latter case demonstrates a primary recurrence after initial treatment, while the former represents secondary recurrence.

Meningiomas that recur after radiosurgery alone are then amenable to surgical resection or reirradiation. These tumors can demonstrate aggressive and rapid rates of regrowth with a wide-ranging latency period of months to decades.[19]

As recurrence rate is highly dependent on tumor histology, it is important to differentiate between tumor grades when discussing tumor control rates. Most studies evaluating the efficacy of SRS following recurrent high-grade meningiomas are sparse and highly variable.[26] At 5-year follow-up, primary and adjuvant radiosurgery showed 93%, 68%, and 0% progression-free survival for benign, atypical, and anaplastic meningiomas, respectively.[19] When looking at recurrence alone, benign meningiomas have a progression-free survival of 93–100% at 5-year follow-up, where atypical meningiomas demonstrated a 60–90% recurrence-free survival at 3-year follow-up, and malignant meningiomas had only a 30–40% local tumor control rate at 3 years.[26] Despite the wide-ranging recurrence rates and variable follow-up periods reported, it is clear that higher grade tumors recur more frequently and at shorter intervals following primary adjuvant, secondary adjuvant, and secondary SRS or SRT administered for meningioma recurrence.

Reirradiation

Reirradiation of recurrent tumors, including meningiomas, is a potential salvage therapy in the setting of recurrence after surgical and SRS/SRT failure. Although multiple rounds of ionizing radiation are never ideal and the risk of adverse radiation effects such as radiation necrosis increases, it remains a viable option in the management of some recurrences. Several large studies have shown the incidence of reirradiation ranges from 3 to 4% in the management of all menigniomas.[20,25] Reirradiation can be in the form of whole brain radiation, fully fractionated SRT, hypofractionated SRS, and targeted SRS.

The indications for reirradiation can be very subjective, most studies advocate reresection for readily accessible lesions and avoiding repeat radiosurgery in the setting of large tumor volumes and situations of rapid local recurrence.[20] For diffuse lesions, and with leptomeningeal seeding or multiple concurrent recurrences, whole brain radiation is an option in the management of recurrent, locally aggressive meningiomas.[20] Whole brain radiation is well-known to cause widespread cognitive decline and significantly decrease quality of life over more limited foci of radiation such as SRS, which should be used whenever possible, even in the setting of multiple radiosurgical targets. Nevertheless, a second session of radiation therapy has demonstrated adequate (80 to 95%) control rates with 3 to 5 year follow-up, that decrease to 50 to 60% with longer term surveillance.[20,27] One study looking at all forms of reradiation of meningiomas,[25] and another focusing on specifically repeat SRS,[20] both demonstrated satisfactory tumor control rates for WHO grade I meningiomas but not for higher WHO II–III grade tumors, where histologic grade was the only significant predictor of decreased progression-free survival.

Kim et al describe a large series where 5 patients also underwent a third session of radiosurgery for recurrent meningioma in the same location. As expected, tumor control rates were lower than with those meningiomas that were successfully treated with fewer rounds of radiation, however, control rates were better than the natural history of these twice recurrent meningiomas.[20]

Brachytherapy

Brachytherapy has been described as a salvage technique in the setting of recurrence with implantation of Iodine 125 (^{125}I) seeds, which secretes a total dose of 100 to 500 Gy at a rate of 0.05 to 0.25 Gy per hour for up to 2 years.[28,29] Although not a first line or often-used treatment modality, brachytherapy is an option in the setting of patients who have already had one or more surgical resections and radiation treatment. It has a small recurrence-free survival advantage over natural history, especially when repeat external SRT is not an option. The use of radioactive seeds in the skull base is limited due to cranial nerve toxicity, causing significant morbidity. Furthermore, up to one-third of patients with brachytherapy have complications including radiation necrosis and wound breakdown.[30] This further limits the application of brachytherapy in the setting of recurrent skull base meningiomas, as reconstruction in these areas can be more tenuous than typical convexity or parasagittal meningiomas.[28]

Particle Therapy

Multiple studies investigating proton-beam and carbon ion radiotherapy have demonstrated good tumor control rates in the management of recurrent meningiomas, especially after multiple prior interventions. These results are comparable to photon radiation.[31,32] Additionally, carbon ion radiotherapy has demonstrated adequate efficacy for atypical and anaplastic meningiomas, which are relatively resistant to photon therapy.[20,31] Thus far, the evidence only demonstrates results comparable to readily-accessible photon-based radiation, and future investigation will need assess the role of particle therapy at earlier phases of care for meningioma patients.[32]

18.3.4 Chemotherapy

The role of adjuvant chemotherapy in the management of meningioma recurrence is still ill-defined. Multiple different agents and therapies have been used in the management of meningioma, especially with recurrent, high grade, aggressive, and invasive tumors. Although several chemotherapeutics have demonstrated growth arrest or minimal tumor regression, no single agent has demonstrated reproducible and sustainable tumor regression.[33] When used in the setting of meningiomas, chemotherapy is reserved for aggressive, recurrent tumors as salvage or palliative therapy.

Hydroxyurea

Hydroxyurea is a ribonucleotide reductase inhibitor that primarily functions by sensitizing cells to radiation by holding them in a radiosensitive reproductive state and preventing DNA repair of damaged cells.[33] Schrell et al in 1997, first described the clinical use of hydroxyurea in recurrent skull base meningioma management, where patients with WHO grade I meningiomas had modest tumor regression while a patient with malignant meningioma demonstrated growth arrest, a minimal but clear benefit over natural history.[34] Subsequent studies have indicated even less success where hydroxyurea has shown some anti-tumor effect, but at best provides growth arrest with delayed disease progression, but without tumor regression.[33,35] Additionally, the most current National Comprehensive Cancer Network (NCCN) guidelines do not advocate the use of hydroxyurea in the management of meningiomas.[36]

Bevacizumab

Bevacizumab is a monoclonal antibody directed against vascular endothelial growth factor (VEGF). It has demonstrated efficacy in the treatment of both recurrent glioblastoma as well as cerebral radiation-necrosis. There is substantial evidence that defines the role of angiogenesis in recurrent meningiomas to be mediated by VEGF, particularly in higher grade (WHO II and III) tumors.[37] These tumors have an increased density of microvessels, VEGF, and VEGF receptors (VEGF-R), however, there was no correlation between VEGF density and WHO I meningiomas.[37,38]

Levels of VEGF and VEGF-R are also correlated with peritumoral brain edema, although biopsy of these regions demonstrates concentrations of VEGF protein without VEGF mRNA, suggesting the VEGF is secreted by the tumor and leaks into the adjacent parenchyma.[37,39] Bevacizumab can be used to decrease peritumoral edema in such cases, and can help decrease steroid-dependence in this cohort of patients where steroids are used liberally.[33] This can, of course, help limit side effects from corticosteroid use (hypertension, diabetes mellitus, weight gain, "Cushing" features).

Ultimately in meningioma patients treated with iterative surgical resection, SRT and/or SRS, the addition of bevacizumab as a salvage technique showed comparable progression-free survival to targeted therapy, octreotide, interferon (IFN)-α therapy, salvage chemotherapy, and hormonal agents. That is to say, the use of bevacizumab demonstrated modest temporary tumor growth arrest and delay of progression in recurrent meningiomas.[37]

Somatostatin Analogs

Some cell proliferation studies have demonstrated significantly impaired DNA synthesis when somatostatin receptors are blocked. Approximately 88% of all meningiomas express one of the subtypes of somatostatin receptors, some of which act on VEGF-mediated pathways. A case report of octreotide administration (a somatostatin analog) in a patient with a meningioma that had dedifferentiated from WHO grade I to a malignant WHO grade III demonstrated growth arrest without tumor regression on MRI.[40] Similarly, a small study evaluating the somatostatin analog, sandostatin LAR, a long-acting form of octreotide, demonstrated long-term disease remission and tumor stabilization, though without regression.[41]

Hormonal Therapy

Sporadic meningiomas are 2 to 3 times more likely to occur in females than males. This ratio is especially high during the child-bearing years of a woman's lifetime. Most low-grade meningiomas express progesterone receptors (PRs), as do most tumors that occur in multiplicity. Mifepristone (RU-486) is an oral progesterone antagonist with a modest affinity for the glucocorticoid receptor, that has been used in the medical management of recurrent low and high-grade meningiomas.[42,43] Several clinical trials of mifepristone conducted with patients with mixed histology in terms of both receptor-status and WHO grade, show heterogeneous results with minimal transient regression in a few patients, tumor stability in most, and tumor progression in up to 40%. Most patients with regression and stability, displayed delay of progression only during active treatment.[42] There is a paucity of studies assessing mifepristone therapy in PR positive meningiomas. A single case series of three postmenopausal women with meningiomatosis demonstrated long-term clinical and radiographic improvement after mifepristone treatment. Although receptor status was largely unknown in this situation, most female patients and those with meningiomatosis present a high density of progesterone receptors, which is likely the basis of tumor regression in this scenario.[43]

Since WHO grade II–III meningiomas have progressively lower rates of PR expression, they are expectedly less susceptible to mifepristone. Furthermore, there are two major subtypes of the PR that have different effects both in disease and non-disease states as well as variable responses to mifepristone. More directed mifepristone clinical trials are warranted, analyzing patients with histologically-proven PR subtype B positive tumors.[42]

Targeted Therapy

Platelet-derived growth factor (PDGF) and its receptors (PDGFR) are frequently expressed in meningiomas, making it another potential therapeutic target. Imatinib mesylate (Gleevec), a PDGFR inhibitor, delivered as monotherapy in a phase II trial had no effect on tumor progression, without any incidences of complete or even partial response, across all histologic grades.[44] Other studies combining imatinib and hydroxyurea treatment in patients with recurrent meningiomas also failed to demonstrate a delay in tumor progression or recurrence.[45,46] Similarly, another phase II trial of targeted molecular therapy with gefitinib and erlotinib, anti-epidermal growth factor receptor (EGFR) drugs, showed disease stability in only one-third of patients with recurrent meningiomas, irrespective of histopathological grade.[47]

Other Chemotherapeutic Agents

Higher grade meningiomas have shown some responsiveness to oral tyrosine kinase inhibitors, with anti-VEGF and PDGFR activity.[37] Another study using IFN-α demonstrated no radiographic response in the recurrent high grade meningiomas, but moderate drug toxicity. Thus far, numerous molecular targets have been identified without significant or sustainable benefit in tumor responsiveness or progression-free survival, though the search for chemotherapeutic agents should continue given the high morbidity and mortality of aggressive meningiomas.

18.4 Conclusion

Recurrent or progressive skull base meningiomas remain a major management challenge for the neurosurgeon. The mainstay of treatment continues to be repeat resection and/or focused radiotherapy with SRS or SRT. When considering reresection, the original approach is often the best approach, however, minimally invasive keyhole and endoscopic routes that minimize tissue and brain manipulation, should be in the armamentarium of the skull base surgeon.

Chemotherapeutic agents, including hydroxyurea, somatostatin analogs, and mifepristone have shown only limited success, with temporary growth arrest and delay of recurrence. Further studies are necessary to increase the chemotherapeutic and directed molecular therapeutic options for recurrent meningioma management. To advance care of these challenging patients, a multidisciplinary approach incorporating specialists in neurosurgery, radiation oncology, otolaryngology, and neuro-oncology as well as translational neuroscientists are needed.

References

[1] Perry A, Louis DN, Budka H, et al. Meningioma. In: Louis DN, Ohgaki H, Wiestler OD, Cavenee WK, eds. WHO Classification of Tumors of the Central Nervous System. Revised 4 t. Herndon, VA: IARC: Lyon; 2016:232–245

[2] Nanda A, Bir SC, Konar S, et al. Outcome of resection of WHO Grade II meningioma and correlation of pathological and radiological predictive factors for recurrence. J Clin Neurosci. 2016; 31:112–121

[3] Nanda A, Vannemreddy P. Recurrence and outcome in skull base meningiomas: do they differ from other intracranial meningiomas? Skull Base. 2008; 18(4):243–252

[4] Jääskeläinen J. Seemingly complete removal of histologically benign intracranial meningioma: late recurrence rate and factors predicting recurrence in 657 patients. A multivariate analysis. Surg Neurol. 1986; 26(5):461–469

[5] da Silva CE, Peixoto de Freitas PE. Recurrence of skull base meningiomas: the role of aggressive removal in surgical treatment. J Neurol Surg B Skull Base. 2016; 77(3):219–225

[6] Gallagher MJ, Jenkinson MD, Brodbelt AR, Mills SJ, Chavredakis E. WHO grade 1 meningioma recurrence: are location and Simpson grade still relevant? Clin Neurol Neurosurg. 2016; 141:117–121

[7] Simpson D. The recurrence of intracranial meningiomas after surgical treatment. J Neurol Neurosurg Psychiatry. 1957; 20(1):22–39

[8] Oya S, Kawai K, Nakatomi H, Saito N. Significance of Simpson grading system in modern meningioma surgery: integration of the grade with MIB-1 labeling index as a key to predict the recurrence of WHO Grade I meningiomas. J Neurosurg. 2012; 117(1):121–128

[9] DeMonte F, Smith HK, Al-Mefty O. Outcome of aggressive removal of cavernous sinus meningiomas. J Neurosurg. 1994; 81(2):245–251

[10] Kano H, Park KJ, Kondziolka D, et al. Does prior microsurgery improve or worsen the outcomes of stereotactic radiosurgery for cavernous sinus meningiomas? Neurosurgery. 2013; 73(3):401–410

[11] Lobo B, Zhang X, Barkhoudarian G, Griffiths CF, Kelly DF. Endonasal endoscopic management of parasellar and cavernous sinus meningiomas. Neurosurg Clin N Am. 2015; 26(3):389–401

[12] Sivakumar W, Lobo B, Zhang X, et al. Endonasal Endoscopic Bony Decompression, Limited Tumor Removal and Stereotactic Radiation Therapy in Invasive Parasellar Meningiomas to Improve Cranial Neuropathy and Endocrinopathy. J Neurol Surg B Skull Base. 2017; 78:S1–S156

[13] Talacchi A, Muggiolu F, De Carlo A, Nicolato A, Locatelli F, Meglio M. Recurrent atypical meningiomas: combining surgery and radiosurgery in one effective multimodal treatment. World Neurosurg. 2016; 87:565–572

[14] Clark VE, Erson-Omay EZ, Serin A, et al. Genomic analysis of non-NF2 meningiomas reveals mutations in TRAF7, KLF4, AKT1, and SMO. Science. 2013; 339(6123):1077–1080

[15] Mukherjee S, Ghosh SN, Chatterjee U, Chatterjee S. Detection of progesterone receptor and the correlation with Ki-67 labeling index in meningiomas. Neurol India. 2011; 59(6):817–822

[16] Umansky F, Shoshan Y, Rosenthal G, Fraifeld S, Spektor S. Radiation-induced meningioma. Neurosurg Focus. 2008; 24(5):E7

[17] Sadetzki S, Flint-Richter P, Ben-Tal T, Nass D. Radiation-induced meningioma: a descriptive study of 253 cases. J Neurosurg. 2002; 97 (5):1078–1082

[18] Kondziolka D, Kano H, Kanaan H, et al. Stereotactic radiosurgery for radiation-induced meningiomas. Neurosurgery. 2009; 64(3):463–469, discussion 469–470

[19] Couldwell WT, Cole CD, Al-Mefty O. Patterns of skull base meningioma progression after failed radiosurgery. J Neurosurg. 2007; 106(1):30–35

[20] Kim M, Cho YH, Kim JH, Kim CJ, Kwon DH. Analysis the causes of radiosurgical failure in intracranial meningiomas treated with radiosurgery. Clin Neurol Neurosurg. 2017; 154:51–58

[21] Borovich B, Doron Y. Recurrence of intracranial meningiomas: the role played by regional multicentricity. J Neurosurg. 1986; 64(1):58–63

[22] Fatemi N, Dusick JR, de Paiva Neto MA, Malkasian D, Kelly DF. Endonasal versus supraorbital keyhole removal of craniopharyngiomas and tuberculum sellae meningiomas. Neurosurgery. 2009; 64(5) Suppl 2:269–284, discussion 284–286

[23] McLaughlin N, Prevedello D, Kelly D, et al. Endoscopic approaches to skull base lesions, ventricular tumors, and cysts. In: Ellenbogen R, Abdulrauf SI, Sekhar L, eds. Principles of Neurological Surgery. 3rd ed. Philadelphia, PA: Elsevier; 2012:681–694

[24] McLaughlin N, Ditzel Filho LFS, Shahlaie K, Solari D, Kassam AB, Kelly DF. The supraorbital approach for recurrent or residual suprasellar tumors. Minim Invasive Neurosurg. 2011; 54(4):155–161

[25] Wojcieszynski AP, Ohri N, Andrews DW, Evans JJ, Dicker AP, Werner-Wasik M. Reirradiation of recurrent meningioma. J Clin Neurosci. 2012; 19(9):1261–1264

[26] Krengli M, Apicella G, Deantonio L, Paolini M, Masini L. Stereotactic radiation therapy for skull base recurrences: Is a salvage approach still possible? Rep Pract Oncol Radiother. 2015; 20(6):430–439

[27] Flannery TJ, Kano H, Lunsford LD, et al. Long-term control of petroclival meningiomas through radiosurgery. J Neurosurg. 2010; 112(5):957–964

[28] Kumar PP, Patil AA, Syh HW, Chu WK, Reeves MA. Role of brachytherapy in the management of the skull base meningioma. Treatment of skull base meningiomas. Cancer. 1993; 71(11):3726–3731

[29] Abou Al-Shaar H, Almefty KK, Abolfotoh M, et al. Brachytherapy in the treatment of recurrent aggressive falcine meningiomas. J Neurooncol. 2015; 124(3):515–522

[30] Ware ML, Larson DA, Sneed PK, Wara WW, McDermott MW. Surgical resection and permanent brachytherapy for recurrent atypical and malignant meningioma. Neurosurgery. 2004; 54(1):55–63, discussion 63–64

[31] Combs SE, Hartmann C, Nikoghosyan A, et al. Carbon ion radiation therapy for high-risk meningiomas. Radiother Oncol. 2010; 95(1):54–59

[32] Combs SE, Welzel T, Habermehl D, et al. Prospective evaluation of early treatment outcome in patients with meningiomas treated with particle therapy based on target volume definition with MRI and 68Ga-DOTATOC-PET. Acta Oncol. 2013; 52(3):514–520

[33] Newton HB. Hydroxyurea chemotherapy in the treatment of meningiomas. Neurosurg Focus. 2007; 23(4):E11

[34] Schrell UM, Rittig MG, Anders M, et al. Hydroxyurea for treatment of unresectable and recurrent meningiomas. II. Decrease in the size of meningiomas in patients treated with hydroxyurea. J Neurosurg. 1997; 86(5):840–844

[35] Mason WP, Gentili F, Macdonald DR, Hariharan S, Cruz CR, Abrey LE. Stabilization of disease progression by hydroxyurea in patients with recurrent or unresectable meningioma. J Neurosurg. 2002; 97(2):341–346

[36] National Comprehensive Cancer Network. Central Nervous System Cancers. NCCN Clin Pract Guidel Oncol. 2017; 2017(1):MENI 1–2

[37] Lou E, Sumrall AL, Turner S, et al. Bevacizumab therapy for adults with recurrent/progressive meningioma: a retrospective series. J Neurooncol. 2012; 109(1):63–70

[38] Maiuri F, De Caro MB, Esposito F, et al. Recurrences of meningiomas: predictive value of pathological features and hormonal and growth factors. J Neurooncol. 2007; 82(1):63–68

[39] Ding Y-S, Wang H-D, Tang K, Hu Z-G, Jin W, Yan W. Expression of vascular endothelial growth factor in human meningiomas and peritumoral brain areas. Ann Clin Lab Sci. 2008; 38(4):344–351

[40] Rammo R, Rock A, Transou A, Raghunathan A, Rock J. Anaplastic meningioma: octreotide therapy for a case of recurrent and progressive intracranial disease. J Neurosurg. 2016; 124(2):496–500

[41] Schulz C, Mathieu R, Kunz U, Mauer UM. Treatment of unresectable skull base meningiomas with somatostatin analogs. Neurosurg Focus. 2011; 30(5):E11

[42] Cossu G, Levivier M, Daniel RT, Messerer M. The role of mifepristone in meningiomas management: A systematic review of the literature. BioMed Res Int. 2015; 2015:267831

[43] Touat M, Lombardi G, Farina P, Kalamarides M, Sanson M. Successful treatment of multiple intracranial meningiomas with the antiprogesterone receptor agent mifepristone (RU486). Acta Neurochir (Wien). 2014; 156(10):1831–1835

[44] Wen PY, Yung WKA, Lamborn KR, et al. Phase II study of imatinib mesylate for recurrent meningiomas (North American Brain Tumor Consortium study 01–08). Neuro-oncol. 2009; 11(6):853–860

[45] Mazza E, Reni M, Lombardi G, et al. A randomized phase II trial of hydroxyurea + imatinib in the treatment of recurrent or progressive meningiomas. Eur J Cancer. 2013; 49:S791

[46] Reardon DA, Desjardins A, Vredenburgh JJ, et al. Phase II study of Gleevec plus hydroxyurea in adults with progressive or recurrent low-grade glioma. Cancer. 2012; 118(19):4759–4767

[47] Norden AD, Raizer JJ, Abrey LE, et al. Phase II trials of erlotinib or gefitinib in patients with recurrent meningioma. J Neurooncol. 2010; 96(2):211–217

19 Natural History and Adjunctive Modalities of Treatment

Peter F. Morgenstern, Jonathan Forbes, Theodore H. Schwartz

Abstract

Follow-up and adjunctive modalities of treatment for meningioma are highly variable. Underlying biology and the expected natural history of meningioma are dependent on the tumor grade, with World Health Organization (WHO) grade I lesions exhibiting the most indolent, benign behavior and WHO grade III tumors behaving most aggressively. Need for, and selection of, adjuvant treatment modality is not standardized, but follow some general guiding principles in considering the goals of achieving long-term tumor control while minimizing neurologic compromise. Radiation, in the form of conventional radiotherapy, stereotactic radiosurgery or brachytherapy, has been employed with success. More recently, trials of medical therapies for more aggressive lesions have been undertaken and yielded promising results but these are not yet the standard of care.

Keywords: meningioma, follow-up, adjuvant treatment, radiotherapy, radiosurgery, chemotherapy

19.1 Introduction

Adjunctive modalities for the treatment of meningioma have advanced substantially over the last 30 years. Recognition of variable underlying tumor biology affecting the aggressiveness of this entity has led to studies of adding radiation and other medical adjuncts to surgical resection, or in some cases independent of surgical intervention. In this chapter, we will review the natural history and recurrence rates for World Health Organization (WHO) grade I, II, and III meningiomas, as well as the current data supporting available adjunctive therapies.

19.2 Natural History

Long-term management of meningiomas is dictated in large part by the natural history of the tumor, which varies substantially by tumor grade and biological behavior, as well as the treatment modality that is applied. Surgery remains the first-line treatment of most meningiomas, and extent of resection as assessed by the Simpson grading scale was identified early on as a method for predicting recurrence (▶ Table 19.1).[1] Although this scale does not account for tumor biology, is subject to surgeon bias, and was formulated before the development of modern microsurgical techniques, it remains an effective predictor of recurrence for grade I meningiomas.[2,3,4] An important consideration, however, is that extent of resection is heavily influenced by tumor location. For example, a complete resection with wide margins may be accomplished relatively easily for a convexity lesion but not for one of the cavernous sinus. Thus, extent of resection combined with a clear understanding of biological behavior, tumor location, and adjuvant modalities can provide a more complete assessment of long-term prognosis and expected outcome, thus guiding the selection of appropriate adjuncts and timing of follow-up.

Tumor location has been presented as an indicator of behavior, but the results are controversial. While some have proposed that skull base meningiomas may follow a more indolent course than previously thought,[5,6] others find that many skull base lesions are aggressive, with a high recurrence rate when complete resection is not achievable.[7] These findings suggest that a multi-pronged approach and an eye toward medical therapies in development for unresectable tumors are critical for improving long-term outcomes in this population. Furthermore, the eloquent structures associated with many skull base lesions, in particular petroclival meningiomas, limit the

Table 19.1 Simpson grading scale for extent of resection of meningioma as a predictor of postoperative recurrence or progression of disease

Grade	Extent of resection	Recurrence/progression (%)
I	Compete tumor resection including dural attachment and abnormal bone	8.9
II	Complete tumor resection with coagulation of dural attachment	15.8
III	Complete intradural tumor resection without removal or coagulation of dural or extradural extension	29.2
IV	Partial resection	39.2
V	Decompression without resection, +/– biopsy	88.9

Adapted from: Simpson D. The recurrence of intracranial meningiomas after surgical treatment. J Neurol Neurosurg Psychiatry. 1957; 20(1):22–39.

surgeon's ability to achieve a gross total resection without significantly increasing morbidity. Although gross total resection is preferred to maximize overall survival, it is often prudent to attempt subtotal resection with adjuvant radiation, an approach that has been shown to yield high rates of local control while minimizing surgical morbidity and maximizing quality of life.[8,9,10,11,12]

Decisions regarding frequency of follow-up imaging and the addition of adjuvants in the post-operative period are affected by predictors of recurrence. The most robust of these predictors are extent of resection as defined by Simpson,[1] the presence of brain invasion and the proliferation rate as observed histologically by MIB-1 (cell proliferation marker) index. However, other factors have been identified in observational data as potential additional data points to predict recurrence and push the practitioner to initiate more frequent follow-up or add adjuvant treatments. These include pial-cortical arterial supply, larger tumor size, presence of edema on preoperative MRI, absence of brain-tumor interface at surgery (a surrogate for brain invasion), and osteolysis.[13]

19.2.1 WHO Grade I

Tumors classified as WHO grade I comprise the largest subset of meningiomas at diagnosis (81%). These tumors are considered benign, with a low recurrence rate (12% at 5 years).[14] Recurrences of WHO I cranial meningiomas may continue to exhibit benign clinical and histologic behavior, but some will demonstrate more aggressive activity at the time of recurrence. It has been suggested that convexity meningiomas behave in this manner more frequently than those of the skull base, though the evidence for this conclusion is limited to retrospective observation.[6]

Despite their benign clinical behavior, the clinical course associated with these tumors is not entirely indolent. Recent evidence has shown that long-term neurocognitive outcomes in patients with WHO I meningioma following surgical resection are impaired when compared to age-matched controls. These patients have higher rates of epilepsy and demonstrate significant impairments in verbal memory, executive functioning, information processing capacity, psychomotor speed, and working memory. Patients with left-sided tumors also exhibit higher rates of verbal memory deficits.[15] All of these factors directly impact quality of life and are critically important components of counseling and decisions to intervene for these patients.

Surgical extirpation is generally accepted as the primary treatment modality for low-grade meningiomas. Simpson I resection remains the goal, with the highest rate of long-term progression-free survival (PFS). However, recent evidence has called into question the importance of wide resections, with limited data suggesting that the differences between Simpson I, II, III, and even IV resections are nonsignificant and perhaps not clinically relevant in the modern era for grade I tumors. This point is supported by the excellent control rates associated with stereotactic radiosurgery (SRS) or radiotherapy (SRT) used as an adjuvant to near total resection.[16] Further prospective study of this question is needed for clarification, but the key guiding principle remains preservation of neurologic function for patients undergoing resection of grade I lesions given the high rates of local control afforded by adjuvant radiation treatment.

As an alternative to surgery, some have proposed radiotherapy alone for small, asymptomatic lesions in difficult locations, particularly for older patients. This approach has yielded long-term PFS rates as high as 90%, though care must be taken to ensure frequent follow-up imaging to ensure that the tumor exhibits benign behavior in the absence of a histologic diagnosis.[17]

19.2.2 WHO Grade II

Compared to benign meningiomas, grade II, or atypical, meningiomas portend a more troublesome course. They represent approximately 15% of all meningiomas and have a 35 to 41% 5-year recurrence rate.[14,18] Their high rate of recurrence and relatively high incidence has allowed for extensive study and a wide array of approaches to improving overall survival for patients with this disease.

Factors contributing to recurrence or progression for atypical meningioma include subtotal resection, advanced age at diagnosis, MIB-1 index more than 8%.[19,20] More recently, attention has been focused on molecular and genetic markers of recurrence risk, with one group finding that a higher rate of copy number alterations correlates with recurrence rates in a cohort of completely resected atypical meningiomas.[21] Other molecular markers and driving pathways for this subtype are under investigation but have not clearly correlated with survival or risk of recurrence.

For these tumors, many recommend adjuvant radiation regardless of extent of resection, in order to reduce recurrence rates. In the optimal case, gross total resection in combination with adjuvant radiotherapy has been shown to achieve high rates of local control.[19,22] However, recently, there has been some controversy over the role of adjuvant radiation to the tumor bed of completely resected grade II tumors. Some suggest immediate postoperative treatment while others advocate a delayed approach, treating only recurrent disease to reduce the radiation burden. The most effective approach is unclear, but most agree that adjuvant radiation is needed if any residual remains.

One potential treatment paradigm based on extent of resection includes MRI of the brain every 3 months for 1 year, then every 6 months for 1-year follow-up by annual follow-up for those undergoing complete resection of an atypical meningioma. Supporters of this approach advocate radiosurgery or resection depending on the nature of recurrence (location, size, and growth rate). Incompletely resected tumors that can undergo radiosurgery are best treated with this adjuvant approach, while those without a target that is amenable to radiosurgery can either be treated with conformal radiation or expectant management. Expectant management of residual disease after surgery is generally reserved, however, for those who are considered high risk radiation candidates (poor wound healing, prior radiation, genetic tumor predisposition) or for whom recurrence at the site could be easily reresected or treated with radiosurgery (i.e., noneloquent convexity tumors).[23]

19.2.3 WHO Grade III

These are the most aggressive meningiomas, occurring in 1 to 4% of cases and accumulating a 56% 5-year recurrence rate.[14,24] Their rarity makes large studies challenging, and outcome data is primarily limited to case series.[18] Based on the limited data available, however, outcomes are quite poor for these tumors, with a 5-year mortality of 40 to 83%, 10-year mortality of 40 to 100% and median survival of 1.5 years.[24,25,26,27,28] The benefits of complete surgical resection for this disease are clear, with more recent data showing those undergoing gross or near-total versus subresection having a 64.5% versus 41.1% 5-year survival rate.[20,24] High mitotic count, proliferation indices, and the presence of brain invasion on histologic analysis have been shown to independently predict poor outcome for this meningioma type, as with the other grades.[29] Younger patients (<60 years) appear to have improved outcomes over older patients as well.[28]

Because of their aggressive behavior and high early recurrence rate, frequent radiographic and clinical follow-up is mandatory for these patients. Most authors agree that adjuvant radiation, either in the form of RT or SRS, is an important component of the clinical paradigm.[25,27,28,30] Although data to support this paradigm is retrospective in nature, the survival differences when compared to historic controls are significant, 40% with radiation versus nearly zero without.[24,25,28] Repeat surgical resection with or without radiation is applied for recurrences. Medical therapies, typically on investigative protocols, are applied for patients with multiply recurrent disease.[27]

19.3 Adjunct Treatment Modalities

19.3.1 Radiation

Meningioma management increasingly employs adjuvant therapies, including radiation, when a curative resection is not possible or when more aggressive pathology is identified. This can include a variety of circumstances, such as eloquent location, aggressive biology, or in cases of recurrence. Although many radiation modalities and

treatment plans exist, those most frequently discussed in the published literature on meningioma management are SRS, conformal external beam radiotherapy (EBRT), and brachytherapy.

Conformal External Beam Radiotherapy

Conformal EBRT is applied in the management of meningioma with the expectation of delaying or arresting tumor growth, rather than reducing tumor size. Some tumors will shrink in a delayed fashion with this modality, and there are reports of dramatic responses to therapy, but this is not typical.[17,31,32,33] This makes it a useful adjunct to prevent or slow recurrence for tumors that have been partially debulked, particularly those adjacent to critical radiosensitive structures, and are therefore, not amenable to radiosurgery. RT may also be useful for patients who are not surgical candidates due to medical comorbidities.

RT dosing and fractionation for meningioma are variable, but doses are typically in the range of 50 to 60 Gy spread over approximately 30 fractions.[32] Postoperative radiotherapy has been attempted in all meningioma types, but the most consistent benefit has been observed in those with grade II and III tumors with incomplete resection. In these patients, RT has been shown to improve local control and survival.[34,35,36]

Radiation sources, in particular particle (proton or carbon) and photon, have been evaluated for efficacy in grade II and III meningiomas, partially resected and recurrent lesions. Both have been shown to achieve higher rates of local control than surgery alone. Small series have suggested that proton beam therapy or combinations of proton and photon beams may be more effective than photon beam alone, though evidence to support this conclusion remains limited. And while proton beams may afford more precise targeting, both sources have been shown to be well-tolerated with low rates of radiation necrosis and other complications.[31,33,35,37,38] The primary benefit of particle therapy is a potential reduction in the rate of secondary malignancy. This, however, is difficult to demonstrate as it requires very long-term follow-up, for which studies are ongoing.[39]

Patients with low-grade lesions may also benefit from fractionated radiation therapy. For example, RT at the time of initial resection, rather than recurrence, has been advanced as an option for patients with pathology predicting higher recurrence rates, such as papillary meningioma and even for other grade I tumors, and has been shown to improve overall survival in a small cohort.[40,41] Recurrent low-grade tumors in difficult surgical locations have also been shown to achieve high local control rates with the addition of radiation therapy (93% at 5 years, 86–91% at 10 years).[39,41]

Complications of conformal radiotherapy are uncommon with careful planning around critical structures. But delayed toxicities including cranial neuropathies, in particular optic neuropathy, and radiation necrosis of healthy brain tissue do occur in 0 to 19% of patients among modern studies of patients with skull base lesions. Patients with convexity lesions experience complications at a lower rate.[32] Patients with convexity lesions experience complications at a lower rate.

Stereotactic Radiosurgery

SRS has been extensively studied for all grades of meningioma, both as a stand-alone treatment and as an adjuvant to surgery. Initially, this modality was applied to unresectable or incompletely resectable skull base lesions with tumor control rates of 85 to 100% using either gamma knife or linear accelerator-based technologies.[42,43,44,45] Margin doses for SRS to meningiomas typically range from 12 to 18 Gy.[9,43,46,47]

This role as an adjuvant or second-line treatment is well-established with strong supportive data when tumor volume and location accommodate this modality. Tumor control rates are improved for higher grade lesions with SRS compared to without radiation, and high rates of control have been achieved for incompletely resected grade I lesions as well.[46,48]

Indications for SRS in the management of meningioma have expanded as technology has improved and impressive tumor control rates with low rates of toxicity have been demonstrated. SRS has been studied as an upfront treatment for surgically inaccessible or difficult lesions, in particular those of petroclival origin. While these studies are inevitably confounded by a lack of histologic data to confirm tumor grade, they do provide some evidence that ablative doses of focused radiation may provide long-term tumor control without surgery. Predictors of good tumor response include small size and no history of prior radiation. Furthermore, careful SRS planning has been shown to preserve cranial nerve function when tumor volumes are small.[46,49,50,51] Thus, for small lesions that, due to location, are difficult to access safely with surgery, SRS may be a useful tool to achieve tumor control.

Limited studies have been undertaken to evaluate hypofractionated stereotactic RT as well, a potentially useful adjunct for patients with skull base lesions that cannot be safely targeted with single fraction ablative doses of radiation. Hypofractionated treatment plans vary widely in both prescribed dose and fraction number depending on morphology of the lesion and proximity to sensitive structures.[52] This approach appears to be safe and well-tolerated and may afford some level of tumor control, though further investigation is needed to confirm this assertion.[53]

Open questions about SRS include its role as an upfront treatment compared to surgery, and its position in multidisciplinary approach to more aggressive lesions. Comparisons of rates of tumor control for low-grade lesions show similar results between conformal EBRT and SRS, while control rates appear to be slightly better with

Table 19.2 Five-year local control rates for radiation modalities used as adjuvants to incomplete surgical resection for meningioma

Meningioma grade	Conformal radiotherapy (%)	Stereotactic radiosurgery (%)
Grade I	85–100[32,33,55]	86.2–98.5[46,56]
Grade II/III	38–61[35,37]	40–74% (3-year)[57,58]

radiosurgery for high grade lesions (▶ Table 19.2). This conclusion is limited, however, as it is based on comparisons of individually published cohorts rather than randomized trials. One comparison of EBRT and SRS for patients with cavernous sinus meningiomas based on a nonrandomized cohort study has been published and showed comparable rates of tumor control but a superior radiographic response for the SRS group. A firm consensus remains elusive, but these authors suggest that SRS is preferred when tumor volumes are small (< 3 cm) and are sufficiently separated from radiosensitive eloquent structures such as the optic apparatus because of the radiographic response benefit and convenience of a single fraction of therapy for the patient.[54] Larger randomized studies with long-term follow-up of each meningioma grade with EBRT and SRS would help answer the question of which is superior.

19.3.2 Brachytherapy

Local implanted radiation sources, or brachytherapy, have been used to treat many systemic tumors and have been investigated for a variety of brain tumors, primary and metastatic.[59,60] This adjuvant treatment was first attempted for recurrent skull base and malignant or atypical meningiomas, with the intention of boosting the dose provided by EBRT. Although promising in initial studies, the approach has been limited by the need for extensive surgical exposure of the tumor in order to effectively implant the radiation source, as well as by a high rate (27%) of radiation necrosis and wound complications.[61,62]

After the initial studies of brachytherapy placement through wide surgical exposure of meningiomas, stereotactic placement of ^{125}I seeds was attempted and has demonstrated improved local control with a reduction in the complication rates seen with open placement, suggesting that this provides a viable adjuvant therapy for higher grade recurrent tumors.[63] The largest long-term study to date, published in 2017, retrospectively examined the placement of ^{125}I seeds at the time of maximal safe resection for atypical or anaplastic meningioma. This study confirmed high rates of local control compared to historical cohorts, and was similarly limited by high rates of radiation necrosis and wound complications requiring reoperation.[64] Although stereotactic and open surgical placement of brachytherapy seeds have shown impressive local control rates over the last 20 to 30 years, improving technology for external beam high dose radiation has limited this adjuvant modality's utility and it has not become a mainstream therapeutic option. It is instead still currently reserved as a salvage option after recurrence of previously resected, and often previously radiated tumors.

19.3.3 Medical Therapies

Medical therapeutic options represent a field of active study for the management of meningiomas, particularly for more aggressive tumor grades and for recurrent disease. While surgery represents the mainstay of treatment for the vast majority of enlarging or symptomatic meningiomas, on occasion, these tumors recur despite multiple attempts at surgery and/or radiation therapy. In the subset of patients with recurrent meningiomas who are no longer candidates for additional surgery and/or radiation, medical treatment is sometimes considered as a method of salvage therapy.[65] Researchers have sought to take advantage of existing traditional chemotherapeutics, as well as hormonal and targeted therapies. While there are many contemporary studies involving laboratory models that may yield novel agents in the future, the subsequent discussion is limited to medical agents that have been evaluated in clinical trials for recurrent meningioma unresponsive to surgical and radiation therapy.

Medical therapies for recurrent meningiomas fall into one of the following categories: cytotoxic, hormonal, and targeted molecular agents—including angiogenesis inhibitors, and immunomodulatory.

Cytotoxic

Cytotoxic agents, by definition, preferentially target rapidly dividing cells. Temozolomide, irinotecan, and hydroxyurea are three such traditional chemotherapeutics that have been formally investigated for use in meningioma.

Temozolomide is an alkylating agent that has shown great efficacy in treatment of glioblastomas.[66] However, in a phase II study in which temozolomide was administered to patients with meningiomas refractory to surgery and RT, zero of 16 patients exhibited a response to therapy.[67] Irinotecan is a topoisomerase-1 inhibitor that had previously been shown to exhibit inhibitory effects in experimental models of malignant meningioma.[68] In a phase II trial of 16 patients with meningiomas refractory to treatment with surgery and RT, the study was stopped prematurely after zero patients demonstrated PFS benefit at 6 months.[65] In initial reports, hydroxyurea—a ribonucleotide reductase inhibitor that arrests the cell cycle in S phase and induces apoptosis—was linked to significant benefit in clinical outcomes in patients with recurrent or unresectable meningiomas.[69,70] However, many of the initial studies that reported efficacy were limited by poor design.[71] A subsequent retrospective series of 60 patients conducted by Chamberlain et al demonstrated a 6-month PFS rate of only 10%. None of the patients demonstrated radiographic regression.[72] Chamberlain et al also reported

the results of treatment with hydroxyurea in 35 patients with grade II and grade III recurrent meningiomas; in this study, a 6-month (PFS) of only 3% was noted.[73] A more recent trial with hydroxyurea and imatinib, a Bcr-Abl tyrosine kinase inhibitor, demonstrated modest antitumor activity a 6-month PFS of 67%.[74] Collectively, these studies have led many to conclude there are no cytotoxic agents that offer consistent efficacy in controlling the growth of recurrent meningiomas.[71,75]

Hormonal

Interest in hormonal therapy for treatment of recurrent meningiomas arose following the discovery of high expression of hormone receptors in these tumor cells. Previous reports have noted the presence of progesterone and estrogen receptors in 76% and 19% of meningiomas, respectively.[76] A number of progesterone antagonists have been investigated for efficacy in treatment of recurrent meningiomas. In a small prospective clinical trial, megestrol did not show any significant antitumor activity.[76] Despite promising results in initial trials, a phase III clinical trial of another oral antiprogestational agent (mifepristone) also failed to demonstrate any significant clinical benefit.[77] This failure was later hypothesized to relate to a loss of progesterone receptor expression noted with progression in meningioma grade.[78] A phase II study of 19 patients investigating tamoxifen, an estrogen receptor antagonist, also demonstrated minimal efficacy.[79]

Among hormonal agents, somatostatin has perhaps generated the most interest. Meningiomas have been found to express a high density of somatostatin receptors—particularly the sst2A subtype.[80] In a study of 16 patients confirmed to have tumor-associated somatostatin receptors using ^{111}In-octreotide single-photon emission computed tomography (SPECT) imaging, 31% of patients demonstrated a partial radiographic response, with 44% achieving PFS at 6 months following treatment with a long-acting somatostatin analog (Sandostatin LA).[80] This algorithm has been associated with positive outcomes following treatment with octreotide in other reports.[75] Initial optimism with pasireotide, a long-acting somatostatin analog with a wider affinity for the spectrum of somatostatin receptors, faded after a phase II trial of 34 patients demonstrated limited to no effect of the number of patients with PFS survival at 6 months. This study did, however, note an increase in PFS in tumors that expressed somatostatin receptor 3, suggesting that further study in this subset of meningiomas may be warranted.[81]

Molecularly Targeted Therapy

Molecularly targeted therapy is a third area of active study today, of particular interest as our understanding of meningioma tumorigenesis continues to grow. Targets of small molecule inhibitors are typically growth factor receptors or downstream signaling molecules in pathways that drive tumor growth.[71] Platelet-derived growth factor (PDGF) and epidermal growth factor (EGF) are two such small molecules that have been identified as antiapoptotic factors in meningioma growth.[82] In a phase II trial of 23 patients, Wen et al evaluated imatinib, an inhibitor of the PDGF receptor pathway, and found that it was well-tolerated but had a minimal effect on tumor control. In this study, 0% PFS at 6 months in the atypical and malignant meningioma groups was noted.[78] In a subsequent trial of imatinib and hydroxyurea, no patient achieved a radiographic response—although 62% of patients were noted to have achieved radiographic PFS at 6 months.[74] Two combination antagonists of PDGF and vascular-endothelial growth factor (VEGF) receptors (VEGFRs) have demonstrated some evidence of clinical efficacy in phase II trials. In 25 patients given the combination antagonist vatalanib, one patient showed a partial radiologic response and 15 remained stable at 6-month evaluation.[83] Recent phase II data has also identified sunitinib as a potential agent for recurrent meningioma, with some patients demonstrating dramatic radiographic response. Treatment with sunitinib resulted in median PFS of 5.2 months; survival was noted to be significantly higher in VEGFR2-positive patients.[84,85] Bevacizumab is a monoclonal antibody that binds to and directly inhibits VEGF, inhibiting angiogenesis. In a retrospective study of 15 patients, this agent was associated with a 6-month

PFS of 43.8% in a cohort of anaplastic and atypical meningiomas.[86] Lastly, EGF receptors have also been studied in meningioma tumorigenesis.[87] However, in two separate phase II trials, no survival benefit was shown with the EGFR antagonists, gefitinib or erlotinib.[71]

Immunomodulatory

Immunomodulators represent the final class of medical therapy directed against recurrent meningiomas. Only one immunomodulator, interferon-alpha 2B, has been evaluated in a phase II trial. In this study, zero of 35 patients with recurrent grade I meningiomas experienced a complete or partial radiographic response. A PFS at 6 months of 54% was reported in this study.[88]

In 2011, the National Comprehensive Cancer Network (NCCN) published guidelines in which the use of three agents (hydroxyurea, interferon-alpha, and sandostatin) for treatment of recurrent meningiomas was advocated. Review of the data in ▶ Table 19.3 supports consideration for sandostatin and interferon-alpha in recurrent meningiomas. However, the phase II clinical data in support of hydroxyurea is less compelling. In addition to the agents referenced in the NCCN report, recent trials assessing targeted molecular antagonists of PDGF and/or VEGF appear to demonstrate promising results. Although an ideal medical therapy for meningioma has not been identified, substantial progress has been made in the study of agents

Table 19.3 Summary of studies evaluating medical treatment of recurrent meningiomas

Study, Year	Phase	Agent	N	Grade I	Grade II	Grade III	% RR	6-m PFS	Summary
Chamberlain, 2004[67]	II	Temozolomide	16	NS	NS	NS	0%	0%	No clinical efficacy shown.
Chamberlain, 2006[65]	II	irinotecan	16	100%	0%	0%	0%	6%	No clinical efficacy shown.
Chamberlain, 2011[72]	N/A	Hydroxyurea	60	100%	0%	0%	0%	10%	Minimal clinical efficacy shown.
Chamberlain, 2012[73]	N/A	Hydroxyurea	35	0%	63%	37%	0%	3%	Minimal clinical efficacy shown.
Ji, 2015[77]	III	Mifepristone	80/84*	NS*	NS	NS	1.4%	NS	No survival benefit shown.
Chamberlain, 2007[80]	Pilot	Somatostatin	16	NS	NS	NS	31%	44%	Some clinical efficacy shown.
Wen, 2009[78]	II	Imatinib	23	57%	22%	22%	0%	29%	Some clinical efficacy shown.
Raizer, 2011[83]	II	Vatalanib	21	0	67%	33%	5%	38%	Some clinical efficacy shown.
Kaley, 2015[85]	II	Sunitinib	36	0%	83%	17%	6%	42%	Some clinical efficacy shown.
Chamberlain, 2008[88]	II	IFN-alpha 2B	35	100%	0%	0%	0%	54%	Some clinical efficacy shown.

*Study included 80 in mifepristone group and 84 in placebo group. Report did note 8 atypical meningiomas in mifepristone group and 9 in placebo group.
6-m PFS: 6-month progression-free survival; IFN, interferon; NS: not specified; RR: radiographic response (e.g., percentage of patients in which medical therapy results in significant decrease in tumor volume.

for recurrent or aggressive disease and the landscape of management options for these tumors is continuing to change over time.

19.4 Conclusion

The long-term management of meningioma is dictated by tumor grade, as WHO grade I, II, and III tumors represent very different illnesses. Low-grade meningioma is best approached as a chronic disease: indolent and potentially recurrent with the ability to affect survival and quality of life over time. High-grade meningioma is an aggressive tumor with poor long-term survival. This knowledge in the simplest sense helps guide frequency of follow-up and the delivery of adjunctive therapies. Additional granularity is added to the calculation of recurrence risk with the index of cellular proliferation, brain invasion, and other intrinsic factors, as well as extent of resection defined by Simpson grade. External delivery of radiation is the mainstay of adjunctive therapies for meningioma when required, either in the form of EBRT or SRS. Brachytherapy remains an experimental option, as do the various medical therapies currently being investigated. Further research in the areas of combination therapies and molecularly targeted therapy is poised to remodel the algorithm for managing meningioma.

References

[1] Simpson D. The recurrence of intracranial meningiomas after surgical treatment. J Neurol Neurosurg Psychiatry. 1957; 20(1): 22–39

[2] Winther TL, Torp SH. Significance of the extent of resection in modern neurosurgical practice of World Health Organization grade I meningiomas. World Neurosurg. 2017; 99:104–110

[3] Gousias K, Schramm J, Simon M. The Simpson grading revisited: aggressive surgery and its place in modern meningioma management. J Neurosurg. 2016; 125(3):551–560

[4] Gallagher MJ, Jenkinson MD, Brodbelt AR, Mills SJ, Chavredakis E. WHO grade 1 meningioma recurrence: are location and Simpson grade still relevant? Clin Neurol Neurosurg. 2016; 141:117–121

[5] Bindal R, Goodman JM, Kawasaki A, Purvin V, Kuzma B. The natural history of untreated skull base meningiomas. Surg Neurol. 2003; 59(2):87–92, discussion 92

[6] McGovern SL, Aldape KD, Munsell MF, Mahajan A, DeMonte F, Woo SY. A comparison of World Health Organization tumor grades at recurrence in patients with non-skull base and skull base meningiomas. J Neurosurg. 2010; 112(5):925–933

[7] Mathiesen T, Lindquist C, Kihlström L, Karlsson B. Recurrence of cranial base meningiomas. Neurosurgery. 1996; 39(1):2–7, discussion 8–9

[8] Li D, Tang J, Ren C, Wu Z, Zhang L-W, Zhang J-T. Surgical management of medium and large petroclivalmeningiomas: a single institution's experience of 199 cases with long-term follow-up. Acta Neurochir (Wien). 2016; 158(3):409–425, discussion 425

[9] Nanda A, Thakur JD, Sonig A, Missios S. Microsurgical resectability, outcomes, and tumor control in meningiomas occupying the cavernous sinus. J Neurosurg. 2016; 125(2):378–392

[10] Ohba S, Kobayashi M, Horiguchi T, et al. Long-term surgical outcome and biological prognostic factors in patients with skull base meningiomas. J Neurosurg. 2011; 114(5):1278–1287

[11] Ichinose T, Goto T, Ishibashi K, Takami T, Ohata K. The role of radical microsurgical resection in multimodal treatment for skull base meningioma. J Neurosurg. 2010; 113(5):1072–1078

[12] Natarajan SK, Sekhar LN, Schessel D, Morita A. Petroclivalmeningiomas: multimodality treatment and outcomes at long-term follow-up. Neurosurgery. 2007; 60(6):965–979, discussion 979–981

[13] Ildan F, Erman T, Göçer AI, et al. Predicting the probability of meningioma recurrence in the preoperative and early postoperative period: a multivariate analysis in the midterm follow-up. Skull Base. 2007; 17(3):157–171

[14] Perry A, Stafford SL, Scheithauer BW, Suman VJ, Lohse CM. Meningioma grading: an analysis of histologic parameters. Am J Surg Pathol. 1997; 21(12):1455–1465

[15] Dijkstra M, van Nieuwenhuizen D, Stalpers LJA, et al. Late neurocognitive sequelae in patients with WHO grade I meningioma. J Neurol Neurosurg Psychiatry. 2009; 80(8):910–915

[16] Sughrue ME, Kane AJ, Shangari G, et al. The relevance of Simpson Grade I and II resection in modern neurosurgical treatment of World Health Organization Grade I meningiomas. J Neurosurg. 2010; 113(5):1029–1035

[17] Mendenhall WM, Morris CG, Amdur RJ, Foote KD, Friedman WA. Radiotherapy alone or after subtotal resection for benign skull base meningiomas. Cancer. 2003; 98(7):1473–1482

[18] Chohan MO, Ryan CT, Singh R, et al. Predictors of treatment response and survival outcomes in meningioma recurrence with atypical or anaplastic histology. Neurosurgery. 2017(June)

[19] Wang Y-C, Chuang C-C, Wei K-C, et al. Skull base atypical meningioma: long term surgical outcome and prognostic factors. Clin Neurol Neurosurg. 2015; 128:112–116

[20] Aizer AA, Bi WL, Kandola MS, et al. Extent of resection and overall survival for patients with atypical and malignant meningioma. Cancer. 2015; 121(24):4376–4381

[21] Aizer AA, Abedalthagafi M, Bi WL, et al. A prognostic cytogenetic scoring system to guide the adjuvant management of patients with atypical meningioma. Neuro-oncol. 2016; 18(2):269–274

[22] Aizer AA, Arvold ND, Catalano P, et al. Adjuvant radiation therapy, local recurrence, and the need for salvage therapy in atypical meningioma. Neuro-oncol. 2014; 16(11):1547–1553

[23] Pearson BE, Markert JM, Fisher WS, et al. Hitting a moving target: evolution of a treatment paradigm for atypical meningiomas amid changing diagnostic criteria. Neurosurg Focus. 2008; 24(5):E3

[24] Sughrue ME, Sanai N, Shangari G, Parsa AT, Berger MS, McDermott MW. Outcome and survival following primary and repeat surgery for World Health Organization Grade III meningiomas. J Neurosurg. 2010; 113(2):202–209

[25] Perry A, Scheithauer BW, Stafford SL, Lohse CM, Wollan PC. "Malignancy" in meningiomas: a clinicopathologic study of 116 patients, with grading implications. Cancer. 1999; 85(9):2046–2056

[26] de Almeida AN, Pereira BJA, Pires Aguiar PH, et al. Clinical outcome, tumor recurrence, and causes of death: A long-term follow-up of surgically treated meningiomas. World Neurosurg. 2017; 102: 139–143

[27] Balasubramanian SK, Sharma M, Silva D, et al. Longitudinal experience with WHO Grade III (anaplastic) meningiomas at a single institution. J Neurooncol. 2017; 131(3):555–563

[28] Durand A, Labrousse F, Jouvet A, et al. WHO grade II and III meningiomas: a study of prognostic factors. J Neurooncol. 2009; 95(3):367–375

[29] Vranic A, Popovic M, Cör A, Prestor B, Pizem J. Mitotic count, brain invasion, and location are independent predictors of recurrence-free survival in primary atypical and malignant meningiomas: a study of 86 patients. Neurosurgery. 2010; 67(4):1124–1132

[30] Chohan MO, Levin AM, Singh R, et al. Three-dimensional volumetric measurements in defining endoscope-guided giant adenoma surgery outcomes. Pituitary. 2016; 19(3):311–321

[31] Noel G, Gondi V. Proton therapy for tumors of the base of the skull. Linchuang Zhongliuxue Zazhi. 2016; 5(4):51

[32] Minniti G, Amichetti M, Enrici RM. Radiotherapy and radiosurgery for benign skull base meningiomas. Radiat Oncol. 2009; 4(1):42

[33] Wenkel E, Thornton AF, Finkelstein D, et al. Benign meningioma: partially resected, biopsied, and recurrent intracranial tumors treated with combined proton and photon radiotherapy. Int J Radiat Oncol Biol Phys. 2000; 48(5):1363–1370

[34] Choi Y, Lim DH, Jo K, Nam DH, Seol H-J, Lee J-I. Efficacy of post-operative radiotherapy for high grade meningiomas. J Neurooncol. 2014; 119(2):405–412

[35] Hug EB, Devries A, Thornton AF, et al. Management of atypical and malignant meningiomas: role of high-dose, 3D-conformal radiation therapy. J Neurooncol. 2000; 48(2):151–160

[36] Talacchi A, Muggiolu F, De Carlo A, Nicolato A, Locatelli F, Meglio M. Recurrent atypical meningiomas: combining surgery and radiosurgery in one effective multimodal treatment. World Neurosurg. 2016; 87:565–572

[37] Boskos C, Feuvret L, Noel G, et al. Combined proton and photon conformal radiotherapy for intracranial atypical and malignant meningioma. Int J Radiat Oncol Biol Phys. 2009; 75(2):399–406

[38] Noël G, Habrand J-L, Mammar H, et al. Highly conformal therapy using proton component in the management of meningiomas. Preliminary experience of the Centre de Protonthérapie d'Orsay. Strahlenther Onkol. 2002; 178(9):480–485

[39] Combs SE, Kessel K, Habermehl D, Haberer T, Jäkel O, Debus J. Proton and carbon ion radiotherapy for primary brain tumors and tumors of the skull base. Acta Oncol. 2013; 52(7):1504–1509

[40] Fong C, Nagasawa DT, Chung LK, et al. Systematic analysis of outcomes for surgical resection and radiotherapy in patients with papillary meningioma. J Neurol Surg B Skull Base. 2015; 76(4):252–256

[41] Soldà F, Wharram B, De Ieso PB, Bonner J, Ashley S, Brada M. Long-term efficacy of fractionated radiotherapy for benign meningiomas. Radiother Oncol. 2013; 109(2):330–334

[42] Zachenhofer I, Wolfsberger S, Aichholzer M, et al. Gamma Knife radiosurgery for cranial base meningiomas: experience of tumor control, clinical course, and morbidity in a follow-up of more than 8 years. Neurosurgery. 2006; 58(1):28–36, discussion 28–36

[43] Igaki H, Maruyama K, Koga T, et al. Stereotactic radiosurgery for skull base meningioma. Neurol Med Chir (Tokyo). 2009; 49(10):456–461

[44] Kreil W, Luggin J, Fuchs I, Weigl V, Eustacchio S, Papaefthymiou G. Long term experience of gamma knife radiosurgery for benign skull base meningiomas. J Neurol Neurosurg Psychiatry. 2005; 76(10):1425–1430

[45] Chuang C-C, Chang C-N, Tsang N-M, et al. Linear accelerator-based radiosurgery in the management of skull base meningiomas. J Neurooncol. 2004; 66(1–2):241–249

[46] Sheehan JP, Williams BJ, Yen CP. Stereotactic radiosurgery for WHO grade I meningiomas. J Neurooncol. 2010; 99(3):407–416

[47] Han JH, Kim DG, Chung H-T, et al. Gamma knife radiosurgery for skull base meningiomas: long-term radiologic and clinical outcome. Int J Radiat Oncol Biol Phys. 2008; 72(5):1324–1332

[48] Santacroce A, Walier M, Régis J, et al. Long-term tumor control of benign intracranial meningiomas after radiosurgery in a series of 4565 patients. Neurosurgery. 2012; 70(1):32–39, discussion 39

[49] Starke R, Kano H, Ding D, et al. Stereotactic radiosurgery of petroclival meningiomas: a multicenter study. J Neurooncol. 2014; 119(1):169–176

[50] Flannery TJ, Kano H, Lunsford LD, et al. Long-term control of petroclival meningiomas through radiosurgery. J Neurosurg. 2010; 112(5):957–964

[51] Starke RM, Nguyen JH, Rainey J, et al. Gamma Knife surgery of meningiomas located in the posterior fossa: factors predictive of outcome and remission. J Neurosurg. 2011; 114(5):1399–1409

[52] Gorman L, Ruben J, Myers R, Dally M. Role of hypofractionated stereotactic radiotherapy in treatment of skull base meningiomas. J Clin Neurosci. 2008; 15(8):856–862

[53] Navarria P, Pessina F, Cozzi L, et al. Hypofractionated stereotactic radiation therapy in skull base meningiomas. J Neurooncol. 2015; 124(2):283–289

[54] Metellus P, Régis J, Muracciole X, et al. Evaluation of fractionated radiotherapy and gamma knife radiosurgery in cavernous sinus meningiomas: treatment strategy. Neurosurgery. 2005; 57(5):873–886, discussion 873–886

[55] Noël G, Bollet MA, Calugaru V, et al. Functional outcome of patients with benign meningioma treated by 3D conformal irradiation with a combination of photons and protons. Int J Radiat Oncol Biol Phys. 2005; 62(5):1412–1422

[56] Pinzi V, Biagioli E, Roberto A, et al. Radiosurgery for intracranial meningiomas: A systematic review and meta-analysis. Crit Rev Oncol Hematol. 2017; 113:122–134

[57] Aboukais R, Zairi F, Lejeune J-P, et al. Grade 2 meningioma and radiosurgery. J Neurosurg. 2015; 122(5):1157–1162

[58] Choi CYH, Soltys SG, Gibbs IC, et al. Cyberknife stereotactic radiosurgery for treatment of atypical (WHO grade II) cranial meningiomas. Neurosurgery. 2010; 67(5):1180–1188

[59] Kumar PP, Good RR, Jones EO, et al. A new method for treatment of unresectable, recurrent brain tumors with single permanent high-activity 125iodine brachytherapy. Radiat Med. 1986; 4(1):12–20

[60] Bernstein M, Gutin PH. Interstitial irradiation of skull base tumours. Can J NeurolSci. 1985; 12(4):366–370

[61] Gutin PH, Leibel SA, Hosobuchi Y, et al. Brachytherapy of recurrent tumors of the skull base and spine with iodine-125 sources. Neurosurgery. 1987; 20(6):938–945

[62] Ware ML, Larson DA, Sneed PK, Wara WW, McDermott MW. Surgical resection and permanent brachytherapy for recurrent atypical and malignant meningioma. Neurosurgery. 2004; 54(1):55–63, discussion 63–64

[63] Kumar PP, Patil AA, Syh HW, Chu WK, Reeves MA. Role of brachytherapy in the management of the skull base meningioma. Treatment of skull base meningiomas. Cancer. 1993; 71(11):3726–3731

[64] Magill ST, Lau D, Raleigh DR, Sneed PK, Fogh SE, McDermott MW. Surgical resection and interstitial Iodine-125 brachytherapy for high-grade meningiomas: A 25-year series. Neurosurgery. 2017; 80(3):409–416

[65] Chamberlain MC, Tsao-Wei DD, Groshen S. Salvage chemotherapy with CPT-11 for recurrent meningioma. J Neurooncol. 2006; 78(3):271–276

[66] Dresemann G. Temozolomide in malignant glioma. Onco Targets Ther. 2010; 3:139–146

[67] Chamberlain MC, Tsao-Wei DD, Groshen S. Temozolomide for treatment-resistant recurrent meningioma. Neurology. 2004; 62(7):1210–1212

[68] Gupta V, Su YS, Samuelson CG, et al. Irinotecan: a potential new chemotherapeutic agent for atypical or malignant meningiomas. J Neurosurg. 2007; 106(3):455–462

[69] Schrell UM, Rittig MG, Anders M, et al. Hydroxyurea for treatment of unresectable and recurrent meningiomas. II. Decrease in the size of meningiomas in patients treated with hydroxyurea. J Neurosurg. 1997; 86(5):840–844

[70] Mason WP, Gentili F, Macdonald DR, Hariharan S, Cruz CR, Abrey LE. Stabilization of disease progression by hydroxyurea in patients with recurrent or unresectable meningioma. J Neurosurg. 2002; 97(2):341–346

[71] Moazzam AA, Wagle N, Zada G. Recent developments in chemotherapy for meningiomas: a review. Neurosurg Focus. 2013; 35(6):E18

[72] Chamberlain MC, Johnston SK. Hydroxyurea for recurrent surgery and radiation refractory meningioma: a retrospective case series. J Neurooncol. 2011; 104(3):765–771

[73] Chamberlain MC. Hydroxyurea for recurrent surgery and radiation refractory high-grade meningioma. J Neurooncol. 2012; 107(2):315–321

[74] Reardon DA, Norden AD, Desjardins A, et al. Phase II study of Gleevec® plus hydroxyurea (HU) in adults with progressive or recurrent meningioma. J Neurooncol. 2012; 106(2):409–415

[75] Rammo R, Rock A, Transou A, Raghunathan A, Rock J. Anaplastic meningioma: octreotide therapy for a case of recurrent and progressive intracranial disease. J Neurosurg. 2016; 124(2):496–500

[76] Grunberg SM, Weiss MH. Lack of efficacy of megestrol acetate in the treatment of unresectable meningioma. J Neurooncol. 1990; 8(1):61–65

[77] Ji Y, Rankin C, Grunberg S, et al. Double-blind phase III randomized trial of the antiprogestin agent mifepristone in the treatment of unresectable meningioma: SWOG S9005. J Clin Oncol. 2015; 33(34): 4093–4098

[78] Wen PY, Yung WKA, Lamborn KR, et al. Phase II study of imatinibmesylate for recurrent meningiomas (North American Brain Tumor Consortium study 01–08). Neuro-oncol. 2009; 11(6):853–860

[79] Goodwin JW, Crowley J, Eyre HJ, Stafford B, Jaeckle KA, Townsend JJ. A phase II evaluation of tamoxifen in unresectable or refractory meningiomas: a Southwest Oncology Group study. J Neurooncol. 1993; 15(1):75–77

[80] Chamberlain MC, Glantz MJ, Fadul CE. Recurrent meningioma: salvage therapy with long-acting somatostatin analogue. Neurology. 2007; 69(10):969–973

[81] Norden AD, Ligon KL, Hammond SN, et al. Phase II study of monthly pasireotide LAR (SOM230C) for recurrent or progressive meningioma. Neurology. 2015; 84(3):280–286

[82] Sherman WJ, Raizer JJ. Chemotherapy: What is its role in meningioma? Expert Rev Neurother. 2012; 12(10):1189–1195, quiz 1196

[83] Raizer JJ, Grimm SA, Rademaker A, et al. A phase II trial of PTK787/ZK 222584 in recurrent or progressive radiation and surgery refractory meningiomas. J Neurooncol. 2014; 117(1):93–101

[84] Raheja A, Colman H, Palmer CA, Couldwell WT. Dramatic radiographic response resulting in cerebrospinal fluid rhinorrhea associated with sunitinib therapy in recurrent atypical meningioma: case report. J Neurosurg. 2016(December):1–6

[85] Kaley TJ, Wen P, Schiff D, et al. Phase II trial of sunitinib for recurrent and progressive atypical and anaplastic meningioma. Neuro-oncol. 2015; 17(1):116–121

[86] Nayak L, Iwamoto FM, Rudnick JD, et al. Atypical and anaplastic meningiomas treated with bevacizumab. J Neurooncol. 2012; 109(1): 187–193

[87] Carroll RS, Black PM, Zhang J, et al. Expression and activation of epidermal growth factor receptors in meningiomas. J Neurosurg. 1997; 87(2):315–323

[88] Chamberlain MC, Glantz MJ. Interferon-alpha for recurrent World Health Organization grade 1 intracranial meningiomas. Cancer. 2008; 113(8):2146–2151

20 Complications in the Management of Skull Base Meningioma

Deopujari CE, Vikram S. Karmarkar

Abstract

Skull base meningiomas pose a formidable surgical challenge to the neurosurgeon. A study of their surgical management offers a window into the evolution of neurosurgical techniques over the last century. Various aspects of skull base meningiomas have been discussed earlier in other chapters of this book. Here we attempt to give an overview of the location and approach related complications during surgical treatment, their avoidance, and strategies for corrections.

Keywords: skull base, meningioma, complications, adverse events, transcranial approach, transnasal endoscopic approach, CSF leak, skull base repair

20.1 Overview

Mastering the art of avoidance of both intraoperative and postoperative problems is a key factor in operative excellence and optimization of outcome.— Michael L. J. Apuzzo.[1]

All disease conditions and their management carry the inherent possibility of complications. Complications may be termed as adverse effects or undesired consequences of a disease, either in the diagnosis or its treatment. There have been differing views of what constitutes a complication after surgery and numerous attempts have been made to classify these events into medical or surgical, minor or major, or to grade them according to severity.[1] This is useful to assess outcomes as well as compare the techniques or treatment methods. A recent addition to this has been the detailed grading of neurosurgical complications by Ibanez L et al.[2]

Meningiomas have always held a special place in the hearts and minds of neurosurgeons. Although the first successful surgical excision of an olfactory groove meningioma is credited to Durante F in 1885,[3] it was in the era of Cushing and others, that many of our current concepts have crystallized. Harvey Cushing, in his Cavendish lecture of 1922, stated, "There is today, nothing in the whole realm of this surgery, more gratifying than the successful removal of meningioma with subsequent functional recovery, especially should a correct pathological diagnosis have been previously made. The difficulties are admittedly great, sometimes insurmountable and though the disappointments still are many, another generation of neurological surgeons will unquestionably see them largely overcome."[4]

With modern imaging, a correct pathological diagnosis for the meningioma (a term coined by Cushing) has been possible in majority of cases. Several generations of neurological surgeons have tried to surmount the challenges with technical advances in hemostasis, drilling techniques for access and microscope or endoscopic visualization, resulting in remarkable improvements in morbidity and mortality. Although, the majority of complications related to the surgery and postoperative period have considerably reduced, newer techniques of access to various locations have posed new challenges. This chapter aims to describe and analyze the location and approach related complications in skull base meningioma surgery, along with possible measures of avoidance and treatment.

The surgical goal is complete elimination of the tumor along with involved dura and bone followed by monitoring for residual or recurrent disease, and then tackling this with repeat surgery or adjunctive treatment. To this end, several classifications have been proposed and validated. The Simpsons grading[5] is the most common grading scheme for extent of resection and predicting of recurrence, whereas the Levine-Sekhar classification and its variants have been validated for prediction of resectability of skull base meningiomas.[6] Most neurosurgeons have their own philosophy for treatment of this lesion, from the very aggressive to the more cautionary.[7] Meningiomas at the base of the skull are particularly challenging for preservation of the nerves and vessels running along the base, as also for the reconstruction of the skull base.

20.2 Preoperative Factors for Prediction of Complications

20.2.1 Clinicoradiological Factors

Skull base meningiomas can arise from a wide variety of locations from the olfactory bulb anteriorly to the foramen magnum inferiorly. These lesions come to notice if they cause focal deficits, convulsions, or lobar dysfunction (usually frontal). Unfortunately, in many parts of the world, some of the early symptoms like headache, retro-orbital pain are considered nonspecific, and hence may be ignored by the patients. Therefore, these lesions may attain a large size and multicompartmental involvement may be present by the time they seek medical care.

Larger lesions cause raised intracranial pressure and present with generalized headaches, visual disturbance, and papilledema. Localized headache, seen with convexity meningioma is usually missing in skull base lesions. However, sellar/parasellar tumors can cause an ill localized headache and retro-orbital pain. This is thought to be caused by dural stretch. Sometimes, lesions at the skull base may be found incidentally with no apparent clinical features, during a scan for other reasons, viz., head injury or magnetic resonance (MR) evaluation of the cervical spine. The challenge here is to decide if treatment is needed, what approach and strategies to follow for minimizing complications and optimizing outcomes. Nakamura et al[8] studied the natural history of 47 incidental (majority—skull base) meningiomas and concluded that the rate of growth of these tumors was slow. Most could be followed with serial imaging. Younger patients and higher signal intensity on T2 images were predictive factors for faster growth rate while the presence of calcium and lower signal on T2 suggested lower rates of growth. Others have advocated an observation only policy if the lesion is asymptomatic, reserving the surgical option for patients younger than 65 years of age who have increased in size or become symptomatic on follow-up. Patients older than 65 years, with symptomatic tumors smaller than 3 cm, tend to be treated with stereotactic radiosurgery; symptomatic patients with a larger tumors are usually treated with surgery and adjuvant radiotherapy if necessary.[9] We have usually followed the policy of observation in asymptomatic patients over 65 years in difficult locations.

Radiologic assessment is an integral part of the management and many imaging factors need to be assessed to predict possible complications. **Perilesional edema** is a harbinger of a higher-grade lesion and possible seizures in the perioperative period. The so called "lions mane" which is bifrontal edema due to an anterior skull base meningioma has been shown to extend the postoperative stay (▶ Fig. 20.1). It is also associated with more frontal lobar dysfunction in the perioperative period.[10] The so-called "brain cuff" which is brain edema or a rim of gliotic brain around an anterior skull base meningioma is considered by some a more challenging lesion to manage, especially through the transnasal route.[11,12] More recently, a meta-analysis by Schwartz et al[13] have not found this to be uniformly applicable.

Neural canal involvement must be looked for especially at the optic canal in clinoidal, tuberculum, sellar, and parasellar lesions. Other foramina which can be affected include the foramen rotundum, foramen ovale, internal acoustic meatus, jugular foramen, and hypoglossal canal.

Tumors arising in the cavernous sinus or extending into the cavernous sinus need careful evaluation as vascular and nerve compromise can be expected with aggressive excision. Tumors medial to the carotid are amenable for transnasal endoscopic excision while tumors lateral to the carotid require more extensive skull base transcranial approaches.

CT reveals the degree of hyperostosis, in cases of skull base meningiomas, which needs to be drilled to achieve a more complete excision and decompression. It also reveals the degree of bone erosion, especially of the petrous bone in cases of petroclival or sphenopetroclival meningiomas. This is essential to prevent damage to the

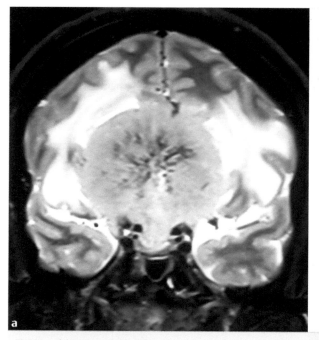
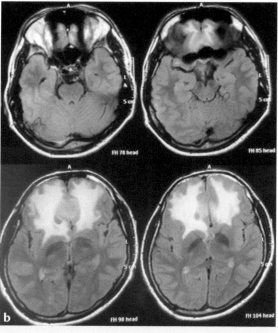

Fig. 20.1 (a) T2-weighted MRI brain (coronal view) showing peritumoral edema in a case of olfactory groove meningioma ("lion's mane appearance"). (b) Fluid-attenuated inversion recovery (FLAIR) images of MRI brain (axial view) showing peritumoral edema of moderate degree in a case of small tuberculum sellae meningioma.

petrous internal carotid artery (ICA) and greater superficial petrosal nerve during tumor resection.

An important component of noninvasive vascular imaging is the CT angiography (CTA) or the MR angiography (MRA). Encasement or displacement of the major arteries and their branches can then be anticipated. This impacts the operative strategy. Imaging should also be carefully analyzed to identify involvement of the adventitia of the ICA to prevent catastrophic bleeding. Identification of a dominant and hypoplastic vertebral artery helps in deciding the safer surgical corridor in cases of anterior foramen magnum meningiomas (▶ Fig. 20.2).

To summarize, the following radiological parameters should be carefully evaluated for avoiding complications during surgery of a skull base meningioma, namely, presence of arterial encasement or invasion, invasion of cavernous sinus, involvement of cranial nerves, orbital invasion, dural or brain invasion, and involvement of the other dural venous sinuses. These factors are not only helpful in selecting a suitable corridor but also to predict and prevent intra- and postoperative complications.

Digital subtraction angiography (DSA) and preoperative embolization of skull base meningiomas has been a strategy in many neurosurgical units. In our opinion today, DSA should be done only if there is a possibility and need for preoperative embolization or carotid sacrifice is being planned. Though a common practice in our department till 2000 was to embolize these tumors; currently, we do not practice the same and our strategy is to begin by detaching the tumor from the skull base, reducing the major blood supply. The supply from the external carotid

artery (ECA) is usually the most amenable for embolization. Variations, "dangerous anastomoses" between ECA and ICA are a potential hazard during embolization and need to be recognized and avoided to prevent cranial nerve deficits.[14]

20.2.2 Multidisciplinary Approach

It is important to emphasize the need of a team approach to tackle these difficult tumors. Ideally, these cases should be performed at a center which has sufficient experience dealing with these tumors. Close collaboration with otorhinolaryngologists, radiologists, interventional radiologists/endovascular surgeons, oncologists, stereotactic radiosurgeons, craniofacial surgeons etc. may be necessary in cases of large and invasive tumors.

20.2.3 Surgeon Factors

Many skull base meningiomas can be treated with equal efficacy using endoscopic skull base approaches instead of the transcranial route. In these cases, surgeon's preference and experience also play a key role in selection of a surgical approach. Availability of intraoperative navigation, micro-Doppler to identify vascular structures, intraoperative electrophysiological monitoring has helped us achieve more radical resections with safety. We have no access to intraoperative MRI and/or CT which may be useful to assess the degree of resection.

20.2.4 Patient Factors

Significant medical comorbidities, prior radiotherapy, prior surgery pose significant challenges in achieving a safe and complete resection of a skull base meningioma.

20.3 Perioperative, Operative Complications and Prevention

20.3.1 Anesthesia Considerations

Anticipation and avoidance of anesthesia related complications needs vigilance and prompt actions. Preoperative assessment and optimization of cardiorespiratory, renal, hepatic, and hematologic parameters is vital. Proper positioning and padding of the pressure points is necessary to prevent position related compression neuropathies. In the supine position, slight flexion of the knees prevents hyperextension and locking of the knee joint. Padding under the elbow prevents damage to the ulnar nerve and padding below the ankle/Achilles tendon is necessary to prevent pressure injury. The head is usually fixed in a skull clamp or supported by soft gel pillow if pin fixation is not used. In the prone position, adequate padding is needed for the chest, pelvis, patellae, and the forefoot. The skull rests on a gel pillow if not immobilized in a skull

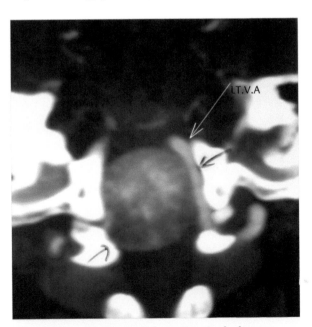

Fig. 20.2 Computed tomography angiogram of a foramen magnum meningioma showing hypoplastic right vertebral artery and displaced left vertebral artery.

clamp. If a gel pillow/horseshoe head holder is used, extreme vigilance is required to ensure there is no pressure on the globes of the eyes. This is to ensure a potentially disastrous pressure induced visual compromise.[15] Lateral positions need care for the dependent part of the body, especially the arm, brachial plexus, and peroneal nerves of the bent, dependent lower limb. For the sitting position, excessive flexion of the neck must be avoided. Occasionally, this can lead to quadriparesis postoperatively.[16] Other possible complications seen with the sitting position include hypotension, air embolism, pneumocephalus, and increased incidence of subdural hemorrhages.

Induction of anesthesia needs to be smooth as some these patients have compensated intracranial pressure. There is a role for a lumbar drain, especially for extended endoscopic skull base procedures. In this case, care must be taken to prevent excess drainage of cerebrospinal fluid (CSF) prior to the excision. This may cause brain shifts and herniation syndromes in larger tumors. Similar vigilance should be exercised with external ventricular drainage.

End tidal carbon dioxide monitoring (EtCO$_2$), oxygenation (SpO$_2$), and blood pressure maintenance are vital for optimal brain perfusion. Strategies where intraoperative neurophysiological monitoring is used include maintaining the level of anesthesia on inhalational agents, intravenous anesthetics, and to avoid paralyzing agents.

20.3.2 Operative Complications

Brain Swelling

For the transcranial approaches, preoperatively, steroids may be started if significant brain edema is noted on the MRI. In these cases, a bolus of 20% mannitol with or without furosemide can be administered during craniotomy to avoid brain swelling. After completion of the bone work, on opening the dura, if brain swelling persists then the following strategy checklist should be used:

- *Position of patient:* Extreme twisting or awkward position of head and neck can hamper venous return and may lead to a full brain. It is best to position the head around 30° above the heart level and to avoid extreme twisting of the neck.
- *Depth of anesthesia and ventilation:* The patient must be adequately under anesthesia. This aids brain relaxation avoiding brain swelling. Various monitoring devices and scales like the bispectral index quantify the depth of anesthesia. Maintenance of carbon dioxide tension also contributes to a lax brain.
- *Bone removal:* Sometimes, additional osteotomies may need to be performed in cases of persistent brain swelling to improve tumor visualization. Some of these manoeuvres include performing at orbitozygomatic osteotomy, orbital bar osteotomies etc. in cases of anterior skull base meningiomas.

- *CSF release:* Early release of CSF from a cistern or the Sylvian fissure can reduce the brain swelling. Alternatively, release of CSF from the lumbar drain or the external ventricular drain has a similar effect.
- *Prevention of venous injury:* It is important to plan and perform the craniotomy meticulously to prevent damage to the dural venous sinuses and major draining veins. The transverse and sigmoid sinuses are at risk while performing a retrosigmoid approach for a posterior petrous meningioma, while the vein of Labbe and the Sylvian veins, sphenoparietal sinus may be at risk while performing a subtemporal approach and fronto-orbitozygomatic osteotomy, respectively.
- *Brain retraction:* Once the brain is lax after the manoeuvres, a brain retractor may be used primarily to provide a clear surgical trajectory.[17]

In case all the above fail, it may be sometimes necessary to resect some part of the brain to create a clear surgical corridor, viz., temporal or frontal polectomy or resection of lateral one-third of cerebellum, which is seldom necessary these days because of excellent anesthetic drugs and monitoring. Some consider it prudent to abandon the procedure and to re-explore after an interval.

During the endonasal approaches, the skull base meningioma is usually directly accessed at the end of skull base drilling and dural opening and then gradually debulked. Hence, brain swelling is usually not a problem. Larger tumors are usually not amenable to transnasal excision.

Hemorrhage

The best way to tackle intraoperative hemorrhage is to anticipate the possibility of hemorrhage. Adequate arrangements for blood transfusion should be made based on the radiological features. Preoperative embolization should be considered in selected cases. Sequential coagulation and disconnection of the lesion usually devascularize the skull base meningioma almost completely, however, pial parasitization of small branches may be seen occasionally. This coupled with internal tumor debulking is the most commonly used technique for excision. Careful dissection from the pial surface is essential to prevent damage to the normal vasculature of the brain. Maintaining the pial-arachnoid plane is the key to prevent "en passant" vessels as well as perforators.

Damage to Neural and Vascular Structures

Meningiomas at the skull base have close contact with one or more cranial nerves, the basal surface of the brain or the brainstem and intracranial blood vessels. Arachnoid is the best protective cover for a cranial nerve and the neuraxis including the brainstem. Careful dissection should be done to dissect the tumor from the cranial nerves and the brainstem, whilst preserving the pia arachnoid layers. Special attention must be paid to the nerves running through the posterior fossa, in cases of posterior fossa skull base meningiomas. Occasionally, some part of these tumors is closely adherent to the adventitia of major blood vessels. Here, it may be prudent to leave some tumor behind to prevent neural/vascular damage (▶ Fig. 20.3). Intraoperative monitoring is extremely useful in these cases to identify the cranial nerves and prevent iatrogenic injury.

Cerebrospinal Fluid Leak

This is probably the most common complication especially following transnasal surgery. This is also seen when the air sinuses are opened in the cranial approaches. Prevention by appropriate approach and reconstruction planning is the best way to avoid this complication. If there is leak despite this, the initial treatment may be conservative, with positioning, lumbar drainage of CSF, and bed rest. If the patient fails conservative treatment, or if there is a high flow leak, re-exploration and repair is

necessary. Strategies for this include multilayer fascia, fat repair, fresh vascularized nasal mucosal flaps, and use of tissue fibrin glue.[18,19] Sometimes, novel methods need to be used, like a pericranial rotation flap or a pedicled free flap.[20] Following transcranial surgery, CSF leaks must be prevented at the time of the primary surgery. For the frontal sinus breach, removing the mucosa, plugging the frontal ostium, and using a pericranial flap to cranialize the sinus is necessary. Similarly, the opened ethmoid, sphenoid sinuses need to be covered with a long enough vascularized pericranial flap from the inferior aspect. For middle and posterior fossa lesions where there is breach of the mastoid cells or internal auditory meatus, there may be a paradoxical CSF rhinorrhea with CSF traversing the eustachian canal into the nasopharynx and then out the nose. In these situations, care must be taken to obliterate the opened mastoid air cells or the internal auditory canal with bone wax, fat, or muscle.[21]

In case of previous surgery or radiation, harvesting of a local pericranial flap may be difficult, in such cases, fascia lata or other artificial dural substitutes may be used.

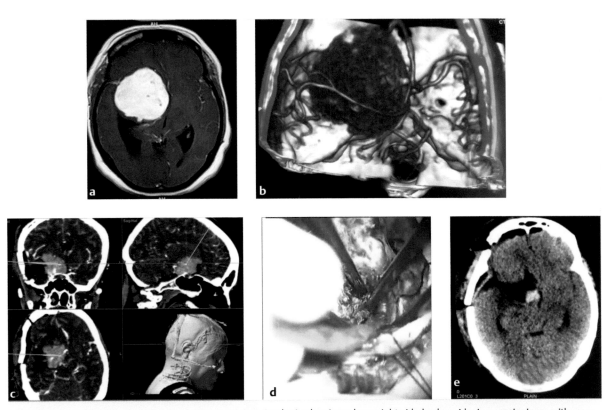

Fig. 20.3 **(a)** Axial postcontrast magnetic resonance imaging brain showing a large right sided sphenoid wing meningioma with mass effect and midline shift to left. **(b)** CT angiogram depicting the meningioma encasing the middle cerebral artery (MCA). **(c)** Navigation snapshots to guide in localization and understanding relationship of major vessels traversing/running around tumor. **(d)** Intraoperative image of the MCA coursing through the meningioma. **(e)** Postoperative CT brain plain showing part of the tumor encasing the MCA left behind.

20.4 Postoperative Complications and Prevention

In the immediate postoperative period, there may systemic disturbances like electrolyte imbalance, drop in hemoglobin in case of bleeding during surgery, etc. These need to be looked for and corrected in the intensive care setting.

Brain edema and hemorrhage and hydrocephalus are concerns after skull base surgery. A control imaging study along with clinical assessment following surgery can help localize these. Minor tumor bed hemorrhage may be left alone and edema needs to be controlled with corticosteroids and dehydrating agents like mannitol and diuretics like furosemide or acetazolamide.

Deep vein thrombosis (DVT) is a known complication of any supratentorial tumor surgery. The rates of DVT are higher in meningiomas and upto 10% rates have been reported, though it may be variable depending upon concurrent medical factors.[22] This study found a positive correlation with higher body mass index, older age, and more than 4 hours of surgical time. Another significant factor for DVT was prolonged immobilization of the patient following surgery. The grade of the tumor did not seem to influence the rates of DVT.

Does a higher grade of tumor mean a higher complication rate? Peritumor brain edema was studied by was studied by Osawa et al.[23] They found that the uncommon grade I meningiomas have more edema than the common grade I or grade II or III tumors.[23] The fact that another therapy modality, radiotherapy is sometimes needed, may increase the morbidity. Is radiation therapy necessary post-surgery for higher grade meningiomas? There is some literature that recommends a wait and watch policy after higher grade tumor excision.[24] Hence, post-surgery complications need not be higher for higher grade tumors if a safe maximal resection can be done. The potential for recurrence though is higher than for lower grade lesions.

Is hydrocephalus a common complication following surgery for skull base meningiomas? Burkhardt et al[25] tried to analyze this question in a large series of cases. They analyzed many possible causes for the development of communicating hydrocephalus after skull base meningioma surgery. The two factors they found significant were age and the duration of the procedure (▶ Fig. 20.4). There have been case reports where patients with small meningiomas have developed communicating hydrocephalus.[26] The hypothesis for this was thought to be a high protein content in the CSF leading to impaired absorption.

Craniovertebral (CV) junction instability is known to occur especially when the tumor at the CV junction has eroded the occipital condyle or the procedure (especially far lateral approaches) has destabilized the occipito-atlantal joints.[27] The images must be analyzed preoperatively, and CV junction stabilization done if instability is anticipated or encountered during surgery (▶ Fig. 20.5).

20.5 Approach-related Problems

These meningiomas may be approached from above the skull base and in selected cases from the inferior aspect through the endoscopic transnasal route.

20.5.1 Transcranial Approaches (▶ Table 20.1, ▶ Table 20.2, and ▶ Table 20.3)

These include:
- Frontal approaches—bifrontal, unifrontal, pterional, supraorbital keyhole.
- Lateral—Temporal, cavernous sinus approaches, petrosectomies, presigmoid.
- Posterior—Lateral posterior or retromastoid and its variants, paramedian and midline suboccipital approach. Foramen magnum lesions can be approached by posterior, posterolateral (far lateral and its variants).
- Combined approach.

CSF leak is possible in any of these. This may manifest as a rhinorrhea, paradoxical rhinorrhea, otorrhea, or may leak from the wound itself. To reiterate, attention needs to be paid to cranializing the frontal sinus, sealing the

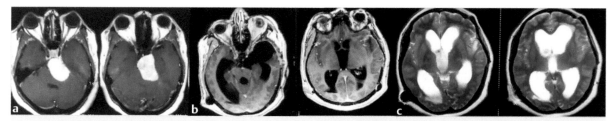

Fig. 20.4 (a) MRI brain post contrast (axial view) showing a petroclival meningioma which was excised by posterior, followed by temporal approach. (b) Follow-up post contrast and (c) T2 weighted magnetic resonance imaging scan after 3 months of definitive surgery showing a delayed onset hydrocephalus after complete excision of the tumor.

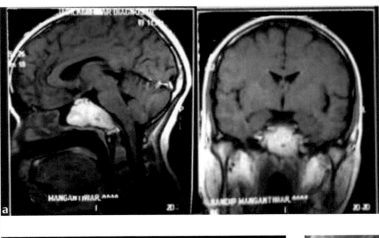
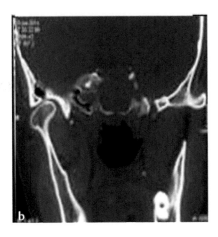
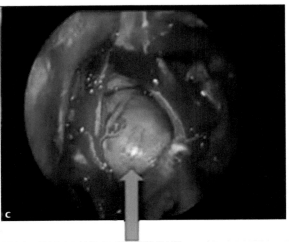
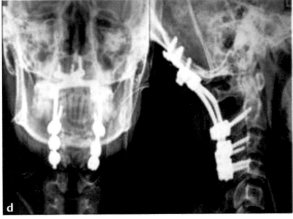

Fig. 20.5 **(a)** Magnetic resonance imaging brain post contrast scan (sagittal and coronal views) showing an enhancing, large, expansile lesion of the clivus involving the sella. **(b)** Computed tomography scan showing involvement of the occipital left condyle. **(c)** Intraoperative image of the tumor protruding into the sphenoid (*arrow*). **(d)** Decision to do occipito-cervical fusion till C4 level taken. Postoperative X-ray cervical spine showing the same.

mastoid air cells, the internal acoustic meatus. Also, careful closure of the dura helps preventing a pseudomeningocele and CSF leak (▶ Fig. 20.6). Tension pneumocephalus may need further intervention. Fortunately, this complication is not very commonly seen except in some cases where the sitting position has been used (▶ Fig. 20.7).

Optic nerve decompression is necessary and decompression is necessary when the optic canal/nerve is involved. Strategies like extradural opening of the optic canal, section of the falciform ligament, and carful sharp dissection of the tumor from the nerve are necessary. During drilling of the optic canal, if the sphenoid sinus or the supraoptic ethmoid air cell (Onodi cell) is opened, it needs repair at the end of the procedure with fat/muscle plug, fascia, and fibrin glue.[28] A technical note to be remembered is, while drilling the skull base especially near the cranial nerve foramina, it is essential to adequately cool the burr with saline irrigation. This is important to prevent thermal injury to the nerves. Preservation of the ophthalmic artery is mandatory and care must be taken of the vascular supply of the chiasm and retrochiasmatic structures. The smaller branches of the ICA like the posterior communicating and the anterior choroidal if damaged can lead to severe focal deficits following internal capsule and brainstem ischemia. The pituitary stalk needs to be recognized and preserved. It can be identified by the vessels that run in it in a longitudinal fashion. Arachnoidal planes need to be preserved where possible. They act as natural barriers and protect their contents.

In the cavernous sinus and lateral approaches, the III, IV, V, and VI nerves need to be recognized. Similarly, in the posterior fossa, the fifth through twelfth nerves need protection as do the branches of the vertebrobasilar trunk. There is usually a layer of arachnoid over the brainstem and the tumor can be separated from it. Rarely,

Table 20.1 Transcranial anterior and anterolateral approaches (frontal uni/bifrontal, supraorbital, frontolateral, transcavernous approaches)

Complication	Prevention	Management
Brain swelling	Planning of craniotomy, durotomy, placement of lumbar drain/EVD where feasible	CSF drainage-cisterns or ventricular tap. Dehydrating agents like mannitol, furosemide Last resort-resection of the pole if safe
Olfactory nerve damage	Avoid direct stretch especially near cribriform plate. Oxidized cellulose and fibrin glue over this point described	
Optic nerve and chiasm	Early identification as nerve may be distorted by lesion. Preservation of vasculature, especially inferior surface	
Oculomotor, trochlear, abducens—these converge in the cavernous sinus lateral wall (except VI)	Avoid tumor dissection in the cavernous sinus if possible. Identification and preservation of nerves. Cisternal segments need to be identified and preserved (IIIrd-lateral to ICA and IV below free edge of tentorium)	Direct repair if both ends visible and accessible or fibrin glue to approximate ends
Trigeminal nerve	Recognition of nerves exiting through the skullbase foramina (SOF, rotundum, ovale) and avoidance of dissection in the cavernous sinus	
Vascular injury—carotid and branches, perforators, veins	Arachnoidal dissection to preserve the adventitia. Leaving behind tumor firmly adherent to the adventitia. Dissection to save perforators	For large vessels, consider low power coagulation for perforator avulsion injury. Direct suture of tear if large. Augmentation of flow with bypass from ECA branches
CSF leak. Unrecognized dural and skull base breach. Alternatively, intentional drilling of skull base to remove pathology	To obliterate the frontal, ethmoid air sinuses if opened during approach. Dural repair with natural substitute like pericranium, fascia, or artificial substitutes like collagen sheets	For unrecognized leaks, attempt to localize leak site (CT/MR Cisternography). May try conservative treatment. If fails re-explore and plug leak
Dural tears during craniotomy, facial nerve injury and temporalis injury	Anticipation of adherent dura and use of high speed drills. Interfascial dissection to avoid frontalis branch of facial nerve. Careful dissection of temporalis muscle and gentle retraction prevent temporalis atrophy	Meticulous dural repair

Abbreviations: CSF, cerebrospinal fluid; ECA, external carotid artery; EVD, external ventricular drain; ICA, internal carotid artery; SOF, superior orbital fissure.

there is pial invasion of the brainstem. Thus, it may be prudent to leave behind tumor adherent to perforators, major blood vessels or cranial nerves than to attempt resection and cause damage to these structures. Injury to branches of facial nerve (frontalis division) during the frontolateral and temporal approaches is possible. This can be prevented by dissecting below the fat pad of the temporalis.[29] Elevation of the temporalis muscle without much thermal energy is important to prevent temporalis muscle atrophy and cosmetic changes postoperatively.[30]

20.5.2 Transnasal Endoscopic Skull Base Approaches (▶ Table 20.4)

The most significant complication of this approach is CSF leak. Prevention requires meticulous planning of the reconstruction before the start of the procedure. Reconstruction can be done by multilayer fat fascia bone/cartilage or using fascia fat and vascularized nasal

mucosal flaps. Care must be taken not to pack the defect with too much fat, especially near the optic apparatus. Vascular injury is the other major complication in these approaches. The course of the internal carotid artery is important to map in these approaches. Adjuncts that help preserve them are image guidance and micro-Doppler probes to insonate the carotid artery. Other structures at risk include the abducens nerve in the cavernous sinus and in the Dorello's canal when doing transclival approaches. All the other cranial nerves and the vertebrobasilar system branches are at risk during intradural dissection.

20.6 Location-related Complications

20.6.1 Olfactory Groove

Meningiomas here pose special challenges transcranially with opening of the frontal sinuses, and potential CSF

Table 20.2 Transcranial lateral and posterolateral approaches (including temporal, petrosal, combined middle and posterior fossa approaches)

Complications	Prevention	Management
Intratemporal damage including ICA, facial nerve and GSPN, inner/middle ear structures	Sound knowledge of anatomy, drybone/cadaver dissection necessary. Image guidance useful during surgery	
Trochlear nerve injury The cisternal portion of the nerve travels under the free edge of the tentorium	Tentorial cuts need to planned. Small caliber nerve—easily stretched or damaged	Direct repair or glue repair if approximation of both ends satisfactory
Trigeminal cisternal portion begins in the posterior fossa and arches over to the Gasserian ganglion and posterior cavernous sinus	Usually a large structure and less prone to complete section	The patient may require tarsorrhaphy, especially if concomitant facial nerve involvement
Venous sinus and vein damage	Venous imaging (MRV and DSA helpful to decide drainage pattern) preserve the temporal lobe draining veins including the superficial MCV, vein of Labbe, basal veins. The transverse/sigmoid sinus should be protected during the exposure and approach	Avoid direct coagulation of the veins; repair venous sinus with suture or patch graft. Where the sinus invaded and blocked, can resect sinus with tumor
CSF leak	This may happen through the mastoid air cells, eustachian tube, nasopharynx, and the nose (paradoxical rhinorrhea). Proper sealing of the opened mastoid cells with bone wax/fat/muscle and fibrin glue required. Dural repair is necessary	Initial conservative treatment, if leak persists, re-exploration and sealing defect to be considered
Arterial injury. petrous carotid artery	Bony landmarks—arcuate eminence. Image guidance in cases where petrous canal eroded/involved	Temporary balloon occlusion with a Fogarty embolectomy catheter inflated proximal to bleed in the canal. Emergency bypass procedure
Dural tears during craniotomy	Anticipation of adherent dura and appropriate use of high speed drills	Meticulous dural repair

Abbreviations: CSF, cerebrospinal fluid; DSA, digital subtraction angiography; GSPN, greater superficial petrosal nerve; ICA, internal carotid artery; MCV, middle cerebral vein; MRV, magnetic resonance venography.

Table 20.3 Transcranial posterior approaches (retromastoid suboccipital, midline suboccipital, far lateral and variants and supracerebellar approaches)

Complications	Prevention	Management
Vascular injury including venous sinus (torcula, transverse, sigmoid), petrosal vein damage	Careful dissection of the dura from the bone and use of high speed drills as necessary	Pressure, gelatin sponge, fibrin glue, other flowable hemostatic agents, suture of sinus walls
Cranial nerve injury (abducens, facial, vestibulocochlear, glossopharyngeal, vagus, accessory, and hypoglossal)	Anatomic landmarks for exit and entry in skull base. Image guidance. Neurophysiological monitoring Preserve arachnoid plane over brainstem	Direct suture or approximation with glue if ends close
Major arterial injury	Best avoided with adequate visualization, anticipation, and dissection. Avoid excessive coagulation over the capsule of the lesion	
CSF leak and pseudomeningocele	Meticulous dural closure and closing all open air cells with bone wax/fat/muscle	Conservative treatment followed by re-exploration and closure of defect

Abbreviation: CSF, cerebrospinal fluid.

leak. Saving olfactory function is variously described by Kanno et al[31] with use of dissection to get length and gluing to the skull base to prevent avulsion during retraction. Brain edema in larger tumors and rarely venous compromise during cutting of the superior sagittal sinus is known. CSF leak from transnasal endoscopic approaches has reduced remarkably using pedicled mucosal flaps.

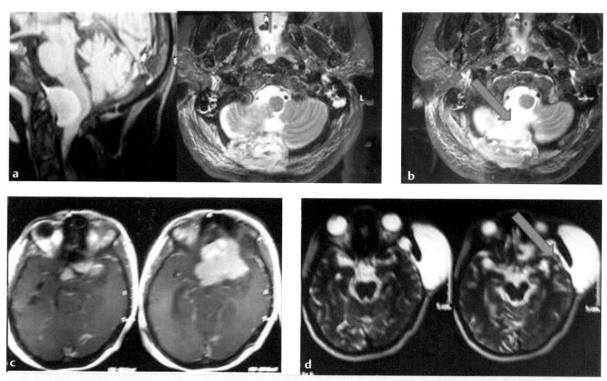

Fig. 20.6 (a) MRI craniovertebral junction post contrast (sagittal view) showing a large foramen magnum meningioma causing brainstem compression. (b) Follow-up T2-weighted image of MRI brain (axial view) showing a postoperative pseudomeningocele with the site of cerebrospinal fluid (CSF) leak seen (arrow). (c) MRI brain post contrast (axial view) showing a left medial sphenoid wing meningioma. (d) Follow-up MRI brain T2-weighted image showing pseudomeningocele with the site of CSF leak (arrow).

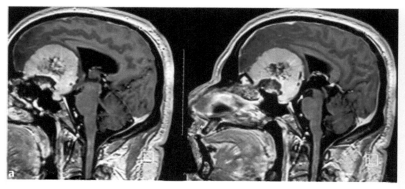

Fig. 20.7 (a) Magnetic resonance imaging brain post contrast (sagittal view) showing an olfactory groove meningioma with calcification and bony hyperostosis. (b) Postoperative computed tomography brain plain showing pneumocephalus.

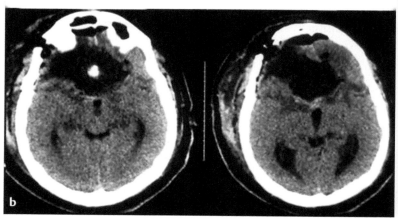

Table 20.4 Endoscopic endonasal methods (planum to C2, and midline to middle fossa in coronal plane)

Complications	Prevention	Management
CSF leak	Planning reconstruction with vascularized mucosal flaps or multilayered closure. Flaps include nasoseptal, lateral nasal, turbinate flaps, nasopharyngeal flap	Lumbar drainage and if significant re-exploration and repair of leak, using different flap or pericranial flaps. Occasionally, free flaps may be used
Vascular injury ICA at risk. Basilar, branches when working on intradural aspect of the meningioma	Thorough knowledge of the vascular anatomy. Use of diamond burr to drill over the artery. Use of micro-Doppler to insonate and locate Careful dissection of the large vessels	If major arterial bleed in skull base, pack and wait. If bleeding from small perforator, may be coagulated with bipolar coagulation Early angiography to look for pseudoaneurysm. If seen, needs treatment (commonly endovascular)
Cranial nerve injury (olfactory, optic, trigeminal, abducens)	Copious saline irrigation while drilling the base near the exiting cranial nerves. Use diamond burrs for skull base drilling near nerve foramina. Dissecting tumor away from the nerve. Maintain vascularity of the chiasm. Avoid dissection in the cavernous sinus lateral to the carotid artery	

Abbreviations: CSF, cerebrospinal fluid; ICA, internal carotid artery.

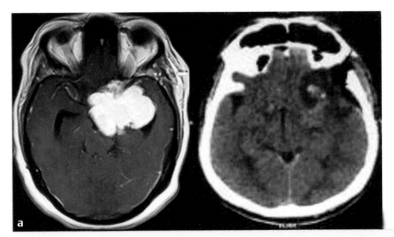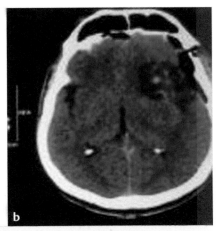

Fig. 20.8 (a) Magnetic resonance imaging brain post contrast (axial view) showing a left medial sphenoid wing meningioma with mass effect. **(b)** Postoperatively patient developed transient Broca's aphasia due to cerebral edema seen on computed tomography brain plain. Aphasia resolved completely over 2 weeks.

20.6.2 Planum and Tuberculum Sellae

During transcranial approaches, the optic nerve or chiasm may be prone to injury as also the large arteries at the base of the skull. Special care of the pituitary stalk must be ensured to prevent long-term hormone and electrolyte imbalances. In the endoscopic approaches, the normal pituitary gland, infundibulum, and arteries are at risk.

20.6.3 Cavernous Sinus/Parasellar

Special care must be taken of the cranial nerves and the ICA in either approach as the cavernous sinus and parasellar space is densely filled with vital neurovascular structures.

20.6.4 Sphenoid Wing Meningioma

These are usually treated with the transcranial approaches and cerebral edema, middle cerebral artery (MCA) injury, optic nerve injury (clinoidal meningioma) must be anticipated and avoided (▶ Fig. 20.8).

20.6.5 Middle Cranial Fossa Meningioma

Again, the transcranial approach is the commonly utilized path and injury to the trigeminal nerve and the ICA and its branches must be avoided. Traction on the greater superficial petrosal nerve is to be avoided as this is known to stretch the facial nerve with resultant morbidity.

20.6.6 Petroclival Meningioma

In both the endoscopic (selected cases) and transcranial approaches, abducens damage and vascular injury is to be prevented.

20.6.7 Petrous-tentorial

At risk during the transcranial route, the trochlear and trigeminal branches are at risk and careful dissection is required to avoid damage to the nerves.

20.6.8 Foramen Magnum Meningioma

When transcranial corridors are used, the lower cranial nerves are at risk; vertebral artery injury must be avoided. CSF leak is the major worry in the endoscopic approach. CV instability is a concern in both approaches.

20.7 Conclusion

Skull base meningiomas are one of the most formidable challenges faced by a neurosurgeon. Many centers specializing in treatment of these lesions have emphasized the concept of team work. Endonasal approaches to skull base have added new possibilities in this millennium, along with its challenges.

Though indications are getting much better defined and imaging has evolved to empower us with greater knowledge of safe corridors and tumor resectability (▶ Fig. 20.9), a surgeon should be prepared with all the tricks to avoid complications during and after surgery. Complications arising from surgery for these lesions can be unforgiving. However, complications should not be considered as a failure but rather as proof of challenge posed by the lesion.

Complication avoidance is the key in trying to achieve a "cure" in skull base meningiomas. Proper case selection, awareness of natural history, team approach for selection

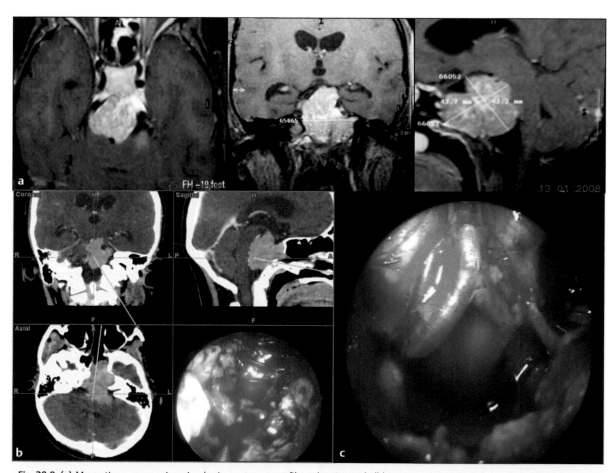

Fig. 20.9 (a) Magnetic resonance imaging brain post contrast films showing a skull base meningioma involving clivus. (b) Lesion accessed via transnasal transclival approach. Intraoperative navigation snapshot of the same showing the safest corridor for approach. (c) Post lesion excision intraoperative image.

of treatment modality and its execution, and a dedicated team of anesthesiologists and intensivists with vigilant nursing is a big help towards that goal.

20.8 Acknowledgment

The authors acknowledge the assistance of Dr. C. Mohanty, Dr. R. Patil, and Dr. S. Shaikh from the Department of Neurosurgery at Bombay Hospital during the preparation of the manuscript.

References

[1] Apuzzo MLJ, ed. Brain Surgery: Complication Avoidance and Management. New York: Churchill Livingstone; 1993

[2] Landriel Ibañez FA, Hem S, Ajler P, et al. A new classification of complications in neurosurgery. World Neurosurg. 2011; 75(5–6): 709–715, discussion 604–611

[3] Tomasello F, Germanò A. Francesco Durante: the history of intracranial meningiomas and beyond. Neurosurgery. 2006; 59(2): 389–396, discussion 389–396

[4] Cushing H. The meningiomas (dural endotheliomas): their source and favored seats of origin (Cavendish Lecture). Brain. 1922; 45: 282–316

[5] Simpson D. The recurrence of intracranial meningiomas after surgical treatment. J Neurol Neurosurg Psychiatry. 1957; 20(1):22–39

[6] Levine ZT, Buchanan RI, Sekhar LN, Rosen CL, Wright DC. Proposed grading system to predict the extent of resection and outcomes for cranial base meningiomas. Neurosurgery. 1999; 45(2):221–230

[7] Goel A, Kothari M. Meningiomas: Are they curable? J Craniovertebr Junction Spine. 2016; 7(3):133–134

[8] Nakamura M, Roser F, Michel J, Jacobs C, Samii M. The natural history of incidental meningiomas. Neurosurgery. 2003; 53(1):62–70, discussion 70–71

[9] Chamoun R, Krisht KM, Couldwell WT. Incidental meningiomas. Neurosurg Focus. 2011; 31(6):E19

[10] Li MS, Portman SM, Rahal A, Mohr G, Balasingam V. The lion's mane sign: surgical results using the bilateral fronto-orbito-nasal approach in large and giant anterior skull base meningiomas. J Neurosurg. 2014; 120(2):315–320

[11] Gardner PA, Kassam AB, Thomas A, et al. Endoscopic endonasal resection of anterior cranial base meningiomas. Neurosurgery. 2008; 63(1):36–52, discussion 52–54

[12] Kassam AB, Prevedello DM, Carrau RL, et al. Endoscopic endonasal skull base surgery: analysis of complications in the authors' initial 800 patients. J Neurosurg. 2011; 114(6):1544–1568

[13] Khan OH, Anand VK, Schwartz TH. Endoscopic endonasal resection of skull base meningiomas: the significance of a "cortical cuff" and brain edema compared with careful case selection and surgical experience in predicting morbidity and extent of resection. Neurosurg Focus. 2014; 37(4):E7

[14] Geibprasert S, Pongpech S, Armstrong D, Krings T. Dangerous extracranial-intracranial anastomoses and supply to the cranial

nerves: vessels the neurointerventionalist needs to know. AJNR Am J Neuroradiol. 2009; 30(8):1459–1468

[15] St-Arnaud D, Paquin MJ. Safe positioning for neurosurgical patients. AORN J. 2008; 87(6):1156–1168, quiz 1169–1172

[16] Samii M, Ammirati M. Surgery of the Skull Base: Meningiomas. 1st ed. Springer, Berlin; 1992

[17] Deopujari CE, Karmarkar VS. Textbook of operative neurosurgery. 1st ed Vol 2. New Delhi: B. I. Publication Co; 2005

[18] Cavallo LM, Messina A, Esposito F, et al. Skull base reconstruction in the extended endoscopic transsphenoidal approach for suprasellar lesions. J Neurosurg. 2007; 107(4):713–720

[19] Hadad G, Bassagasteguy L, Carrau RL, et al. A novel reconstructive technique after endoscopic expanded endonasal approaches: vascular pedicle nasoseptal flap. Laryngoscope. 2006; 116(10): 1882–1886

[20] Zanation AM, Snyderman CH, Carrau RL, Kassam AB, Gardner PA, Prevedello DM. Minimally invasive endoscopic pericranial flap: a new method for endonasal skull base reconstruction. Laryngoscope. 2009; 119(1):13–18

[21] Cusimano MD, Sekhar LN. Pseudo-cerebrospinal fluid rhinorrhea. J Neurosurg. 1994; 80(1):26–30

[22] Hoefnagel D, Kwee LE, van Putten EH, Kros JM, Dirven CM, Dammers R. The incidence of postoperative thromboembolic complications following surgical resection of intracranial meningioma. A retrospective study of a large single center patient cohort. Clin Neurol Neurosurg. 2014; 123:150–154

[23] Osawa T, Tosaka M, Nagaishi M, Yoshimoto Y. Factors affecting peritumoral brain edema in meningioma: special histological subtypes with prominently extensive edema. J Neurooncol. 2013; 111(1):49–57

[24] Lee KD, DePowell JJ, Air EL, Dwivedi AK, Kendler A, McPherson CM. Atypical meningiomas: is postoperative radiotherapy indicated? Neurosurg Focus. 2013; 35(6):E15

[25] Burkhardt JK, Zinn PO, Graenicher M, et al. Predicting postoperative hydrocephalus in 227 patients with skull base meningioma. Neurosurg Focus. 2011; 30(5):E9

[26] Ahmed H, Mohamed ED. Could meningiomas at certain locations at the skull base have a higher incidence of post-operative pseudomeningocele and consequent communicating hydrocephalus than others? (A Retrospective Analysis). Egyptian journal of Neurosurgery. 2013; 28(4)

[27] Vishteh AG, Crawford NR, Melton MS, Spetzler RF, Sonntag VK, Dickman CA. Stability of the craniovertebral junction after unilateral occipital condyle resection: a biomechanical study. J Neurosurg. 1999; 90(1) Suppl:91–98

[28] Patterson RH, Jr, Danylevich A. Surgical removal of craniopharyngiomas by the transcranial approach through the lamina terminalis and sphenoid sinus. Neurosurgery. 1980; 7(2):111–117

[29] Yaşargil MG, Reichman MV, Kubik S. Preservation of the frontotemporal branch of the facial nerve using the interfascial temporalis flap for pterional craniotomy. Technical article. J Neurosurg. 1987; 67(3):463–466

[30] Oikawa S, Mizuno M, Muraoka S, Kobayashi S. Retrograde dissection of the temporalis muscle preventing muscle atrophy for pterional craniotomy. Technical note. J Neurosurg. 1996; 84(2):297–299

[31] Kanno T, Kato S, Kumar S, Kiya N. Brain tumor surgery. 1st ed. Tokyo: Neuron Publishing Co; 1995

Index

Note: Page numbers set **bold** or *italic* indicate headings or figures, respectively.